Neuromusculoskeletal Examination and Assessment

To my parents, Alfred Holdsworth and Vera Petty

For Elsevier:

Senior Commissioning Editor: Sarena Wolfaard
Development Editor: Claire Wilson
Project Manager: Morven Dean
Designer: Stewart Larking

Neuromusculoskeletal Examination and Assessment

A Handbook for Therapists

Nicola J Petty MSc MCSP MMPA MMACP

Principal Lecturer, School of Health Professions, University of Brighton, UK

Foreword by

Agneta Lando

THIRD EDITION

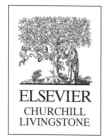

ELSEVIER
CHURCHILL
LIVINGSTONE

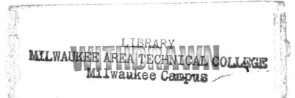
EDINBURGH LONDON NEW YORK OXFORD PHILADELPHIA ST LOUIS SYDNEY TORONTO 2006

ELSEVIER
CHURCHILL
LIVINGSTONE

An imprint of Elsevier Limited

First edition 1997
Second edition 2001
Third edition 2006

ISBN 0443 10204X

British Library Cataloguing in Publication Data
A catalogue record for this book is available from the British Library

Library of Congress Cataloging in Publication Data
A catalog record for this book is available from the Library of Congress

Notice
Neither the Publisher nor the Author assume any responsibility for any loss or
injury and/or damage to persons or property arising out of or related to any use
of the material contained in this book. It is the responsibility of the treating
practitioner, relying on independent expertise and knowledge of the patient, to
determine the best treatment and method of application for the patient.

The Publisher

Printed in China by RDC Group Limited

Contents

Foreword

Do we need textbooks with lengthy, detailed and precise descriptions of clinical examination and assessment? Is it worthwhile for a clinician/academic to spend countless hours putting together a text that will, in part, contain information that will no longer be the latest information available by the time it goes to press? Perhaps you think that I should not be posing these questions in the foreword of a textbook, and that this is the time for praise of the author? Let me assure you that this will come later, now let me deal with the questions.

Learning is a life event without space and time limitations, and with no single 'right' way. Different learning processes work for different individuals; however, most of us require a structure to enable the first steps to take place. We must all start somewhere, and if we are lucky enough to have a wide-based structure as our springboard it gives us a solid foundation upon which to build the rest of our lives' work experience. For example, take undergraduate students with no concept of the process of clinical reasoning; they can easily understand why they have to learn the structure of the body, the workings and pathological patterns of those structures. To arrive at what has gone wrong in specific clinical presentations and to formulate a management programme tailored to the patient's individual situation and needs, the students are required to incorporate many areas of knowledge combined with their own life experience. 'Fortune favours the prepared mind', yes, but not in order to limit what information we take on board, instead to be discerning, critical and questioning to an appropriate degree. Without the

knowledge of how to technically examine, why we perform these tests specifically and how to interpret them, the clinician would be lost.

This textbook provides the way forward. The detail with which the examinations are described and the possible interpretation for a wide variety of findings will be invaluable for any student of manual therapy at under- or post-graduate level. It is gratifying to see that the author allows for variation in body size and shape, both of the therapist and the patient, in her suggestions of manual examination. This textbook has a greater global approach than many of its predecessors (as indicated in its title) and is successful in reflecting the multifaceted approach taken by contemporary expert clinicians. It is for these reasons that the answer to my first question has to be yes.

In the last 15 years the UK has seen an explosive growth in manual therapy-related research. In some countries research in this area was prolific much earlier, and in some they are just starting. The emerging information from these studies is increasingly easier to access via the internet and, therefore, available to a far greater number of practitioners than ever before. This gives us no excuse for not being well informed and up to date. For the student the situation is different. The nature of being at the beginning of the learning process means that it is not always possible to know which questions to ask to get the most informed answer. Questions arising from clinical examination may not be answered by the most recent studies. Some of the information most frequently used by clinicians is patterns of referred pain. The definitive texts in this area were published following research in the 1940s and 1950s. Ergo it is necessary for the student to utilize information from a multitude of sources, produced by professionals from a variety of areas relevant to manual therapy and at different times periods in the development of this clinical field.

This textbook provides information for the beginning of the learning process and beyond. It utilizes up-to-date information combined with previous studies, providing that broad base essential for the 'probing' and critical clinician. The text takes the student through a logical sequence of questioning, examination and assessment, providing an open-minded approach to the diagnosis. It sets out possible management pathways and encourages further exploration and learning by providing ample references for each chapter. Again, the answer to the second question has to be yes.

Nikki Petty is to be congratulated on this mammoth task and clinicians of the future will thank her for her dedication and commitment to detail and be grateful for the ease with which she initiated their learning.

Agneta Lando, August 2005

Preface

Since the previous edition, I have continued to develop my understanding of neuromusculo-skeletal examination and assessment. We are all on a journey, and writing textbooks signifies that journey in a very explicit and public way! This new edition reflects some changes to my thinking, often reflected in subtle changes in language. As well as de-cluttering my home and office, which apparently is characteristic of someone of my age(!), I have also tried to de-clutter parts of the examination process by converging some of the tests into a reduced number of more user-friendly headings, and increased the number of tables.

On re-reading the text, I noticed it was rather dogmatic in places and biased towards joint; I have tried to address this throughout the chapters. I have also attempted to emphasize a patient-centred approach. I have made a number of other alterations to the presentation of the material: some line drawings have been replaced by photographs, the examination charts have been re-written and the references have been updated.

A shift in my thinking has been underpinned by reading some philosophy and coming to realize that the certainty that we want in answer to the big questions of life (and, within that, in our day-to-day lives which include treating patients with neuromusculoskeletal dysfunction), is unrealistic. The concept of absolute certainty is no longer viable. Students, however, often want absolutes and a sense of certainty with their patients and with the science of their profession. The clinician is required to work therapeutically alongside another person and facilitate their rehabilitation. Each of us is made up of a physical body, as well as intellect, will, emotion and spirit, and these in a unique combination. The clinician must act as one person to another person, respecting their intuition as well as their clinical reasoning and theoretical and research knowledge. Clinical practice will always be an art and there will always be uncertainty. While this text emphasizes the skills required to identify a physical dysfunction, it is to be seen within this wider context.

Eastbourne 2005   Nicola J Petty

Acknowledgements

Firstly I would like to thank Ann Moore for her valuable input into the first two editions of this textbook. I would also like to thank the colleagues and friends who were thanked by name for their help in developing the first two editions of the book.

For this third edition, there are some new people I would like to acknowledge. Firstly, thanks to Jonathan Odura and Neeta Gohil who acted as models for over 300 photographs. Thank you, once again, to Bob Seago for another day of photography and Flynn for sorting out the lighting on a dull November day.

I would like to thank the staff at Elsevier, Sarena, Claire and Morven, for their patience, good humour and professional expertise.

Thanks to Christopher Miller, a 3rd year physiotherapy student, for suggesting an additional research paper on neurodynamics and to Kishore Garikipati for information on cranial nerve testing. Finally, thanks to Chris Murphy for comments on a few chapters and for his encouragement to complete this edition.

Glossary of terms

Accessory movement Any movement that cannot be performed actively but that can be performed by an external force, for example antero-posterior glide, medial glide, lateral glide.

Assessment The interpretation of the examination findings, and can be considered synonymous with clinical reasoning.

Asterisks The main findings from the subjective and physical examination.

End-range resistance The resistance that occurs towards the end of the range of physiological or accessory movement.

Examination It is the process of data collection from the patient, and can be divided into subjective and physical examination to separate the interview with the patient from the physical testing procedures.

Movement diagram A method of recording physiological or accessory movement in terms of range, resistance to movement, pain and muscle spasm.

PAIVMs Passive accessory intervertebral movements.

Physiological movement Any movement that can be performed actively, for example flexion, extension, abduction, adduction, medial or lateral rotation.

PPIVMs Passive physiological intervertebral movements.

Through-range resistance The resistance felt during passive, physiological or accessory range of movement.

Chapter 1

Introduction

This text aims to provide guidance to the examination and assessment of patients with neuro-musculoskeletal dysfunction and focuses on the technical skills and clinical reasoning involved. It could be said that this text emphasizes a system of examination that addresses the biological basis of symptoms, as opposed to the psychosocial factors. I have attempted to include the psychological and social aspects of the examination and assessment of patients; however, they are not covered in detail and the reader will need to draw on other literature to cover these gaps.

The text provides a step-by-step approach to the subjective and physical examination of the various regions in the body. Chapter 2, on subjective examination, provides a general guide to the way in which questions might be asked as well as the clinical relevance of questions. Chapter 3, on physical examination, provides a guide to performing the testing procedures and to understanding the relevance of the tests. The following chapters divide the body into regions and provide specific details of the subjective and physical examination and assessment for each particular region. There is a deliberate repetition of information from the first two general chapters into each of the regional chapters to help reinforce the information and to avoid excessive page-turning. The attempt is to provide a user-friendly handbook, where clinicians can go directly to the relevant chapter for information. The body is divided into the following regions: temporomandibular, upper cervical spine, cervicothoracic spine, thoracic spine, shoulder, elbow, wrist/hand, lumbar spine,

pelvis, hip, knee and foot/ankle. Anatomically, biomechanically, functionally and clinically, this is a false and contrived division of the body. More realistic regions might, for example, be the cervico-thoracic-shoulder region and the lumbo-pelvic-hip region. So, while readers are here introduced to the individual regions, they should maintain an awareness of the wider regional areas that are clinically and functionally relevant.

I have used the previous editions of this text to support my undergraduate teaching and have been surprised at how much weight students give a published piece of work. They seem to consider everything in the text as absolutely 'right', and attempt to replicate the procedures shown in the photographs. I would like to comment on this approach. I am a little over 5 ft (1.5 m) tall, weigh 7.5 stone (47.6 kg) and have small hands; so the examination techniques shown in this text are often carried out in a way that is possible for a small person! If you are larger than I – and you probably are – you may well want to adapt the techniques shown in this text; indeed you may be able to perform the techniques with much greater ease.

Another comment worth making at this point is that what you see in this text is *one* way of doing a technique and is not the *only* way. For every technique shown here, there will be a number of alternative ways in which it could be carried out. This text provides an example of how one clinician might perform a physical testing procedure on a particular model; it is up to readers to find alternative ways of carrying out the technique, making adaptations for themselves and for their patients. Clinicians can determine whether or not their adapted technique is *effective* and *efficient* by asking themselves whether it is easy and comfortable to perform, comfortable for the patient, and achieves what it intends to achieve. A technique is easy and comfortable when posture is carefully considered to produce forces easily; the position of the feet, legs, trunk and arms, as well as the position of the patient and plinth height, will all contribute to the ease with which a technique is carried out. When learning, an easy way of checking whether a technique is easy to do is to maintain your position and force applied much longer than it needs to be, and see whether it continues to feel easy. If it becomes tiring, small alterations may be needed. While learning, it can be helpful for the model to imagine that he or she is a patient in pain, so that the standard of comfort required is raised, and then provide honest and constructive feedback to the partner. A technique achieves what it is intended to achieve when it is comfortable, accurate, specific, controlled, appropriate, and handling is sensitively adapted to the tissue response. It is helpful, whenever a technique is being carried out, to ask whether you think you are achieving what you are intending to achieve, and if not, then change your technique. This is not just for novices as they learn techniques; normal everyday clinical practice requires clinicians to adapt examination procedures to individual patients. For those learning these examination procedures for the first time, here are some tips on how handling might be improved:

- Practise, practise, practise! There is no substitute for plenty of good quality practice.
- When practising, split the task into bite-sized chunks, building up into a whole. For example, practise hand-holds, then application of force, then the hand-hold and force on different indi-

viduals, then the communication needed with your model, then all of this together on different individuals.
- Imagine what is happening to the tissues when you are carrying out an examination procedure.
- Tell your model, very specifically, what you want in terms of feedback; model feedback should be honest and constructive.
- Verbalize to your model what you are doing.
- When you do a technique, evaluate it and predict the feedback you will receive from your model, so that you learn to become independent of your model's feedback.
- Act as a model and feel what is happening.
- Act as an observer; if you can see a good technique this can help you to perform a good technique.
- Use a video to observe yourself.
- Imagine yourself doing the examination procedures in your mind in any spare moments.

It is perhaps worth mentioning at the outset that clinicians examining patients with neuromusculoskeletal dysfunction may not be able to identify a particular pathological process. In one patient, for example, the clinician may suspect a meniscal tear or a medial collateral ligament tear of the knee, or a lateral ligament sprain of the ankle. However, in another patient, when current knowledge of pain mechanisms is integrated, and these effects on the presenting symptoms are considered, the goal of identifying exact pathology is clouded. When the detailed analysis of movement dysfunction is considered in conjunction with the psychosocial factors highlighted previously, the clinician is then in a position to establish a reasoned treatment and management strategy. Readers are referred to the companion text for further information on the principles of treatment and management of patients with neuromusculoskeletal dysfunction (Petty 2004).

Reference

Petty N J 2004 Principles of neuromusculoskeletal treatment and management, a guide for therapists. Churchill Livingstone, Edinburgh

Chapter **2**

Subjective examination

INTRODUCTION

This chapter and Chapter 3 cover the general principles and procedures of examination of the neuromusculoskeletal system. This chapter is concerned with the subjective examination, during which information is gathered from the patient and from their medical notes, while Chapter 3 covers the objective or physical examination. This examination system can be adapted to fulfil the examination requirements for people with neuromusculoskeletal problems in various clinical settings – for instance, it might be used in cold orthopaedic and rheumatology ward settings, in gymnasia, e.g. when dealing with children and adolescents with postural problems, as well as in outpatient departments.

It is very difficult to determine the exact pathology of conditions involving the neuromusculoskeletal system, since for many, there are no clear-cut diagnostic tests available. In the lumbar spine, for example, a patient who presents with a set of signs and symptoms that indicate a nerve root irritation may have one of six possible diagnoses confirmed at surgery; conversely, a patient with a confirmed diagnosis at surgery may have had one of many different sets of signs and symptoms (Macnab 1971). This difficulty led Maitland et al (2001) to develop the concept of the 'permeable brick wall', which involves a two-compartment model of reasoning (Box 2.1). It clearly acknowledges the separation of the clinical presentation and the theoretical knowledge that could underpin a diagnosis. The wall is permeable

---

Box 2.1   Permeable brick wall (after Maitland et al 2001, with permission)

The clinician	The patient
	Clinical presentation:
Beliefs	Beliefs
Values	Values
Experience	Experience
Skill	Skill
Anatomy	Anatomy
Biomechanics	Biomechanics
Physiology	Physiology
Pathology	Pathology
Diagnosis	Diagnosis
Theories	Theories
Research findings	Research findings

---

to allow for the fact that some clinical presentations will match the 'textbook' diagnosis, but the bricks of the wall acknowledge that other patients will not fit a known diagnosis. In either case, the clinician manages the patient according to the clinical presentation rather than the diagnosis. In addition, the permeability of the brick wall allows for modification of the diagnosis as more facts become known. The notion of the brick wall may be broadened to incorporate, for both the clinician and the patient, their beliefs, values, experience and skill, as well as their knowledge of theories and research findings (Box 2.1).

By the end of the subjective examination the clinician will have developed the following hypotheses categories (adapted from Jones & Rivett 2004):

- Function abilities and restrictions: what activities the patient is able and unable to do, e.g. walking, lifting, sitting, as well as sport, leisure, family and work activities.
- Patients' perspectives on their experience. This has recently been given a category in its own right, because of its importance; previously it was within contributing factors hypothesis.
- Source of symptoms. This includes the structure or tissue that is thought to be producing the patient's symptoms, the nature of the structure

or tissues in relation to the healing process, and the pain mechanisms involved.

- Contributing factors to the development and maintenance of the problem. There may be environmental, psychosocial, behavioural, physical or heredity factors. Environmental factors may include a patient's work station or work environment, home, car, etc. Psychosocial factors may include the patient's belief that pain or exercise is 'bad', or misunderstanding the nature of their problem. Behavioural factors may include what they do at work or at home, their choice of activities; they may, for example, avoid movement. Physical contributing factors include reduced range of movement, muscle weakness, etc. Heredity plays a part in the development of some musculoskeletal conditions, such as ankylosing spondylitis, osteoarthritis (Solomon et al 2001).
- Precautions/contraindications to physical examination, treatment and management. This includes the severity and irritability of the patient's symptoms and the nature of the patient's condition.
- Management strategy and treatment plan
- Prognosis – this can be affected by factors such as the stage and extent of the injury as well as the patient's expectation, personality and lifestyle. Psychosocial (yellow flags) risk factors, patient's perceived stress at work (blue flags) and work conditions including employment and sickness policy as well as type and amount of work (black flags) are considered to strongly influence the outcome of treatment (Jones & Rivett 2004, Main & Spanswick 2000).

Information from the subjective examination can often give clues as to the most appropriate treatment; for instance, a movement that eases the pain may be adapted as a treatment technique.

The accuracy of the information gained in the subjective examination depends to a large extent on the quality of the communication between the clinician and patient. Clear communication is difficult to achieve and some of the errors that can occur during a question and answer are shown in Figure 2.1. The clinician should speak slowly and

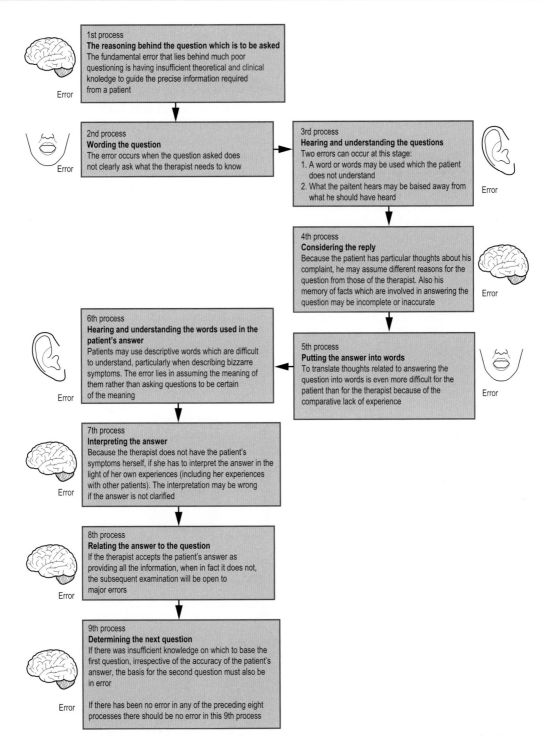

Figure 2.1 The areas for mistakes in verbal communication. (From Maitland et al 2001.)

deliberately, keep questions short and ask only one question at a time (Maitland et al 2001). For further details, readers are directed to an excellent chapter on interviewing skills by Maitland et al (2001).

The usefulness of the information gained in the subjective examination depends to a large extent on the clinician understanding the relevance and pertinence of all the questions asked. This chapter aims to give this background on the questions asked, so that clinicians are able to question effectively and obtain a wealth of useful information on which to base the physical examination.

The most common symptom allied to neuromusculoskeletal dysfunction is pain. Pain is a subjective phenomenon and is different for each individual. It is therefore difficult to estimate the extent of another's psychological and emotional experiences of pain. Pain is a complex experience and includes many dimensions, as shown in Figure 2.2 (McGuire 1995).

In the examination described in this chapter and the next, all these dimensions are investi-

gated, giving the clinician a fairly comprehensive understanding of the patient's pain experience. This is important in order to gain the most from the subjective examination.

This chapter outlines a very detailed subjective examination, which will not be required for every patient. Not every question will need to be asked to the same depth – the clinician must tailor the examination to the patient. An illuminating text on the theoretical concepts underlying the subjective and physical examination can be found in Refshauge & Gass (2004).

The most important findings in the subjective examination are highlighted with asterisks (*) for easy reference and are used at subsequent treatment sessions to evaluate the effects of treatment intervention.

The aim of the subjective examination is to obtain sufficient information about the patient's symptoms so as to be able to plan an efficient, effective and safe physical examination. A summary of the subjective examination is shown in Table 2.1.

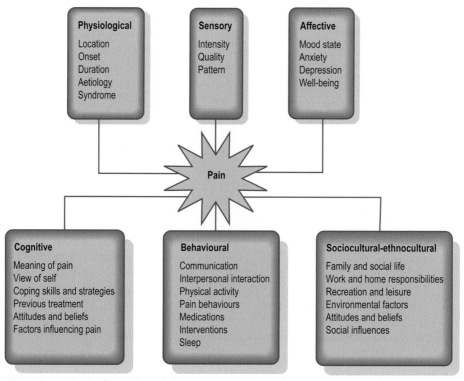

Figure 2.2 Dimensions of pain. (From Petty & Moore 2001, adapted from McGuire 1995.)

<table>
<tr><td colspan="2">**Table 2.1** Summary of subjective examination</td></tr>
</table>

Area of examination	Information gained
Body chart	Type and area of current symptoms, depth, quality, intensity, abnormal sensation, relationship of symptoms
Behaviour of symptoms	Aggravating factors, easing factors, severity and irritability of the condition, 24-hour behaviour, daily activities, stage of the condition
Special questions	General health, drugs, steroids, anticoagulants, recent unexplained weight loss, rheumatoid arthritis, spinal cord or cauda equina symptoms, dizziness, recent X-rays
History of present condition	History of each symptomatic area – how and when it started, how it has changed
Past medical history	Relevant medical history, previous attacks, effect of previous treatment
Social and family history	Age and gender, home and work situation, dependants and leisure activities

THE SUBJECTIVE EXAMINATION STEP BY STEP

Body chart

A body chart (Fig. 2.3) is a useful and quick way of recording information about the area and type of symptoms the patient is experiencing, and its completion is usually the first step in the subjective examination of the patient. Various elements are recorded as follows.

Area of current symptoms

The exact area of the symptoms can be mapped out. A clear demarcation between areas of pain, paraesthesia, stiffness or weakness will distinguish symptoms and their relationship to each other (see Figs 2.11 and 2.12 in Appendix 2.2).

The area of the symptoms does not always identify the structure at fault, since symptoms can be felt in one area but emanate from a distant area; for example, pain felt in the elbow may be locally produced or may be due to pathology in the cervical spine. When the manifestation of symptoms is distant to the pathological tissue this is known as referred pain. The more central the lesion, the more extensive is the possible area of referral; for example, the zygapophyseal joints in the lumbar spine can refer symptoms to the foot (Mooney & Robertson 1976), the hip joint classically refers symptoms as far as the knee, and the joints of the foot tend to produce local symptoms around the joint.

Two explanations have been given for the phenomenon of referred pain (Taylor et al 1984). The first is that axons in peripheral sensory nerves supplying different structures have the same cell body in the dorsal root ganglion (Fig. 2.4). The second explanation is that separate peripheral sensory nerves converge into one cell in the dorsal horn of the spinal cord (Fig. 2.5). The clinician needs to be aware that symptoms can be referred in this way from the spine to the periphery; from the periphery more peripherally or centrally; from the viscera to the spine; or from the spine to the viscera.

The areas of referred symptoms from the viscera are shown in Figure 2.6 (Lindsay et al 1997). In addition, the uterus is capable of referring symptoms to the T10–L2 and S2–S5 regions (van Cranenburgh 1989). The mechanism is explained in Figure 2.7, whereby the visceral afferents converge upon the same posterior horn cells in the spinal cord as the somatic efferents. The patient 'projects' pain from the viscera to the area supplied by corresponding somatic afferent fibres. Referral of symptoms to the viscera is usually from the vertebral column rather than the periphery (Maitland 1991). Symptoms referred from the viscera can sometimes be distinguished from those originating in the neuromusculoskeletal system, as the symptoms are not usually aggravated by activity or relieved by rest.

The clinician ascertains which is the worst symptom (if more than one area). This can help to focus the examination to the most important area and may help to prioritize treatment.

In addition, the patient is asked where s/he feels the symptoms are coming from: 'If you had

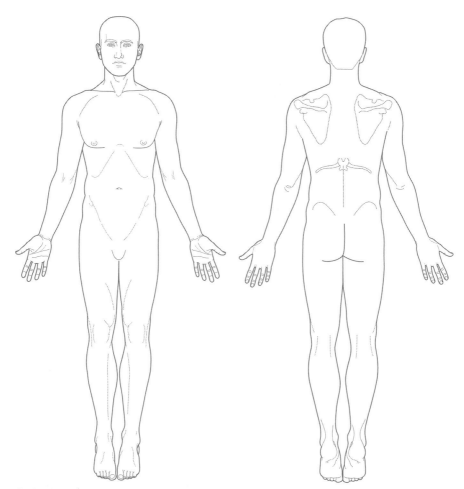

Figure 2.3 Body chart. (Redrawn from Grieve 1991, with permission.)

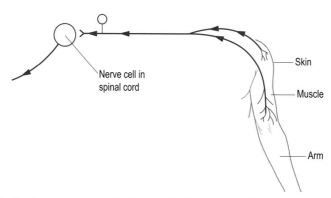

Figure 2.4 Referred pain due to convergence of afferents in the periphery. (After Wells et al 1994, with permission.)

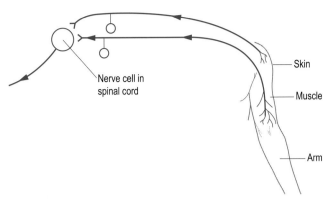

Figure 2.5 Referred pain due to convergence of afferents in the spinal cord. (After Wells et al 1994, with permission.)

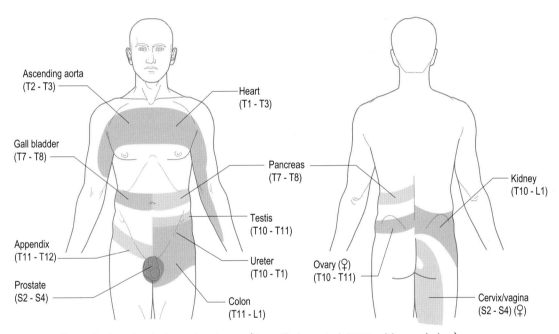

Figure 2.6 Sites of referred pain from the viscera. (From Lindsay et al 1997, with permission.)

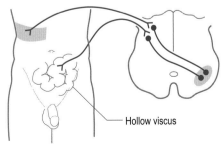

Figure 2.7 The mechanism of referred pain from the viscera. (From Lindsay et al 1997, with permission.)

to put your finger on one spot where you feel it is coming from, where would you put it?' When the patient is able to do this, it can help to pinpoint the source of the symptoms. Care is needed, however, as it may simply be an area of pain referral.

Areas relevant to the region being examined

All other relevant areas are checked for symptom. It is important to ask about pain or even stiffness, as this may be relevant to the patient's main symptom. The unaffected areas are marked with ticks (✓) on the body chart. A patient may only describe the worst symptom, not thinking that it is important to mention an area of slight discomfort – but this may be highly relevant to the understanding of the patient's condition. The cervical and thoracic spinal segments can, for example, give rise to referred symptoms in the upper limb; and the lumbar spine and sacroiliac joints can give rise to referred symptoms in the lower limb. Quite frequently, patients can present with classical signs and symptoms of a peripheral condition such as tennis elbow, but on examination the symptoms are found to emanate from the spine, which is confirmed when palpation or other diagnostic tests of the spine relieve or aggravate the symptoms.

A patient may demonstrate signs of illness behaviour, also called non-organic signs, in the way they report symptoms of pain and record them on a body chart. Pain may be widespread or follow a non-anatomical distribution. The drawing may be very dense and excessively detailed and may spread outside the outline of the body. For an overview of illness behaviours see Box 2.2. The clinician should apply the criteria for illness behaviour with care and be aware of the following (Waddell 2004):

- Need to examine the patient fully
- Avoid observer bias
- Isolated behavioural symptoms mean nothing; only multiple findings are relevant
- Illness behaviour does not explain the cause of the patient's pain, nor does it suggest that the patient has no 'real' pain
- Illness behaviour does not mean that there is no physical disease; most patients have both a physical problem and a degree of illness behaviour

---

Box 2.2 Illness behaviours (Keefe & Block 1982, Waddell 2004)

- Pain drawing
- Pain adjectives and description
- Non-anatomic or behavioural descriptions of symptoms
- Non-organic or behavioural signs
- Overt pain behaviours:
  - Guarding – abnormally stiff, interrupted or rigid movement while moving from one position to another
  - Bracing – a stationary position in which a fully extended limb supports and maintains an abnormal distribution of weight
  - Rubbing – any contact between hand and back, i.e. touching, rubbing or holding the painful area
  - Grimacing – obvious facial expression of pain that may include furrowed brow, narrowed eyes, tightened lips, corners of mouth pulled back and clenched teeth
- Sighing – obvious exaggerated exhalation of air, usually accompanied by the shoulders first rising and then falling; the cheeks may be expanded first
- Use of walking aids
- Down-time
- Help with personal care

- Illness behaviour is not in itself a diagnosis
- Illness behaviour does not mean that the patient is faking or malingering.

The mechanism of pain production can be broadly categorized into nociceptive, peripheral neurogenic and central sensitization. The characteristics for each mechanism are given in Box 2.3.

Quality of the pain

The clinician can ask the patient: 'How would you describe the pain?' The quality of the pain may give a clue as to the anatomical structure at fault (Table 2.2), although this can often be misleading (Austen 1991, Dalton & Jull 1989). The adjective the patient uses to describe their pain may be of an emotional nature, such as tearing,

Box 2.3 Characteristics of pain mechanisms (Doubell, Mannion & Woolf 2002, Fields 1995, Gifford 1996)

Nociceptive pain
- Tends to be localized
- Predictable response, e.g. to stretch, compression or movement
- Responds to simple painkillers and anti-inflammatories
- Improves with appropriate passive treatment

Peripheral neurogenic pain
- Anatomical distribution (spinal segment or peripheral/cranial nerve)
- Burning, sharp, shooting, like electric shock
- Allodynia, dysaesthesia, paraesthesia, possibly a mixture of these
- Provoked by nerve stretch, compression or palpation
- Possible associated muscle weakness and autonomic changes
- Poor response to simple painkillers and anti-inflammatories
- Response to passive treatments varies

Central sensitization
- Widespread, non-anatomical distribution
- Hyperalgesia, allodynia
- Inconsistent response to stimuli and tests
- Pain seems to have 'a mind of its own'
- Drug treatment ineffective
- Unpredictable or no response to passive treatments

Table 2.2 Type of pain thought to be produced by various structures (Magee 1997, Newham & Mills 1999)

Structure	Pain
Bone	Deep, nagging, dull
Muscle	Dull ache
Nerve root	Sharp, shooting
Nerve	Sharp, bright, lightning-like
Sympathetic nerve	Burning, pressure-like, stinging, aching
Vascular	Throbbing, diffuse

analogue scale (VAS), the patient is asked to mark on a 10-cm line the point that best represents the intensity of their pain, where 0 denotes 'no pain' and 10 denotes 'pain as bad as it could possibly be'. The distance of the mark from the left end of the line is measured in millimetres and then becomes a numerical value, which can be recorded. The Present Pain Intensity, which is part of the McGill Pain Questionnaire (Melzack & Wall 1996), measures intensity of pain by asking the patient to choose the word listed below that best describes the intensity of their pain now, at its worst and at its least:

1. Mild
2. Discomforting
3. Distressing
4. Horrible
5. Excruciating.

For comparison, the patient is also asked to score their worst ever toothache, headache and stomach ache. Only the descriptors are shown to the patient, to ensure that they do not choose a numerical value to match their pain. The numbers are strictly for recording purposes only.

It is important to realize that the various pain scales are not interchangeable. Someone who marks their pain at 80 mm on the Visual Analogue Scale will not necessarily give the pain a description of 8 out of 10 on the Numerical Scale, or a Present Pain Intensity of 4. A score can only be compared with another score on the same scale. The intensity of pain score can be repeated several times a day or during a period of treatment, thereby developing a pain diary. This can then be

miserable or terrifying. This suggests that a behavioural component may play a role in this patient's problem.

Intensity of pain

The intensity of pain can be measured by the use of a descriptive, numerical or visual analogue rating scale (Hinnant 1994). These are outlined in Figure 2.8. To complete the descriptive and numerical rating scales, the patient is asked to indicate the description or number which best describes the intensity of their pain. For the visual

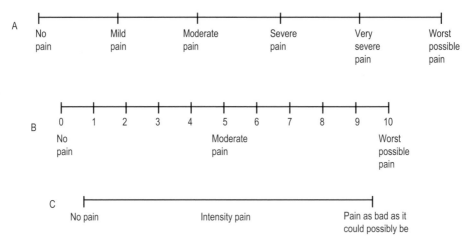

Figure 2.8 Pain intensity rating scales. **A** Simple descriptive pain intensity scale. **B** 1–10 numerical pain intensity scale. **C** Visual analogue scale. (From Hinnant DW 1994 Psychological evaluation and testing. In: Tollinson CD (ed) Handbook of pain management, 2nd edn. © Williams and Wilkins.)

used to construct a pain profile from which the behaviour of pain or the effectiveness of a treatment upon pain can be judged. This is particularly useful with chronic pain sufferers, to determine pain patterns and triggering factors.

Depth of pain

The clinician can ask: 'Is the pain deep down or is it on the surface?' The depth of pain may give some indication as to the structure at fault but, like quality, this can be misleading (Austen 1991). Muscles are thought to produce deep pain (Mense 1993), while joints tend to refer superficially (Mooney & Robertson 1976).

Abnormal sensation

Areas of abnormal sensation are mapped out on the body chart and include paraesthesia (abnormal sensation), anaesthesia (complete loss of sensation), hypoaesthesia (reduced touch sensation), hyperaesthesia (heightened perception to touch), allodynia (pain provoked by stimuli that are normally innocuous), analgesia (absence of appreciation of pain), hypalgesia (reduced appreciation of pain) and hyperalgesia (increased sensitivity to pain). Paraesthesia includes sensations of tingling,

pins and needles, swelling of a limb, tight bands tied around part of the body and water trickling over the skin.

The sensory changes listed above can be generated anywhere along a peripheral or cranial nerve, including the nerve root. A common cause is ischaemia of the nerve, e.g. when part of the brachial plexus is compressed by a cervical rib or when a median nerve compression causes carpal tunnel syndrome. Knowledge of the cutaneous distribution of nerve roots (dermatomes), brachial and lumbosacral plexuses and peripheral nerves enables the clinician to distinguish the sensory loss resulting from a root lesion from that resulting from a peripheral nerve lesion. The cutaneous nerve distribution and dermatome areas are shown in Chapter 3 (Figs 3.18–3.21).

Neurogenic symptoms may also have their origin in the central nervous system. A spinal cord lesion or stroke can cause a variety of sensory changes and long-term pain can sensitize or modify structures like the dorsal horn. Characteristics of central neurogenic symptoms are widespread non-anatomical distribution, change for no apparent reason, lack of consistency in the response to stimulation and passive treatment, and resistance to drug treatment.

Constant or intermittent symptoms

The word 'constant' is used here to mean symptoms that are felt unremittingly for 24 hours a day; any relief of symptoms even for a few minutes would mean that the symptoms were intermittent. The frequency of intermittent symptoms is important as there may be wide variations, from symptoms being felt once a month to once an hour. Specific details are useful at this stage, so that progress can be clearly monitored at subsequent treatment sessions. Constant pain that does not vary is characteristic of malignancy. Constant pain that varies in intensity may be suggestive of inflammatory or infective processes or may occur following trauma due to chemical irritation. Intermittent pain is suggestive of a mechanical disturbance such that forces sufficient to stimulate free nerve endings are producing pain that stops when the force is removed (McKenzie 1981).

Relationship of symptoms

The question of the relationship of symptomatic areas to each other is very important as it helps to establish links between symptoms and gives clues as to the structure(s) at fault. For example, if posterior leg pain is felt when back pain is made worse, then it suggests that the leg pain and the back pain are being produced by the same structure. If, on the other hand, the symptoms occur separately, so that the patient can have back pain without leg pain and leg pain without back pain, then different structures would be thought to be producing these two symptoms.

This completes the information that can be documented on the body chart. An example of a completed body chart is shown in Figures 2.11 and 2.12 in Appendix 2.2.

Behaviour of symptoms

The behaviour of symptoms provides a valuable contribution to the subjective assessment of the patient. It is used in the reassessment strategy to give some indication as to the structure(s) at fault, to give an indication of functional impairment and to allow the therapist to come to a decision on the severity (S), irritability (I) and nature (N) of the condition. This gives valuable information as to the ease/difficulty the therapist may have in reproducing the patient's symptom(s), an indication as to whether a full examination is going to be possible, and lastly an indication as to the vigour which may be required for effective treatment.

Aggravating and easing factors

Aggravating and easing factors are used in the first instance to establish an idea of the severity, irritability and nature of the problem, and the behaviour of symptoms can be further assessed by in-depth questioning as described below.

Aggravating factors. These are movements or postures that produce or increase the patient's symptoms. The exact movement or posture and the time it takes to bring on the symptoms (or make them worse) are established. These indicate how difficult or easy it may be to reproduce the patient's symptoms in the physical examination and how irritable the condition is. For example, symptoms that are felt after 2 hours of hard physical exercise may well be harder to reproduce than symptoms provoked by one single movement such as elbow flexion. The clinician analyses in detail the aggravating movement or posture in order to hypothesize what structures are being stressed and thereby causing the symptoms.

Aggravating factors are determined for each symptomatic area. The effect of aggravating one symptom on the other symptoms is established, as this helps to confirm the relationship between the symptoms. If different symptoms are aggravated by the same position or movement, it suggests that the symptoms are being produced by the same structural dysfunction.

The clinician asks the patient about theoretically known aggravating factors for structures that could be a source of the symptoms, e.g. squatting and going up and down stairs for suspected hip and knee problems, and lifting the head to look upwards for cervical spine problems. A list of common aggravating factors for each joint and for muscle and neurological tissue can be found in Table 2.3. Some worked examples can be found in Appendix 2.2.

The clinician ascertains how the symptoms affect function, such as: static and active postures,

Table 2.3 Common aggravating factors – for each region or structure, examples of various functional activities and a basic analysis of the activity are given

	Functional activity	Analysis of the activity
Temporomandibular joint	Yawning	Depression of mandible
	Chewing	Elevation/depression of mandible
	Talking	Elevation/depression of mandible
Headaches	Stress, eye strain, noise, excessive eating, drinking, smoking, inadequate ventilation, odours	
Cervical spine	Reversing the car	Rotation
	Sitting reading/writing	Sustained flexion
Thoracic spine	Reversing the car	Rotation
	Deep breath	Extension
Shoulder	Tucking shirt in	Hand behind back
	Fastening bra	Hand behind back
	Lying on shoulder	Joint compression
	Reaching up	Flexion
Elbow	Eating	Flexion/extension
	Carrying	Distraction
	Gripping	Flexion/extension
	Leaning on elbow	Compression
Forearm	Turning key in a lock	Pronation/supination
Wrist/hand	Typing/writing	Sustained extension
	Gripping	Extension
	Power gripping	Extension
	Power gripping with twist	Ulnar deviation and pro/supination
	Turning a key	Thumb adduction with supination
	Leaning on hand	Compression
Lumbar spine	Sitting	Flexion
	Standing/walking	Extension
	Lifting/stooping	Flexion
Sacroiliac joint	Standing on one leg	Ipsilateral upward shear, contralateral downward shear
	Turning over in bed	Nutation/counternutation of sacrum
	Getting out of bed	Nutation/counternutation of sacrum
	Walking	Nutation/counternutation of sacrum
Hip	Squat	Flexion
	Walking	Flexion/extension
	Side-lying with painful hip uppermost	Adduction and medial rotation
	Stairs	Flexion/extension
Knee	Squat	Flexion
	Walking	Flexion/extension
	Stairs	Flexion/extension
Foot and ankle	Walking	Dorsiflexion/plantarflexion, inversion/eversion
	Running	Dorsiflexion/plantarflexion, inversion/eversion
Muscular tissue		Contraction of muscle
		Passive stretch of muscle
Nervous tissue		Passive stretch or compression of nervous tissue

e.g. sitting, standing, lying, bending, walking, running, walking on uneven ground, walking up and down stairs, washing, driving, lifting and digging, work, sport and social activities. Note details of the training regimen for any sports activities. The clinician finds out if the patient is left- or right-handed as there may be increased stress on the dominant side.

Detailed information on each of the above activities is useful in order to help determine the structure(s) at fault and identify functional restrictions. This information can be used to determine the aims of treatment and any advice that may be required. The most notable functional restrictions are highlighted with asterisks (*), explored in the physical examination, and reassessed at subsequent treatment sessions to evaluate treatment intervention.

If the patient has changed or abandoned activities in response to their symptoms it is important that this is not at the cost of overall function, particularly if the symptoms are chronic or recurrent. For example, temporary avoidance of some activities can be an effective strategy to overcome an injury, but avoiding most activities for more than a few days may lead to a decline in function and possible chronicity. Regular and wide-ranging help with personal care from family or partner can be a sign of illness behaviour.

Maladaptive coping strategies can easily perpetuate the patients' problem and compromise their treatment (Harding & Williams 1995, Shorland 1998). Coping strategies include:

- Activity avoidance – disuse, lack of fitness, strength and flexibility. May also lead to withdrawal from social activities and interfere with work.
- Underactivity/overactivity cycles (activity avoidance on days with pain, very active on days with less pain). Reduced activity tolerance due to disuse on 'bad' days leads to tissue overload on 'good' days. Over time there may be a gradual increase in pain and decrease in activity.
- Long-term use of medication leads to side-effects such as constipation, indigestion, drowsiness. This may interfere with general function and hinder recovery, as well as perhaps causing the patient to become drug-dependent.

- Visiting a range of therapists and specialists in the pursuit of a diagnosis or cure. The patient is not willing to take control, not willing to apply adaptive coping strategies.

Easing factors. These are movements or positions that ease the patient's symptoms. As with the aggravating factors, the exact movement or posture and the time it takes to ease the symptoms are established. This indicates how difficult or easy it may be to relieve the patient's symptoms in the physical examination and, more importantly, in treatment, and gives an indication of irritability. Symptoms that are readily eased may respond to treatment more quickly than symptoms that are not readily eased. The clinician analyses in detail the easing movement or posture in order to hypothesize which structure(s) are being released from stress. This may indicate the structure(s) that are causing the symptoms.

Again, easing factors are determined for each symptomatic area. The effect of the easing of one symptom on the other symptoms is established as this helps to confirm the relationship between symptoms. If different symptomatic areas ease with the same position or movement, it suggests that the symptoms are being produced by the same structural dysfunction.

The clinician asks the patient about theoretically known easing factors for structures that could be a source of their symptoms; for instance, crook lying for a painful lumbar spine eases pain by reducing intradiscal pressure (Nachemson 1992) and reduces the forces produced by muscle activity (Jull 1986). However, if the patient feels that they can only manage the pain by lying down regularly for long periods this may indicate possible illness behaviour.

Severity and irritability of symptoms

The severity and irritability of symptoms must be determined in order to identify patients who will not be able to tolerate a full physical examination and also to establish guidelines concerning the vigour of the examination strategy. Generally speaking, the tests carried out in the physical examination require the patient to move and sustain positions that provoke symptoms. Sometimes the intensity of the provoked symptoms are too great for these positions to be sustained, i.e. the patient's symptoms are severe. At other times, the symptoms gradually increase with each movement tested until eventually they may become intolerable to the patient and the examination may have to be stopped until the symptoms subside; in this case the patient's symptoms are said to be irritable. The clinician must know before starting the physical examination whether the patient's symptoms are severe and/or irritable so that an appropriate examination is carried out in a way that avoids unnecessary exacerbation of the patient's symptoms.

The clinician asks about specific active physiological movements such as knee flexion, cervical rotation, etc., in order to assess subjectively the severity and irritability of the patient's symptoms.

Severity of the symptoms. The severity of the symptoms is the degree to which symptoms restrict movement and/or function and is related to the intensity of the symptoms. If a movement at a certain point in range provokes pain and this pain is so intense that the movement must immediately be ceased, then the symptoms are defined as severe. If the symptoms are severe then the patient will not be able to tolerate overpressures, and movements must be performed just short of, or just up to, the first point of pain. If the intensity is such that the patient is able to maintain or increase a movement that provokes the symptoms, then the symptoms are not considered to be severe and in this case overpressures can be performed.

In order to determine the severity of the condition, the clinician chooses an aggravating movement and asks, for example, when examining a patient with symptoms emanating from the cervical spine: 'When you turn your head around to the left and you get your neck pain (or you get more pain), can you stay in that position or do you have to bring your head back straight away because the pain is too severe?' If they are able to stay in the position, the symptoms are considered non-severe; if, however, they are unable to maintain the position, the symptoms are deemed to be severe.

Irritability of the symptoms. The irritability of the symptoms is the degree to which symptoms increase and reduce with provocation. Using the

same aggravating movement as for severity, the clinician finds out how long it takes for the provoked symptom to ease. When a movement is performed and pain, for example, is produced (or increased) and continues to be present for a period of time, then the symptom is considered to be irritable. Anything more than a few seconds would require a pause between testing procedures, to allow symptoms to return to their resting level. If the symptom disappears as soon as the movement is stopped, then the symptom is considered to be non-irritable.

Using the same example as above, the clinician might ask: 'When you turn your head around to the left and feel the sharp pain and then immediately turn your head back, does that sharp pain ease immediately or does it take a while to go?' The clinician needs to make sure that the patient has understood by asking: 'You mean that sharp pain, that extra pain that was felt at the end of the movement, takes 10 minutes to go?' If the pain eases immediately, the symptoms are considered to be non-irritable and all movements can be examined. If the symptoms take a few minutes to disappear then the symptoms are irritable and the patient may not be able to tolerate all movements as the symptoms may gradually get worse. The clinician may choose to carry out movements just to the onset of symptom provocation, reduce the number of movements carried out and allow a pause for the symptoms to settle after each movement. Alternatively, the clinician may choose to carry out all movements just short of the onset of symptom provocation, so that all movements can be carried out and no pauses are needed.

Occasionally, latent irritability may occur where a movement or position may induce symptoms that are delayed by some minutes and often continue for a considerable length of time. Careful management is required with these patients to avoid unnecessary exacerbation of their symptoms.

A patient's condition may be severe or irritable or it may be both severe and irritable.

Twenty-four-hour behaviour of symptoms

Night symptoms. The following information is gathered from the patient:

- Does the patient have difficulty getting to sleep because of the symptom(s)? Lying may in some way alter the stress on the structure(s) at fault and provoke symptoms. For example, weight-bearing joints such as the spine, sacroiliac joints, hips, knees and ankles have reduced compressive forces in lying compared with upright postures.
- Which positions are most comfortable and uncomfortable for the patient? The clinician can then analyse these positions to help confirm the possible structures at fault.
- Is the patient woken by symptoms, and, if so, which symptoms and are they associated with movement, e.g. turning over in bed?
- To what extent is the patient disturbed at night:
  - How many nights in the past week?
  - How many times in any one night?
  - How long does it take to get back to sleep?
- It is useful to be as specific as possible as this information can then be used at subsequent attendances to determine the effect of treatment on the condition.
- How many and what type of pillows are used by the patient? For example, foam pillows are often uncomfortable for patients with cervical spine symptoms because their size and non-malleability creates highly flexed or highly side-flexed sleeping positions.
- Does the patient use a firm or soft mattress, and has it recently been changed? Alteration in sleeping posture caused by a new mattress is sometimes sufficient to provoke spinal symptoms.

Morning symptoms. What are the patient's symptoms like in the morning immediately on waking before movement and also after getting up? Prolonged morning pain and stiffness that improves minimally with movement suggests an inflammatory process (Magee 1997). Minimal or absent pain with stiffness in the morning is associated with degenerative conditions such as osteoarthrosis.

Evening symptoms. The patient's symptoms at the beginning of the day are compared with those at the end of the day. Symptoms may depend upon the patient's daily activity levels. Pain that is aggravated by movement and eased by rest generally indicates a mechanical problem of the musculoskeletal system (Corrigan & Maitland

1994). Pain that increases with activity may be due to repeated mechanical stress, an inflammatory process or degenerative process (Jull 1986). Pain may be worse in the evening when the person has been at work all day, compared to when they are off work; the clinician would then explore the activities involved at work to identify what may be aggravating the symptoms.

Stage of the condition

Knowing whether the symptoms are getting better, getting worse or remaining static gives an indication as to the stage of the condition and helps the clinician to determine the time for recovery. Symptoms that are deteriorating will tend to take longer to respond to treatment than symptoms that are resolving.

Special questions

The clinician needs to determine the nature of the patient's condition, differentiating between benign neuromusculoskeletal conditions that are suitable for manual therapy and systemic, neoplastic or other non-neuromusculoskeletal conditions, which are not suitable for treatment. It is important that the clinician realizes that serious conditions may masquerade as neuromusculoskeletal conditions. This is discussed at length by Grieve (1994a) and a published paper by the same author (Grieve 1994b) is reproduced in Appendix 2.3 of this chapter. A number of questions are asked to enable the clinician to establish the nature of the patient's condition and to identify any precautions or absolute contraindications to further examination and application of treatment techniques. Table 2.4 identifies the precautions to neuromusculoskeletal examination and treatment. Some of this information has been obtained from pathology textbooks, for example, Goodman & Biossonnault (1998), and some is simply suggested by the author; readers should note this limitation.

For all patients, the following information is gathered.

General health. Ascertain the general health of the patient, as poor general health can be suggestive of various systemic disease processes. The clinician asks about any feelings of general malaise or

Table 2.4 Precautions to spinal and peripheral passive joint mobilizations and nerve mobilizations

Aspects of subjective examination	Subjective information	Possible cause/implication for examination and/or treatment
Body chart	Constant unremitting pain	Malignancy, systemic, inflammatory cause
	Symptoms in the upper limb below the acromion or symptoms in the lower limb below the gluteal crease	Nerve root compression. Carry out appropriate neurological integrity tests in physical examination
	Widespread sensory changes and/or weakness in upper or lower limb	Compression on more than one nerve root, metabolic (e.g. diabetes, vitamin B12), systemic (e.g. RA)
Aggravating factors	Symptoms severe and/or irritable	Care in treatment to avoid unnecessary provocation or exacerbation
Special questions	Feeling unwell	Systemic or metabolic disease
	General health:	
	– history of malignant disease, in remission	Not relevant
	– active malignant disease if associated with present symptoms	Contraindicates neuromusculoskeletal treatment, may do gentle maintenance exercises
	– active malignant disease not associated with present symptoms	Not relevant
	– hysterectomy	Increased risk of osteoporosis
	Recent unexplained weight loss	Malignancy, systemic
	Diagnosis of bone disease (e.g. osteoporosis, Paget's brittle bone)	Bone may be abnormal and/or weakened. Avoid strong direct force to bone, especially the ribs
	Diagnosis of rheumatoid arthritis or other inflammatory joint disease	Avoid accessory and physiological movements to upper cervical spine and care with other joints
	Diagnosis of infective arthritis	In active stage immobilization is treatment of choice
	Diagnosis of spondylolysis or spondylolisthesis	Avoid strong direct pressure to the subluxed vertebral level
	Systemic steroids	Osteoporosis, poor skin condition requires careful handling, avoid tape
	Anticoagulant therapy	Increase time for blood to clot. Soft tissues may bruise easily
	HIV	Check medication and possible side-effects
	Pregnancy	Ligament laxity, may want to avoid strong forces
	Diabetes	Delayed healing, peripheral neuropathies
	Bilateral hand/feet pins and needles and/or numbness	Spinal cord compression, peripheral neuropathy
	Difficulty walking	Spinal cord compression, peripheral neuropathy, upper motor neurone lesion
	Disturbance of bladder and/or bowel function	Cauda equina syndrome
	Perineum (saddle) Anaesthesia/paraesthesia	Cauda equina syndrome
	For patient's with cervicothoracic symptoms: dizziness, altered vision, nausea, ataxia, drop attacks, altered facial sensation, difficulty speaking, difficulty swallowing, sympathoplegia, hemianaesthesia, hemiplegia	Vertebrobasilar insufficiency, upper cervical instability, disease of the inner ear
	Heart or respiratory disease	May preclude some treatment positions
	Oral contraception	Increased possibility of thrombosis – may avoid strong techniques to cervical spine
	History of smoking	Circulatory problems – increased possibility of thrombosis
Recent history	Trauma	Possible undetected fracture, e.g. scaphoid

fatigue, fever, nausea or vomiting, stress, anxiety or depression. Feeling unwell or tired is common with systemic, metabolic or neoplastic disease (O'Connor & Currier 1992); malaise, lassitude and depression is often associated with rheumatoid arthritis (Dickson & Wright 1984). For the presence of malignant disease which is in remission, there are no precautions to examination or treatment. If, on the other hand, there is active malignancy, then the primary aim of the day-one examination will be to clarify whether or not the presenting symptoms are being caused by the malignancy or whether there is a separate neuromusculoskeletal disorder. If there is a separate neuromusculoskeletal disorder then there are no precautions to examination and treatment. If the symptoms are thought to be associated with the malignancy then this may contraindicate most neuromusculoskeletal treatment techniques, although gentle maintenance exercises may be given. Diabetes can cause delayed healing and so affect the patient's prognosis.

Weight loss. Has the patient noticed any recent weight loss? This may be due to the patient feeling unwell, perhaps with nausea and vomiting. If there is no explanation for rapid weight loss, it may be indicative of malignancy and systemic diseases.

Rheumatoid arthritis. Has the patient ever been diagnosed as having rheumatoid arthritis (RA)? The clinician also needs to find out if a member of the patient's family has ever been diagnosed as having this disease, as it is hereditary and the patient may be presenting with the first signs. Manual treatment of the cervical spine is avoided in patients with RA and other joints are not treated with manual therapy during the acute inflammatory stage of the disease (Grieve 1991). Common symptoms of RA are red swollen joints, pain that is worst in the morning and systemic symptoms.

Drug therapy. In this area, there are three relevant questions.

What drug therapy has the patient been prescribed? This can give useful information about the pathological process and may affect treatment. For example, the strength of any painkillers indicates the intensity of the patient's pain. A neurogenic or central pain component does not tend to respond to analgesic or anti-inflammatory drugs. Care may be needed if the patient attends for treatment soon after taking painkillers as the pain will be temporarily masked and may cause exacerbation of the patient's condition. In addition, the clinician needs to be aware of any side-effects of the drugs taken.

Has the patient been on long-term medication/ steroids? High doses of corticosteroids for a long period of time can weaken the skin and cause osteoporosis. In this case, the patient requires careful handling and avoidance of tape so that the skin is not damaged. Because of the osteoporosis, strong direct forces to the bones may be inadvisable.

Long-term use of medication leads to side-effects such as constipation, indigestion, drowsiness. This may interfere with general function and hinder recovery, as well as perhaps causing the patient to become drug-dependent.

Has the patient been taking anticoagulants? If so, care is needed in the physical examination in order to avoid trauma to tissues and consequent bleeding.

X-rays and medical imaging. Has the patient been X-rayed or had any other medical tests? X-rays are useful to diagnose fractures, arthritis and serious bone pathology such as infection, osteoporosis or tumour and to determine the extent of the injury following trauma. X-rays can provide useful additional information but the findings must be correlated with the patient's clinical presentation. This is particularly true for spinal X-rays, which may reveal the normal age-related degenerative changes of the spine that do not necessarily correlate with the patient's symptoms. For this reason, routine spinal X-rays are no longer considered necessary for non-traumatic spinal pain (Clinical Standards Advisory Report 1994).

Other imaging techniques include computed tomography, magnetic resonance imaging, myelography, discography, bone scans and arthrography. The results of these tests can help to determine the nature of the patient's condition. Further details of these tests and their diagnostic value can be found in Refshauge & Gass (2004).

Neurological symptoms. For spinal conditions, the following information is acquired:

- Has the patient experienced symptoms of spinal cord compression (i.e. compression of the spinal cord that runs from the foramen magnum to L1)? Positive spinal cord symptoms are bilateral tingling in hands or feet and/or disturbance of gait due to disturbance of the sensory and motor pathways of the spinal cord. This can occur at any spinal level but most commonly occurs in the cervical spine (Adams & Logue 1971), causing cervical myelopathy. Recent onset of spinal cord compression may require a prompt referral to a medical practitioner. These symptoms can be further tested in the physical examination by carrying out neurological integrity tests, including the plantar response.
- Has the patient experienced symptoms of cauda equina compression (compression below L1) such as saddle (perineum) anaesthesia/paraesthesia and bladder or bowel sphincter disturbance (loss of control, retention, hesitancy, urgency or a sense of incomplete evacuation) (Grieve 1991)? These symptoms may be due to interference of S3 and S4 nerve roots (Grieve 1981). Prompt surgical attention is required to prevent permanent sphincter paralysis.

Vertebrobasilar insufficiency (VBI). For symptoms emanating from the cervical spine, the clinician should ask about symptoms that may be caused by vertebrobasilar insufficiency. VBI symptoms include: dizziness (most commonly), altered vision (including diplopia), nausea, ataxia, 'drop attacks', altered facial sensation, difficulty speaking, difficulty swallowing, sympathoplegia, hemianaesthesia and hemiplegia (Bogduk 1994). If present, the clinician determines the aggravating and easing factors in the usual way. These symptoms can also be due to upper cervical instability and diseases of the inner ear.

History of the present condition (HPC)

For each symptomatic area, the clinician should ascertain:

- How long the symptom has been present
- Whether there was a sudden or slow onset of the symptom
- Whether there was a known or unknown cause that provoked the onset of the symptom.

These questions give information about the nature of the problem, in other words, the possible pathological processes involved and whether trauma was a feature in the production of symptoms.

To confirm the relationship of symptoms, the clinician asks when the symptoms began in relation to other symptoms. If, for example, anterior knee joint pain started 3 weeks ago and increased 2 days ago when anterior calf pain developed, it would suggest that the knee and calf pain are associated and that the same structure may well be at fault. If there was no change in the knee pain when the calf pain began, the symptoms may not be related and different structures may be producing the two pain areas.

Past medical history (PMH)

The following information is obtained from the patient and/or medical notes:

- Details of any medical history that is relevant to the patient's condition.
- History of any previous attacks, e.g. the number of episodes, when they occurred, the cause, the duration of the episodes and whether the patient fully recovered between episodes. If there have been no previous attacks, has the patient had any episodes of stiffness?
- Results of any past treatments for the same or similar problem. Past treatment records, if available, may then be obtained for further information. It may well be the case that a previously successful treatment modality will be successful again, but greater efforts may be needed to prevent a recurrence. Physical, psychological or social factors may need to be examined in more detail as they may be responsible for the recurrence of the problem.

Social and family history (SH, FH)

Social and family history that is relevant to the onset and progression of the patient's problem is recorded. This includes the patient's perspectives, experience and expectations, age, employment, home situation, and details of any leisure activities. In order to treat appropriately, it is important that the condition is managed within the context of the patient's social and work environment.

The following factors are considered to predict poor treatment outcome in patients with low back pain (Waddell 2004):

- Belief that back pain is harmful or potentially severely disabling
- Fear avoidance behaviours and reduced activity levels
- Tendency to low mood and withdrawing from social interaction
- Expectation that passive treatment will help, rather than active treatment.

The clinician may therefore ask the following types of questions to elucidate these psychosocial risk factors, or 'yellow flags' (Waddell 2004):

- Have you had time off work in the past with back pain?
- What do you understand to be the cause of your back pain?
- What are you expecting will help you?
- How is your employer/co-workers/family responding to your back pain?
- What are you doing to cope with your back pain?
- Do you think you will return to work? When?

Readers are referred to Waddell's excellent text for further information on psychosocial risk factors for patients with low back pain. While these factors have been identified for low back pain, it seems reasonable to suggest that they would be useful for patients with cervical and thoracic spine pain, as well as pain in the periphery. For this reason these questions have been incorporated in each regional chapter.

Plan of the physical examination

When all the subjective information has been collected it is useful to highlight with asterisks for easy reference important findings from the subjective examination and particularly symptomatic areas and one or more functional restrictions. These can then be reassessed at subsequent treatment sessions to evaluate the effects of treatment on the patient's condition. A summary of this first part of the patient examination can be found in Figure 2.9.

In order to plan the physical examination, the following hypotheses should be developed from the subjective examination:

Which joints, muscles and nerves could be a source of the symptoms and need to be examined? Often it is not possible to complete the entire examination on the first day and so examination of structures must be prioritized over subsequent appointments.

What other factors need to be examined? This may include environmental (e.g. inadequate work station), behavioural (e.g. change in tennis serve), emotional (e.g. stress), physical (e.g. poor posture) or biomechanical (e.g. unequal leg length) factors (Jones 1994). There is a range of validated questionnaires to assess these factors and help to remove bias, see Williams (1994, 1995) and Waddell (2004) for further information.

In what way should the physical tests be carried out? Will it be easy or hard to reproduce each symptom? Will it be necessary to use combined movements, repetitive movements, etc. to reproduce the patient's symptoms? Are symptom(s) severe and/or irritable? If symptoms are severe, physical tests may be carried out to just before the onset of symptom production or just to the onset of symptom production; no overpressures will be carried out, as the patient would be unable to tolerate this. If symptoms are irritable, physical tests may be examined to just before symptom production or just to the onset of provocation with less physical tests being examined to allow for rest period between tests.

Are there any precautions and/or contraindications to elements of the physical examination that need to be explored further, such as a possible fracture, early signs of inflammatory joint disease, spinal cord compression, etc?

From the information obtained during the subjective examination, the clinician decides which tests need to be included in the physical examination to confirm or refute the above hypotheses. In addition, the clinician must use the information to prioritize the examination procedures, which may be spread over two or more appointments.

A planning form for the physical examination, such as the one shown in Figure 2.10, can be useful for inexperienced clinicians, to help guide them through the often complex clinical reasoning process. Appendix 2.1 shows an advanced clinical reasoning form for more experienced clinicians.

Body chart	Name
	Age
	Date

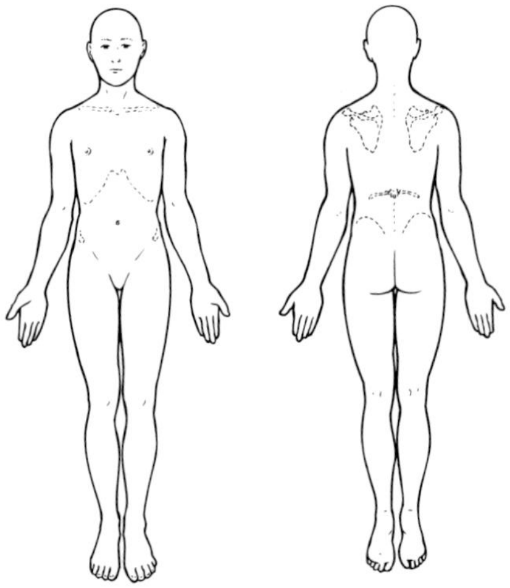

	24-hour behaviour
	Improving static worsening

Relationship of symptoms	Special questions General health Weight loss RA Drugs Steroids Anticoagulants X-ray Cord symptoms Cauda equina symptoms VBI symptoms

Aggravating factors and function	HPC
	PMH
Severe Irritable	
Easing factors	SH & FH (Patient's perspective, experience, expectations. Yellow, blue, black flags)

Figure 2.9   Subjective examination chart.

	Symptom	Symptom	Symptom	Symptom
Is it severe?				
Is it irritable?				
Will you move: – short of production? – point of onset/increase in resting symptoms? – partial reproduction? – total reproduction?				
How will you reproduce symptom: – repeat? – alter speed? – combine? – sustain? – other? (state)				

Are there any precautions or contraindications?   Yes   No State
What other factors contributing to the patient's symptom(s) need to be examined?

Figure 2.10   Physical examination planning form.

APPENDIX 2.1: CLINICAL REASONING FORM

At the end of the subjective examination start to complete the form.
At the end of the physical examination answer the questions in *bold*.

1.1 Source of symptoms

Symptomatic area	Structures under area	Structures which can refer to area	Supporting evidence

1.2 What is the mechanism of each symptom? Explain from information from the subjective and *physical examination findings*

	Symptom	Symptom	Symptom	Symptom
Subjective				
Physical				

1.3 Following the physical examination, what is your clinical diagnosis?

2. Contributing factors

2.1   What factors need to be examined/explored in the physical examination?

2.2 How will you address each contributing factor?

3. Precautions and contraindications

3.1   Are any symptoms severe?   Yes   No
     Which symptoms, and explain why

3.2   Are any symptoms irritable?   Yes   No
     Which symptoms, and explain why

3.3   How much of each symptom are you prepared to provoke in the physical examination?

Symptom	Short of P1	Point of onset or increase in resting symptoms	Partial reproduction	Total reproduction

3.4   Will a neurological examination be necessary in the physical?

yes   no   Explain why

3.5   Following the subjective examination, are there any precautions or contraindications?

yes   no   Explain why

4   Management

4.1   What tests will you do in the physical and what are the expected findings?

Physical tests	Expected findings

4.2   *Were there any unexpected findings from the physical? Explain*

4.3   *What will be your subjective and physical reassessment asterisks?*

4.4   *What is your first choice of treatment (be exact) and explain why?*

4.5   *What do you expect the response to be over the next 24 hours following the first visit? Explain*

4.6   *How do you think you will treat and manage the patient at the 2nd visit, if the patient returns?:*

Same

Better

Worse

4.7   *What advice and education will you give the patient?*

4.8   What needs to be examined on the 2nd and 3rd visits?

2nd visit	3rd visit

5   Prognosis

5.1   List the positive and negative factors (from both the subjective *and physical examination findings*) in considering the patient's prognosis

	Positive	Negative
Subjective		
Physical		

5.2   Overall, is the patient's condition:

    improving   *worsening*   *static*

5.3   What is your overall prognosis for this patient? Be specific

6. After third attendance

6.1 Has your understanding of the patient's problem changed from your interpretations made following the initial subjective and physical examination? If so, explain

6.2 On reflection, were there any clues that you initially missed, misinterpreted, under- or over-weighted? If so, explain

7. After discharge

7.1 Has your understanding of the patient's problem changed from your interpretations made following the third attendance? If so, explain how

7.2 What have you learnt from the management of this patient which will be helpful to you in the future?

APPENDIX 2.2: CASE SCENARIOS

The main aim of the examination and assessment is to determine the structures at fault, and this process begins at the outset of the subjective examination with the body chart and behaviour of symptoms. Two examples of the clinical reasoning process during the first part of the subjective examination are given below.

Patient A

The symptoms are depicted in the body chart in Figure 2.11.

The relationship of the symptoms is as follows. The left and right cervical spine pains come and go together; they appear to be a single area of pain. When the cervical pain worsens, the headache becomes apparent, but the cervical pain can be present without the headache. The left arm pain and paraesthesia in the left hand always come and go together, and these symptoms can be present without any neck pain or headache.

This suggests that one structure is producing the left and right neck pain, another structure is producing the arm pain and paraesthesia in the hand, and, possibly, a third structure is producing the headache.

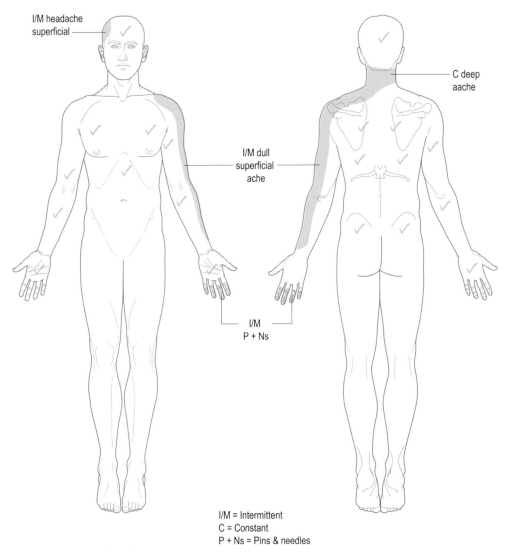

I/M headache superficial

C deep aache

I/M dull superficial ache

I/M
P + Ns

I/M = Intermittent
C = Constant
P + Ns = Pins & needles

Figure 2.11   Body chart patient A.

The information gathered so far from the body chart suggests various structures giving rise to each symptom and these are listed in Table 2.5. The clinician then uses the behaviour of symptoms to further localize which structures may be at fault.

Table 2.5 Structures suspected to be a source of the symptoms

Symptom	Structure
Left cervical spine pain	Cervical spine*
Right cervical spine pain	Cervical spine
Right headache	Cervical spine
	Spine and cerebral dura mater
Left arm pain	Cervical spine
	Neural tissue
	Individual joints – shoulder, elbow and wrist
	Individual muscles around shoulder, elbow, wrist and hand
Paraesthesia in left hand	Cervical spine
	Neural tissue
	Entrapment of brachial plexus around first rib
	Entrapment of nerve at wrist

*Note that, because of the complex anatomy of the spine and the fact that most structures are pain-sensitive, it is very difficult to isolate specific structures in the spine at this stage in the examination. For the purposes of this part of the examination, the region is therefore dealt with as one structure.

Behaviour of symptoms

Aggravating factors. The clinician asks the effect on symptoms of specific aggravating movements and positions for each structure suspected to be a source of symptoms. Table 2.6 illustrates the possible responses of symptoms to aggravating factors.

The logical interpretation of the information on aggravating factors would be that the cervical spine is producing the left and right cervical spine pain and the headache. Abnormal neurodynamics are producing the left arm pain and paraesthesia in the left hand, since the aggravating positions put the nervous system on a stretch.

Easing factors. The relationship of symptoms and the structures at fault may be further confirmed by establishing the easing factors. The patient may find, for example, that keeping the cervical spine still eases the neck pain, that the headaches are eased by avoiding extreme neck positions, and that the left arm pain and pins and needles in the fingers of the left hand are eased by supporting the left arm with the shoulder girdle elevated. This information would confirm the findings from the body chart and aggravating factors.

Patient B

The symptoms are depicted in the body chart in Figure 2.12.

Table 2.6 Possible aggravating factors for each of the symptoms

Symptoms	Cervical spine			Nervous tissue (includes first rib)		Shoulder	Elbow	Wrist
	Extension	Rotation	Sustained flex	Depression of shoulder girdle	Carrying loads	Hand behind back	Flexion/ extension	Flexion/ extension
Cervical spine pain	+	+	+	–	+	–	–	–
Right headache	–	–	+	–	–	–	–	–
Left arm pain	–	–	–	+	+	–	–	–
Pins and needles in left hand	–	–	–	+	+	–	–	–

+, reproduction of symptoms; –, no production of symptoms.

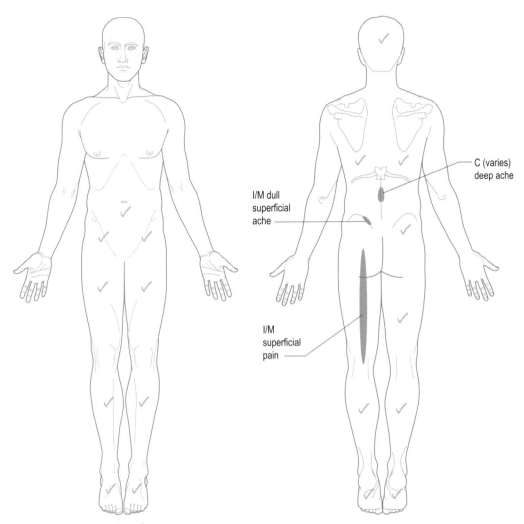

C (varies)
deep ache

I/M dull
superficial
ache

I/M
superficial
pain

Figure 2.12 Body chart patient B.

The relationship of symptoms is as follows. When the lumbar spine pain gets worse (it is constant but varies in intensity), there is no change in any of the other pains. The buttock and thigh pains come and go together. The iliac crest pain, buttock and posterior thigh pain come on separately; the patient can have the iliac crest pain without the buttock and thigh pain, and similarly the buttock and thigh pain can come on without the iliac crest pain.

Since none of the symptoms seem to be associated, this would suggest that there are three different structures at fault, each causing one of the three areas of pain.

The information gathered so far from the body chart suggests that various structures are giving rise to each symptom; these are listed in Table 2.7. The clinician then uses the behaviour of symptoms to further localize which structures are at fault.

Behaviour of symptoms

Aggravating factors. The clinician asks the effect on symptoms of specific aggravating movements and positions for each structure suspected to be a source of symptoms. Table 2.8 illustrates the possible responses of symptoms to aggravating factors.

The logical interpretation of the information on aggravating factors would be that the lumbar spine is producing the central lumbar spine pain, the left sacroiliac joint is producing the left iliac crest pain, and abnormal neurodynamics are producing the posterior buttock and left thigh pain.

Easing factors. The relationship between symptoms may be further confirmed by establishing the easing factors. The patient may find that the lumbar spine pain is eased by lying supine and that the iliac crest pain is eased by applying a tight belt around the pelvis. Provocation of the buttock and posterior thigh pain is reduced by avoiding any stretch to the sciatic nerve, such as in long sitting or getting in or out of a car. This information would confirm the findings from the body chart and aggravating factors.

Table 2.7 Structures suspected to be a source of the symptoms

Symptom	Structure
Central low back pain	Lumbar spine
Left iliac crest pain	Lumbar spine
	Sacroiliac joint
Left buttock and thigh pain	Lumbar spine
	Sacroiliac joint
	Nervous tissue
	Muscles

APPENDIX 2.3: COUNTERFEIT CLINICAL PRESENTATIONS (from Grieve 1994b)

Since physiotherapists are now 'first contact' clinicians, we have assumed greater responsibilities. While those interested in manipulation and allied treatments energetically improve their competence in the various techniques and applications, we might profitably spend a little time considering what we are doing all this to.

If we take patients off the street, we need more than ever to be awake for those conditions that may be other than benign neuromusculoskeletal. This is not 'diagnosis', only an enlightened awareness of when manual or other physical therapy may be more than merely foolish and perhaps dangerous.

There is also the factor of delaying more appropriate treatment. It is not in the patients' best interest to foster the notion that 'first contact clinician' also means 'diagnostician' (Grieve 1991). Pain distribution might confuse unwary or overconfident therapists, who may assume familiarity with a syndrome they recognize and then perhaps find themselves confronting the tip of a very different kind of iceberg.

Distribution of pain from visceral conditions, especially, can easily mislead, unless one maintains a lively awareness of how they can present. Some examples follow:

- Angina can affect face, neck and jaw only, and true anginal pain can on occasions be posterior thoracic as well as precordial. Simple thoracic joint problems often simulate angina, of course.

Table 2.8 Possible aggravating factors for each of the symptoms

Symptoms	Lumbar spine		Sacroiliac joint			Nervous tissue	Hip
	Flexion	Walking	Sitting	Standing on one leg	Rolling over in bed	Long sit	Squat
Lumbar spine pain	+	–	+	–	–	–	–
Iliac crest pain	–	+	–	+	+	–	–
Buttock and posterior thigh pain	–	–	–	–	–	+	–

+, reproduction of symptoms; –, no production of symptoms.

- Hiatus hernia may present with chest and bilateral shoulder pain, as may oesophageal spasm with, in this case, added radiation to the back.
- Virtually anything in the abdomen can present with back pain; examples are peptic ulcer, cancer of the colon or rectum, retroperitoneal disease (e.g. cancer of the pancreas) or abdominal arterial disease (Grieve 1994a). Some suggest that a peptic ulcer must be a gross lesion to refer pain to the back, yet individuals with an ulcer shallow enough to escape barium meal examination may have back pain from the ulcer. Even when the ulcer is healing a glass of milk will ease the backache that follows gardening (Brewerton, personal communication, 1990). It is important to quickly identify non-neuromusculoskeletal conditions so these patients can receive appropriate treatment.

Provocation and relief

A common opinion is that benign neuromusculoskeletal conditions of the spine are recognizable because the clinical features are provoked by certain postures and activities (such as coughing and sneezing) and lessened by other (antalgic) postures and activities; this pattern of provocation and relief being the distinguishing factor. By contrast, the features of systemic, neoplastic or other (non-neuromusculoskeletal) conditions are said, in broad terms, to be identifiable in being less influenced by postures or activity.

This rule of thumb is too simplistic; many conditions, in either category, do not behave in this way.

The writer recalls two patients: one who, with a clear history of recent trauma to the left upper thorax, developed the classic features of a simple rib joint lesion, and another who presented with a watertight history of bouts of low back pain, closely related to prolonged periods of sitting and stooping. In each case, the physical signs confirmed the opinion that these were simple benign lesions. Both were neoplasms. Both patients soon succumbed. Fortunately, treatment was not aggressive or enthusiastic and soon stopped.

Malignant testicular tumours in young men

The reason for writing in a little detail about this tumour is that, while infrequent, it is the most common form of cancer in young men by reason of its age-specific incidence, i.e. 20–35 years. The incidence is steadily increasing in many countries. In Scotland, for example, the frequency has doubled from 2.5 males per 100 000 to 5.0 per 100 000 in the last two decades (Kaye 1990). Denmark has also reported a significant increase in recent years.

Metastases from the testis occur in the majority of patients with testicular germ-cell tumours, progressing through the lymphatics via the spermatic cord to the para-aortic, retroperitoneal and retrocrural lymph nodes, then through the thoracic duct to the posterior mediastinum and (usually left-sided) supraclavicular lymph nodes. Vascular spread may also occur, usually involving the lungs as well as the lymph nodes.

Clinical features

The characteristically hard-textured mass is painless in 75% of patients, and is usually discovered by self-examination. As a rule, the patient is otherwise healthy and asymptomatic. That is, until the para-aortic lymph nodes become involved, which is declared by backache (Cantwell et al 1989, Cole 1987, Smith et al 1989). Low back pain is the common early symptom of retroperitoneal lymph node metastasis. The pain is provoked by coughing and sneezing, and this feature may well delay diagnosis of the true cause (Cantwell et al 1989), besides initiating time-wasting and ineffectual treatment for a supposed benign lumbar spine condition. In the advanced stage there is anorexia, weight loss and dyspnoea.

Caution

There exists a wide variety of clinical misrepresentations, the signs and symptoms of which are counterfeit and should not be taken at their face value. A few have been mentioned; for others see Grieve (1994a). Physiotherapy is inappropriate (Sicard-Rosenbaum & Danoff 1993). It is wise to remember that radiography will not reveal metastasis of vertebral bone until the involvement is gross or at least well advanced (O'Connor & Currier 1992).

We should be awake for the young man who, in the absence of a history of trauma or stress and otherwise in good health, presents with low back pain which is provoked by coughing and sneezing.

Patients should be encouraged to examine themselves. The finding of a suspicious hard lump indicates the need for prompt referral to a surgeon or oncology department. Happily, chemotherapy is often curative.

References

Adams C B T, Logue V 1971 Studies in cervical spondylotic myelopathy II. The movement and contour of the spine in relation to the neural complications of cervical spondylosis. Brain 94: 569–587

Austen R 1991 The distribution and characteristics of lumbar-lower limb symptoms in subjects with and without a neurological deficit. In: Proceedings of the Manipulative Physiotherapists Association of Australia, 7th biennial conference, New South Wales, pp 252–257

Bogduk N 1994 Cervical causes of headache and dizziness. In: Boyling J D, Palastanga N (eds) Grieve's modern manual therapy, 2nd edn. Churchill Livingstone, Edinburgh, ch 22, p 317

Cantwell B M, McDonald I, Campbell S, Millward M J, Roberts J T 1989 Back pain delaying diagnosis of metastatic testicular tumours. Lancet 2(8665): 739–740

Clinical Standards Advisory Report 1994 Report of a CSAG committee on back pain. HMSO, London

Cole R P 1987 Low back pain and testicular cancer. British Medical Journal 295: 840–841

Corrigan B, Maitland G D 1994 Musculoskeletal and sports injuries. Butterworth-Heinemann, Oxford

Dalton P A, Jull G A 1989 The distribution and characteristics of neck-arm pain in patients with and without a neurological deficit. Australian Journal of Physiotherapy 35(1): 3–8

Dickson R A, Wright V 1984 Musculoskeletal disease. Heinemann, London

Doubell T P, Mannion R J, Woolf C 2002 The dorsal horn: state-dependent sensory processing, plasticity and the generation of pain. In: Melzack R, Wall P (eds) Textbook of pain, 4th edn. Churchill Livingstone, Edinburgh, ch 6, p 165

Fields H (ed) 1995 Core curriculum for professional education in pain, 2nd edn. IASP, Seattle, WA

Gifford L 1996 The clinical biology of ache and pains (course manual), 5th edn. Neuro-Orthopaedic Institute UK, Falmouth

Goodman C C, Boisonnault W G 1998 Pathology: implications for the physical therapist. W B Saunders, Philadelphia

Grieve G P 1981 Common vertebral joint problems. Churchill Livingstone, Edinburgh

Grieve G P 1991 Mobilisation of the spine, 5th edn. Churchill Livingstone, Edinburgh

Grieve G P 1994a The masqueraders. In: Boyling J D, Palastanga N (eds) Grieve's modern manual therapy, 2nd edn. Churchill Livingstone, Edinburgh, ch 63, p 841

Grieve G P 1994b Counterfeit clinical presentations. Manipulative Physiotherapist 26: 17–19

Harding V, Williams A C de C 1995 Extending physiotherapy skills using a psychological approach: cognitive-behavioural management of chronic pain. Physiotherapy 81(11): 681–688

Hinnant D W 1994 Psychological evaluation and testing. In: Tollison C D (ed) Handbook of pain management, 2nd edn. Williams & Wilkins, Baltimore, MD, ch 4, p 18

Jones M A 1994 Clinical reasoning process in manipulative therapy. In: Boyling J D, Palastanga N (eds) Grieve's modern manual therapy, 2nd edn. Churchill Livingstone, Edinburgh, ch 34, p 471

Jones M A, Rivett D A 2004 Clinical reasoning for manual therapists. Butterworth-Heinemann, Edinburgh

Jull G A 1986 Examination of the lumbar spine. In: Grieve GP (ed) Modern manual therapy. Churchill Livingstone, Edinburgh, ch 51, p 547

Kaye S B 1990 Testis cancer. In: McArdle C (ed) Surgical oncology. Butterworth, London, ch 10

Keefe F J, Block A R 1982 Development of an observation method for assessing pain behaviour in chronic low back pain patients. Behavioral Therapy 13: 363–375

Lindsay K W, Bone I, Callander R 1997 Neurology and neurosurgery illustrated, 3rd edn. Churchill Livingstone, Edinburgh

McGuire D B 1995 The multiple dimensions of cancer pain: a framework for assessment and management. In: McGuire D B, Yarbro C H, Ferrell B R (eds) Cancer pain management, 2nd edn. Jones & Bartlett, Boston, MA, ch 1, pp 1–17

McKenzie R A 1981 The lumbar spine: mechanical diagnosis and therapy. Spinal Publications, New Zealand

Macnab I 1971 Negative disc exploration, an analysis of the causes of nerve-root involvement in sixty eight patients. Journal of Bone and Joint Surgery 53A(5): 891–903

Magee D J 1997 Orthopedic physical assessment, 3rd edn. W B Saunders, Philadelphia

Main C J, Spanswick C C 2000 Pain management, an interdisciplinary approach. Churchill Livingstone, Edinburgh

Maitland G D 1991 Peripheral manipulation, 3rd edn. Butterworths, London

Maitland G D, Hengeveld E, Banks K, English K 2001 Maitland's vertebral manipulation, 6th edn. Butterworth-Heinemann, Oxford

Melzack R, Wall P 1996 The challenge of pain, 2nd edn. Penguin, London

Mense S 1993 Nociception from skeletal muscle in relation to clinical muscle pain. Pain 54(3): 241–289

Mooney V, Robertson J 1976 The facet syndrome. Clinical Orthopaedics and Related Research 115: 149–156

Nachemson A 1992 Lumbar mechanics as revealed by lumbar intradiscal pressure measurements. In: Jayson M I V (ed) The lumbar spine and back pain, 4th edn. Churchill Livingstone, Edinburgh, ch 9, p 157

Newham D J, Mills K R 1999 Muscles tendons and ligaments. In: Wall P D, Melzack R (eds) Textbook of pain, 4th edn. Churchill Livingstone, Edinburgh, ch 22, p 517

O'Connor M I, Currier B L 1992 Metastatic disease of the spine. Orthopaedics 15: 611–620

Refshauge K, Gass E (eds) 2004 Musculoskeletal physiotherapy clinical science and evidence-based practice. Butterworth-Heinemann, Oxford

Shorland S 1998 Management of chronic pain following whiplash injuries. In Gifford L (ed) Topical issues in pain. Neuro-Orthopaedic Institute UK, Falmouth, ch 8, pp 115–134

Sicard-Rosenbaum L, Danoff J 1993 Cancer and ultrasound: a warning. Physical Therapy 73: 404–406

Smith D B, Newlands E S, Rustin G J, Begent R H, Bagshawe K D 1989 Lumbar pain in stage 1 testicular germ-cell tumour: a symptom preceding radiological abnormality. British Journal of Urology 64: 302–304

Solomon L, Warwick D, Nayagam S 2001 Apley's system of orthopaedics and fractures, 8th edn. Arnold, London

Taylor D C M, Pierau Fr-K, Mizutani M 1984 Possible bases for referred pain. In: Holden A V, Winlow W (eds) The neurobiology of pain. Manchester University Press, Manchester, ch 10, p 143

Van Cranenburgh B 1989 Inleiding in de toegepaste neurowetenschappen, deel 1, Neurofilosofie (Introduction to applied neuroscience, part 1, Neurophysiology), 3rd edn. Uitgeversmaatschappij de Tijdstroom, Lochum

Waddell G 2004 The back pain revolution, 2nd edn. Churchill Livingstone, Edinburgh

Wells P E, Frampton V, Bowsher D 1994 Pain management by physiotherapy, 2nd edn. Butterworth-Heinemann, Oxford

Williams A C de C 1994 Assessment of the chronic pain patient. Clinical Psychology Forum 71: 9–13

Williams A C de C 1995 Pain measurement in chronic pain management. Pain Reviews 2: 39–63

Chapter 3

Physical examination

CHAPTER CONTENTS

INTRODUCTION

The aim of the physical examination is to determine what structure(s) and/or factor(s) are responsible for producing the patient's symptoms. Physical testing procedures are carried out to collect evidence to confirm the clinician's hypotheses and negate other possible hypotheses. As has been clearly stated elsewhere, the physical examination 'is not simply the indiscriminate application of routine tests, but rather should be seen as an extension of the subjective examination . . . for specifically testing hypotheses considered from the subjective examination' (Jones & Jones 1994).

Two assumptions are made when carrying out the physical examination:

- If symptoms are reproduced (or eased) then the test has somehow effected the structures at fault. The word 'structures' is used in the widest sense of the word, and could include anatomical structures or physiological mechanisms. None of the tests stress individual structures in isolation – each test affects a number of tissues, both locally and at a distance. For example, knee flexion will affect the tibiofemoral and patellofemoral intra-articular and periarticular joint structures, surrounding muscles and nerves, as well as joints, muscles and nerves proximally at the hip and spine and distally at the ankle.
- If an abnormality is detected in a structure, which theoretically could refer symptoms to the symptomatic area, then that structure is

suspected to be a source of the symptoms; and is fully examined in the physical examination. The abnormality is described as a comparable sign (Maitland 1991).

The term 'objective' is often applied to the physical examination but suggests that this part of the examination is not prejudiced and that the findings are valid and reliable. This is certainly misleading as most of the tests carried out rely on the skill of the clinician to observe, move and palpate the patient, and as stated earlier, these are not pure tests. The clinician needs to take account of this when making an assessment of a patient based on the findings of the physical examination. The clinician should use all the information obtained from the subjective and physical examination in order to make sense of the patient's overall presentation; that is, making features fit (Maitland et al 2001). The clinician must therefore keep an open mind, thinking logically throughout the physical examination, not quickly jumping to conclusions based on just one or two tests.

The physical examination is summarized in Table 3.1. Some of the tests that are common to a number of areas of the body, such as posture, muscle tests and neurological examination, are described in this chapter, rather than repeating them in each chapter. More specific tests, such as vertebrobasilar insufficiency, are described in the relevant chapters. The order of the testing given

below can, of course, be varied according to the patient and the condition.

PHYSICAL EXAMINATION STEP BY STEP

Observation

Informal and formal observation of static and dynamic postures can give the clinician information about the following:

- The pathology, e.g. olecranon bursitis produces a localized swelling over the olecranon process
- Whether the patient displays overt pain behaviour (see Box 2.2) and the possible factors contributing to the patient's problem, e.g. a difference in the height of the left and right anterior superior iliac spines in standing suggests a leg length discrepancy
- The physical testing procedures that need to be carried out, e.g. strength tests for any muscle that appears wasted on observation
- The possible treatment techniques, e.g. postural re-education for patients who suffer from headaches and who are observed to have a forward head posture.

It should be remembered, however, that the posture a patient adopts reflects a multitude of factors, including not only the state of bone, joint, muscle and neural tissue, but also the pain experienced and the patient's emotions and body awareness or lack thereof.

Table 3.1 Summary of the physical examination

Observation	Informal and formal observation of posture, muscle bulk and tone, soft tissues, gait, function and patient's attitude
Joint integrity tests	For example, knee abduction and adduction stress tests
Active physiological movements with overpressure	Active movements with overpressure
Passive physiological movements	
Muscle tests	Strength, control, length, isometric contraction, diagnostic
Nerve tests	Neurological integrity, neurodynamic, diagnostic
Special tests	Vascular, soft tissue, cardiorespiratory, etc.
Palpation	Superficial and deep soft tissues, bone, joint, ligament, muscle, tendon and nerve
Joint tests	Accessory movements, natural apophyseal glides, sustained natural apophyseal glides, mobilizations with movement

Informal observation

The clinician should observe the patient in dynamic and static situations; the quality of movement is noted, as are the postural characteristics and facial expression. The observation starts at the beginning of the subjective examination but continues throughout the rest of the subjective and physical examinations. It may well be that this informal observation is as informative as the formal assessment, as a patient under such scrutiny may not adopt his/her usual posture. For example the clinician observes whether the patient is using aids (prescribed or non-prescribed) such as collars, sticks and corsets and whether they are being used in an appropriate way. An aid that is used in an overt manner, such as a bandage worn over clothing, is an indication of possible illness behaviour.

Formal observation

Observation of posture. The clinician observes posture by examining the anterior, lateral and posterior views of the patient. The ideal alignment is summarized in Figure 3.1. Typical postures that will be observed include:

- The *upper (or shoulder) crossed syndrome*, shown in Figure 3.2, where there is elevation and protraction of the shoulders, rotation and abduction (winging) of the scapulae and forward head posture (Janda 1994, 2002).

- The *lower (or pelvic) crossed syndrome*, shown in Figure 3.3, where there is an anteriorly rotated pelvis, an increased lumbar lordosis and slight flexion of the hips.

- The *kyphosis–lordosis posture* (Kendall et al 1993). This is shown in Figure 3.4 and is more or less equivalent to the upper and lower crossed syndromes.

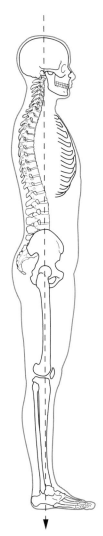

Figure 3.1 Ideal alignment. (From Kendall et al 1993 Muscles testing and function, 4th edn. © Williams and Wilkins.)

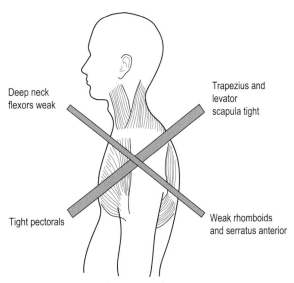

Deep neck flexors weak

Trapezius and levator scapula tight

Tight pectorals

Weak rhomboids and serratus anterior

Figure 3.2 Upper (or shoulder) crossed syndrome. (From Chaitow 1996, with permission.)

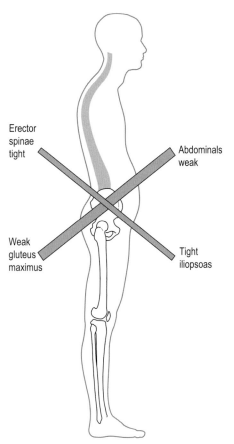

Figure 3.3   Lower (or pelvic) crossed syndrome. (From Chaitow 1996, with permission.)

- *Layer syndrome* (Janda 1994, 2002, Jull & Janda 1987), shown in Figure 3.5, where there are alternate 'layers' of hypertrophic and hypotrophic muscles when the patient is viewed from behind. There is weakness of the lower stabilizers of the scapula, lumbosacral erector spinae, gluteus maximus, rectus abdominis and transversus abdominis; there is hypertrophy of the cervical erector spinae, upper trapezius, levator scapulae, thoracolumbar erector spinae and hamstrings.

- The *flat back posture* (Kendall et al 1993), shown in Figure 3.6, which is characterized by a slightly extended cervical spine, flexion of the upper part of the thoracic spine (the lower part is straight), absent lumbar lordosis, a posterior pelvic tilt and extension of the hip joints and slight plantarflexion of the ankle joints. This is

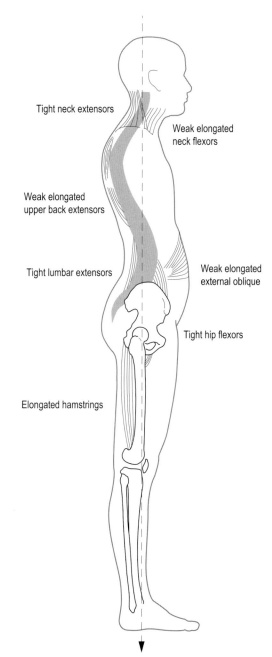

Figure 3.4   Kyphosis–lordosis posture. (After Kendall et al 1993 Muscles: testing and function, 4th edn. © Williams & Wilkins.)

thought to be due to elongated and weak hip flexors and short, strong hamstrings. Sahrmann (1993) additionally considers the lumbar paraspinal muscles to be long.

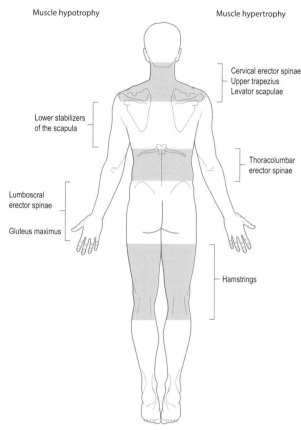

Muscle hypotrophy

Muscle hypertrophy

Cervical erector spinae
Upper trapezius
Levator scapulae

Lower stabilizers
of the scapula

Thoracolumbar
erector spinae

Lumboscral
erector spinae

Gluteus maximus

Hamstrings

Figure 3.5   Layer syndrome. (From Jull & Janda 1987, with permission.)

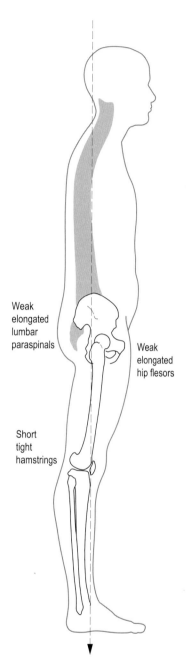

Weak
elongated
lumbar
paraspinals

Weak
elongated
hip flesors

Short
tight
hamstrings

Figure 3.6   Flat back posture. (After Kendall et al 1993 Muscles: testing and function, 4th edn. Williams & Wilkins.)

- The *sway back posture* (Kendall et al 1993), shown in Figure 3.7, which is characterized by a forward head posture, slightly extended cervical spine, increased flexion and posterior displacement of the upper trunk, flexion of the lumbar spine, posterior pelvic tilt, hyper-extended hip joints with anterior displacement of the pelvis, hyperextended knee joints and neutral ankle joints. This posture is thought to be due to elongated and weak hip flexors, external obliques, upper back extensors and neck flexors, short and strong hamstrings and upper fibres of the internal oblique abdominal muscles, and strong, but not short, lumbar paraspinal muscles.

- The *handedness posture* (Kendall et al 1993), shown in Figure 3.8, which is characterized, for right-handed individuals, as a low right shoulder, adducted scapulae with the right scapula depressed, a thoracolumbar curve convex to the left, lateral pelvic tilt (high on the right), right hip joint adducted with slight medial rotation, and the left hip joint abducted with some

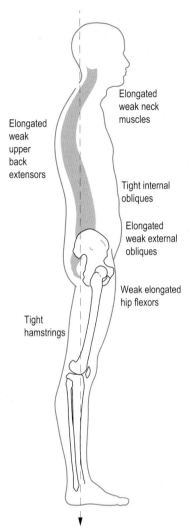

Elongated weak neck muscles

Elongated weak upper back extensors

Tight internal obliques

Elongated weak external obliques

Weak elongated hip flexors

Tight hamstrings

Figure 3.7 Sway back posture. (After Kendall et al 1993 Muscles: testing and function, 4th edn. Williams & Wilkins.)

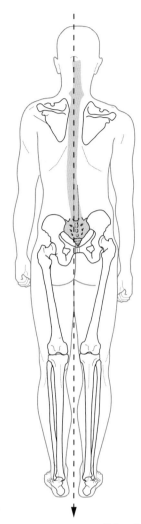

Figure 3.8 Handedness posture. (After Kendall et al 1993 Muscles: testing and function, 4th edn. Williams & Wilkins.)

pronation of the right foot. It is thought to be due to the following muscles being elongated and weak: left lateral trunk muscles, hip abductors on the right, left hip adductors, right peroneus longus and brevis, left tibialis posterior, left flexor hallucis longus and left flexor digitorum longus. The right tensor fasciae latae may or may not be weak. There are short and strong right lateral trunk muscles, left hip abductors, right hip adductors, left peroneus longus and brevis, right tibialis posterior, right flexor hallucis longus and right flexor digitorum longus. The left tensor fasciae latae is usually strong

and there may be tightness in the iliotibial band. There is the appearance of a longer right leg.

Other postural presentations may include skin creases at various spinal levels. A common example would be a crease at the mid-cervical spine indicating a focus of movement at that level; this would be followed up later on in the examination with passive accessory intervertebral movement (PAIVM) and passive physiological intervertebral movement (PPIVM), which would uncover hypermobility at this level. Protracted and downward rotation of the scapula with internal rotation of the humerus is another common presentation; muscle length of rhomboids, levator scapula, pectoralis minor would be indicated as well as muscle control of mid and lower fibres of trapezius and serratus anterior.

Any abnormal asymmetry in posture can be corrected to determine its relevance to the patient's problem. If the symptoms are changed by altering an asymmetrical posture, this suggests that the posture is related to the problem. If the symptoms are not affected then the asymmetrical posture is probably not relevant. Note the resting position of relevant joints as this may be indicative of abnormal length of the muscles (White & Sahrmann 1994).

For further details on examination of posture, readers are referred to Magee 1997, Kendall et al 1993 and other similar textbooks.

The clinician can also observe the patient in sustained postures and during habitual/repetitive movement where these are relevant to the problem. Sustained postures and habitual movements are thought to have a major role in the development of dysfunction (Sahrmann 2002). A patient with neck pain when sitting, for example,

may be observed to have an extended cervical spine and poking chin as well as holding the pelvis in posterior pelvic tilt (Fig. 3.9). When the clinician corrects this posture to determine its relevance to the patient's problem, by guiding the pelvis into anterior pelvic tilt, the poking chin may be lessened and the neck pain reduced.

An example of habitual movement pattern may be a patient with lumbar spine pain who has pain on bending forwards. The patient may flex predominantly at the lumbar spine or predominantly at the hips (Fig. 3.10). If movement mainly occurs at the lumbar spine then this region may be found to be hypermobile (tested by PAIVMs and PPIVMs later on in the examination) and the region where movement is least may be found to be hypomobile.

Observation of muscle form. The clinician observes muscle shape, bulk and tone of the patient, comparing the left and right sides. It must be remembered that handedness and level and frequency of physical activity may produce differences in muscle bulk between sides.

Muscles produce and control movement, and normal movement is dependent on the strength

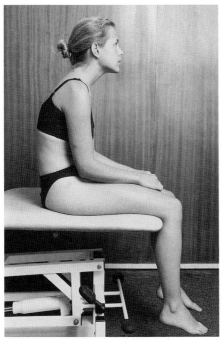 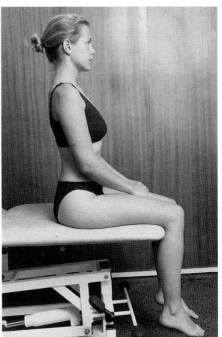

A   B

Figure 3.9 The effect of pelvic tilt on cervical spine posture. **A** In posterior pelvic tilt the cervical spine is extended with a poking chin. **B** When the posterior pelvic tilt is reduced the cervical spine is in a more neutral position.

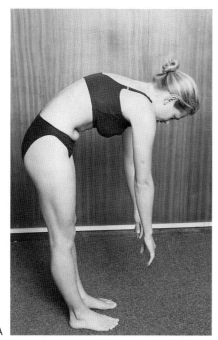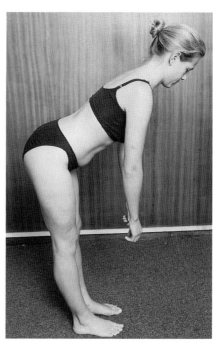

Figure 3.10   On bending forwards the patient may bend predominantly at the lumbar spine (**A**) or at the hips (**B**).

Table 3.2   Reaction of muscles to stress (Comerford & Kinetic Control 2000, Janda 1994, Jull & Janda 1987)

Muscles prone to become tight	Muscles prone to become weak
Masseter, temporalis, digastric and suboccipital muscles, levator scapulae, rhomboid major and minor, upper trapezius, sternocleidomastoid, pectoralis major and minor scalenes, flexors of the upper limb, erector spinae (particularly thoracolumbar and cervical parts), quadratus lumborum, piriformis, tensor fasciae latae, rectus femoris, hamstrings, short hip adductors, tibialis posterior, gastrocnemius	Serratus anterior, middle and lower fibres of trapezius, deep neck flexors, mylohyoid, subscapularis, extensors of upper limb, gluteus maximus, medius and minimus, deep lumbar multifidus, iliopsoas, vastus medialis and lateralis, tibialis anterior and peronei

The reaction of longus colli, longus capitis, rectus capitis anterior, supraspinatus, infraspinatus and teres minor and major is unclear (Janda 1994).

and flexibility of the agonist and antagonist muscles acting over a joint. A concept of muscle imbalance in some individuals has been described by several workers (Jull & Janda 1987, Kendall et al 1999, White & Sahrmann 1994). The postural muscles are thought to shorten under stress, while the phasic muscles become weak (Jull & Janda 1987). In this context, 'phasic' describes muscles that produce movement. These muscles are listed in Table 3.2. More recently, however, White &

Sahrmann (1994) have suggested that the postural muscles tend to lengthen and then appear weak as they are tested in a shortened position.

Observation of soft tissues. The local and general soft tissues can be observed, noting the colour and texture of the skin, the presence of scars, abnormal skin creases suggesting an underlying deformity, swelling of the soft tissues or effusion of the joints. Skin colour and texture can indicate the state of the circulation (a bluish tinge suggesting cyanosis or bruising and redness indicating inflammation), the state of the patient's general health, sympathetic changes such as increased sweating, bruising and the presence of other diseases. For example, peripheral nerve lesions may result in shiny skin that has lost its elasticity and hair, and nails may become brittle and ridged; such as with complex regional pain syndrome (previously called reflex sympathetic dystrophy). Scars may indicate injury or surgery and will be red if recent and white and avascular if old.

Observation of gait. This is often applicable for spinal and lower limb problems. The clinician observes the gait from the front, behind and at the side, looking at the pelvis, hips, knees, ankles and feet. A detailed description of the observation can be found in Magee (1997). Common abnormalities of gait include the following:

- An antalgic gait due to pain at the hip, knee or foot, characterized by a shortened stance phase of the affected limb as compared with the non-affected limb
- An arthrogenic gait, which occurs with hip or knee fusion and is characterized by exaggerated plantarflexion of the opposite ankle and circumduction of the stiff leg to clear the toes
- A gluteus maximus gait due to weakness of this muscle, producing a posterior thoracic movement during the stance phase to maintain hip extension
- Trendelenburg's sign, which is due to weakness of gluteus medius, congenital dislocation of the hip or coxa vara, causing an excessive lateral movement of the thorax towards the affected limb during its stance phase of the gait cycle
- A short leg gait producing a lateral shift of the trunk towards the affected side during the stance phase
- A drop foot gait due to weakness of the ankle and foot dorsiflexors, which causes the patient to lift the knee higher than the unaffected limb
- A stiff knee or hip gait, where the patient lifts the affected leg higher than the unaffected leg in order to clear the ground.

Observation of the patient's attitude and feelings. The age, gender and ethnicity of patients and their cultural, occupational and social backgrounds will all affect the attitudes and feelings they have towards themselves, their condition and the clinician. Patients may feel apprehensive, fearful, embarrassed, restless, resentful, angry or depressed in relation to their condition and/or the clinician. They may, for example, have had several, possibly conflicting explanations of their problem. Unrealistic thoughts and beliefs affect the patients' response to health problems and treatment (Shorland 1998, Zusman 1998). Clinicians should be aware of and sensitive to these attitudes, and empathize and communicate appropriately so as to develop a rapport with their patients and thus enhance their compliance with the treatment.

Joint integrity tests

These are specific tests to determine the stability of the joint and will often be carried out early in the examination, as any instability found will affect, and may contraindicate, further testing. Specific tests are described in the relevant chapters.

Active physiological movements

Active movements are general tests that effect joints, nerves and muscles. In the previous edition of this text, these movements came under the umbrella of 'joint' tests; this can be misleading and is revised here. A detailed examination is made of the quality and range of active and passive (described later) physiological movement. A physiological movement is defined as a movement that can be performed actively – examples include flexion, extension, abduction, adduction, and medial and lateral rotation of the hip or glenohumeral joints. These movements are examined actively; in other words, the patient produces the movement, which tests the function not only of the joint but also of the muscles that produce the movement and the relevant nerves. If the patient's symptoms allow, the clinician then applies an overpressure force to the movement to further assess the movement. In this situation overpressure could be classified as a passive movement; however, normal convention would include overpressure within active movement testing.

The function of a joint is to allow full-range friction-free movement between the bones. A joint is considered to be normal if there is painless full active range of movement and if the resistance to movement felt by the clinician on applying over-pressure is considered to be normal (Maitland 1991). Joint dysfunction is manifested by a reduced (hypomobile) or increased (hypermobile) range of movement, abnormal resistance to movement (through the range or at the end of the range), pain and muscle spasm.

The aims of active physiological movements (Jull 1994) are to:

- Reproduce all or part of the patient's symptoms – the movements that produce symptoms are then analysed to determine which structures are being stressed and these are then implicated as a source of the symptoms
- Determine the pattern, quality, range, resistance and pain response for each movement
- Identify factors that have predisposed to or arisen from the disorder
- Obtain signs on which to assess effectiveness of treatment (reassessment 'asterisks' or 'markers').

This part of the examination offers confirmatory evidence (or not) as to the severity and irritability of the condition that was initially assessed in the subjective examination. The clinician must remain open-minded, as the assessment of severity and irritability has quite commonly to be refined at this stage.

The following information can be noted during the movements, and can be depicted on a movement diagram (described later in the chapter):

- The quality of movement
- The range of movement
- The presence of resistance through the range of movement and at the end of the range of movement
- Pain behaviour (local and referred) through the range
- The occurrence of muscle spasm during the range of movement.

The procedure for testing active physiological movement is as follows.

Resting symptoms prior to each movement should be established so that the effect of the movement on the symptoms can be clearly ascertained.

The active physiological movement is carried out and the *quality of the active physiological move-ment* is observed, noting the smoothness and control of the movement, any deviation from a normal pattern of movement, the muscle activity involved and the tissue tension produced through range. Movement deviation can then be corrected to determine its relevance to the symptoms. A relevant movement deviation is one where symptoms are altered when it is corrected; if symptoms do not change on movement correction, this suggests that the deviation is not relevant to the patient's problem.

The quality of movement can be tested further by altering part of the patient's posture during an active movement (White & Sahrmann 1994). For example, cervical movements can be retested with the clinician passively placing the scapula in various positions to determine the effect of length and stretch of the sternocleidomastoid, upper trapezius and levator scapulae.

An alternative method of testing the quality of movement in more detail is by palpating the proximal joint as the movement is carried out; for example, palpation of the cervical spinous processes during shoulder elevation may reveal excessive or abnormal spinal movement (White & Sahrmann 1994).

Active physiological movements test not only the function of joints but also the function of muscles and nerves. This interrelationship is well explained by a movement-system balance (MSB) theory put forward by White & Sahrmann (1994). It suggests that there is an ideal mode of movement-system function and that any deviation from this will be less efficient and more stressful to the components of the system.

Ideal movement-system function is considered to be dependent on:

- The maintenance of precise movement of rotating parts; in other words, the instantaneous axis of rotation (IAR) follows a normal path. The pivot point about which the vertebrae move constantly changes during physiological movements and its location at any instant is referred to as the IAR. The shape of the joint surfaces and the mobility and length of soft tissue structures (skin, ligament, tendon, muscle and nerves) are all thought to affect the position of the IAR. There is some support for this theory, as several studies have found that some pathological conditions have been associated with an altered IAR (Amevo et al 1992, Frankel et al 1971, Pennal et al 1972).

- Normal muscle length. As mentioned earlier, muscles can become shortened or lengthened and this will affect the quality and range of movement.
- Normal motor control, i.e. the precise and coordinated action of muscles.
- Normal relative stiffness of contractile and non-contractile tissue. It is suggested that the body takes the line of least resistance during movement – in other words, movement will occur where resistance is least. Thus, for instance, areas of hypomobility will often be compensated by movement at other areas, which then become hypermobile. An example of this is seen in patients who have had a spinal fusion that is associated with hypermobility at adjacent segments. In the same way, excessive shoulder girdle elevation will occur at the scapulothoracic complex in patients suffering from chronic capsulitis. With time, these movements become 'learned' and the soft tissues around the joint adapt to the new movement patterns such that muscles may become weak and lengthened or tight and shortened.
- Normal kinetics, i.e. the movement-system function of joints proximal and distal to the site of the symptoms.

A movement abnormality may therefore be due to several factors (White & Sahrmann 1994):

- A shortened tissue, which may prevent a particular movement
- A muscle that is weak and unable to produce the movement
- A movement 'taken over' by a dominant muscle – this may occur with muscle paralysis, altered muscle length-tension relationship, pain inhibition, repetitive movements or postures leading to learned movement patterns
- Pain on movement.

Joint range is measured clinically using a goniometer or tape measure, or more commonly it is done by eye. Readers are directed to other texts on details of joint measurement (American Academy of Orthopaedic Surgeons 1990, Gerhardt 1992). It is worth mentioning here that range of movement is influenced by a number of factors – age, gender, occupation, date, time of day, temperature, emotional status, effort, medication, injury and disease – and there are wide variations in range of movement between individuals (Gerhardt 1992).

Pain behaviour (both local and referred) throughout the joint range is recorded. The clinician asks the patient to indicate the point in the range where pain is first felt or is increased (if there is pain present before moving) and then how this pain is affected by further movement. The clinician can crudely quantify the pain by asking the patient to rate the pain on a scale of 0–10, where '0' represents no pain and '10' represents the maximum pain ever felt by the patient. The behaviour of the pain through the range can be clearly documented using a movement diagram, which is described later in this chapter.

The eliciting of any *muscle spasm* through the range of movement is noted. Muscle spasm is an involuntary contraction of muscle as a result of nerve irritation or secondary to injury of underlying structures, such as bone, joint or muscle, and occurs in order to prevent movement and further injury.

Overpressure is applied at the end of a physiological range (as long as the symptoms are not severe). Overpressure needs to be carried out carefully if it is to give accurate information; the following guidelines may help the clinician:

- The patient needs to be comfortable and suitably supported
- The clinician needs to be in a comfortable position
- The clinician uses body weight or the upper trunk to produce the force, rather than the intrinsic muscles of the hand, which can be uncomfortable for the patient
- For accurate direction of the overpressure force, the clinician's forearm is positioned in line with the direction of the force
- The force is applied slowly and smoothly to the end of the available range
- At the end of the available range, the clinician can then apply small oscillatory movements to feel the resistance at this position.

There are a variety of ways of applying overpressure; the choice will depend on factors such as the size of the clinician, the size of the patient and the health and age of the patient. The over-pressures demonstrated in each of the following chapters are given as examples only; it is the application of the principles that is more important.

While applying overpressure, the clinician will:

- Feel the quality of the movement
- Note the range of further movement
- Feel the resistance through the latter part of the range and at the end of the range
- Note the behaviour of pain (local and referred) through the overpressed range of movement
- Feel the presence of any muscle spasm through the range.

Some clinicians do not add an overpressure if the movement is limited by pain. However, it is argued here that the clinician cannot be certain that the movement is limited by pain unless they apply the overpressure. The other reason why it can be informative to apply overpressure in the presence of pain is that one of three scenarios can occur; the overpressure can cause the pain to ease, to stay the same, or to get worse. This information can help the clinician to understand in more detail the movement and what is limiting it and may also be helpful in selecting a treatment dose. For example, a rather more provocative movement may be chosen when on overpressure the pain eases or stays the same, compared to when the pain increases. What is vital when applying an overpressure to a movement that appears to be limited by pain is to apply the force extremely slowly and carefully, to only minimally increase the patient's pain.

Normal movement should be pain-free, smooth and resistance-free until the later stages of range when resistance will gradually increase until it limits further movement. Poor quality of movement could be demonstrated by the patient's facial expression, e.g. excessive grimacing due to excessive effort or pain; by limb trembling due to muscle weakness; by substitution movements elsewhere due to joint restriction or muscle weakness – for instance, on active hip flexion the clinician may observe lumbar flexion and posterior rotation of the pelvis.

Movement is limited by one or more of a number of factors, such as articular surface contact, limit of ligamentous, muscle or tendon extensibility and apposition of soft tissue, and each of these factors will give a different quality of resistance. For example, wrist flexion and extension are limited by increasing tension in the surrounding ligaments and muscles; knee flexion is limited by soft tissue apposition of the calf and thigh muscles; and elbow extension is limited by bony apposition. Thus different joints and different movements have different end-feels. The quality of this resistance felt at the end of range has been categorized by Cyriax (1982) and Kaltenborn (2002) as shown in Table 3.3. The resistance is considered abnormal if a joint does not have its characteristic normal end-feel, e.g. when knee flexion has a hard end-feel or if the resistance is felt too early or too late in what is considered normal range of movement. Additionally, Cyriax describes three abnormal end-feels: empty, springy and muscle spasm (Table 3.4).

The pain may increase, decrease or stay the same when overpressure is applied. This is valuable information as it can confirm the severity of the patient's pain and can help to determine the firmness with which manual treatment techniques

Table 3.3   Normal end-feels (Cyriax 1982, Kaltenborn 2002)

Cyriax	Kaltenborn	Description
Soft tissue approximation	Soft tissue approximation or soft tissue stretch	Soft end-feel, e.g. knee flexion or ankle dorsiflexion
Capsular feel	Firm soft tissue stretch	Fairly hard halt to movement, e.g. shoulder, elbow or hip rotation due to capsular or ligamentous stretching
Bone to bone	Hard	Abrupt halt to the movement, e.g. elbow extension

Table 3.4 Abnormal end-feels (Cyriax 1982, Kaltenborn 2002). Abnormality is also recognized if a joint does not have its characteristic end-feel or if the resistance is felt too early or too late in what is considered the normal range

Cyriax	Kaltenborn	Description
Empty feel	Empty	No resistance offered due to severe pain secondary to serious pathology such as fractures, active inflammatory processes, neoplasm, etc.
Springy block		A rebound feel at end range, e.g. with a torn meniscus blocking knee extension
Spasm		Sudden hard end-feel due to muscle spasm

Box 3.1 Modifications to the examination of active physiological movements

- Repeated movements
- Speed of movement
- Combined movements
- Compression or distraction
- Sustained movements
- Injuring movements
- Differentiation tests
- Functional ability

can be applied. A patient whose pain is eased or remains the same with overpressure could be treated more firmly than a patient whose pain is increased.

Further information about the active range of movement can be gained in a number of ways (Box 3.1), as described below:

Repeated movements. Repeating a movement several times may alter the quality and range of the movement. There may be a gradual increase in range with repeated movements because of the effects of hysteresis on the collagen-containing tissues such as joint capsules, ligaments, muscles and nerves (Gilmore 1986). If a patient with a Colles fracture who has recently come out of plaster were to repeatedly move the wrist into flexion, the range of movement would probably increase. There may be an increase or decrease in symptoms as the movement is repeated.

The change in symptoms with repeated movements of the spine has been more fully described by McKenzie (1981, 1990). He divides all mechanical joint problems of the spine into three syndromes; postural, dysfunction and derangement.

If movements cause symptoms at the end of range and repeated movements do not significantly alter the symptoms, the condition is classified as a dysfunction syndrome. The syndrome is thought to be caused by shortening of scar tissue such that, when movement puts the shortened tissue on stretch, pain is produced, but is relieved as soon as the stretch is taken off. It will occur whenever there is inadequate mobilization following trauma or spinal surgery where scar tissue has been laid down during the healing process. Of course, this scenario is commonly seen in the peripheral joints following a period of immobilization, e.g. after a fracture.

If repeated movements produce phenomena known as peripheralization and centralization of symptoms, the condition is classified as a derangement syndrome. Peripheralization occurs when symptoms arising from the spine and felt laterally from the midline or distally (into arms or legs) are increased or transferred to a more distal position when certain movements are performed. Centralization occurs when symptoms arising from the spine and felt laterally from the midline or distally (into arms or legs) are reduced or transferred to a more central position when certain movements are performed. A patient will exhibit both phenomena – peripheralization of symptoms on repeating a movement in one direction and centralization on repeated movement in the opposite direction. For example, a patient may develop leg pain (peripheralization) on repetitive lumbar spine flexion that eases on repetitive extension (centralization); similarly, arm pain may be produced on repetitive cervical flexion that eases on repeated extension (Fig. 3.11).

The exact mechanisms underlying these phenomena are unclear. Repeated movements in the spine alter the position of the nucleus pulposus within the intervertebral disc (Shah et al 1978) and it is thought that this increases or decreases pres-sure on pain-sensitive structures. McKenzie (1981, 1990) postulated that the nucleus pulposus may be displaced in any number of directions, and repeated movements have the effect of increasing this displacement. So, for example, it is suggested that if the nucleus pulposus lies anteriorly, then repeated extension would move the nucleus ante-

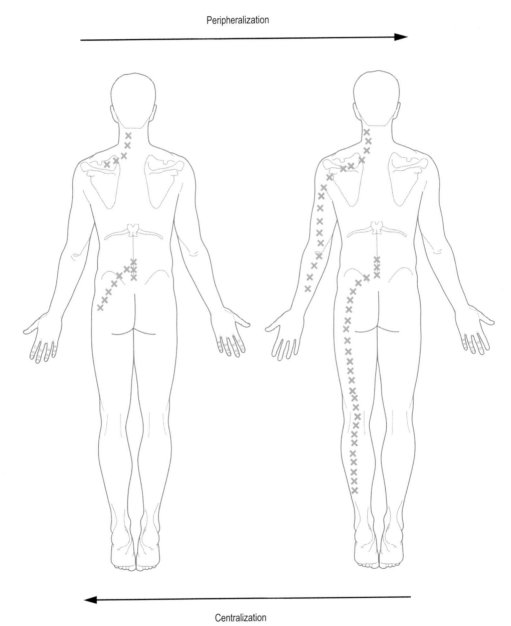

Figure 3.11 Peripheralization and centralization phenomena.

riorly and repeated flexion would move the nucleus posteriorly. The commonest nuclear displacement occurs in the posterior direction following, for example, prolonged periods of flexion; repetitive flexion is thought to then move the nucleus pulposus even more posteriorly. This increases the pressure on the pain-sensitive structures around the posterior aspect of the intervertebral disc and is thought to cause referral of pain into the leg (peripheralization). Repeated extension then causes the nucleus to move anteriorly and thus relieves the pressure on the pain-sensitive structures and eases the leg pain (centralization). While this is a rather simplistic and inaccurate explanation, particularly in the light of recent research on the cervical intervertebral disc (Mercer & Jull 1996), the true mechanism by which repetitive movements alter the patient's pain still remains unclear. There are various degrees of disc derangement and these are discussed in the chapters on the examination of the cervical, thoracic and lumbar spine.

Speed of the movement. Movements can be carried out at different speeds and symptoms are noted. Increasing the speed of movement may be necessary in order to replicate the patient's functional restriction and reproduce the patient's symptoms. For example, a footballer with knee pain may only feel symptoms when running fast and symptoms may only be reproduced with quick movements of the knee, and possibly only when weight-bearing. One of the reasons that the speed of the movement can alter symptoms is because the rate of loading of viscoelastic tissues affects their extensibility and stiffness (Noyes et al 1974).

Combined movements. Combined movements are where movement in one plane is combined with movement in another plane; for example, shoulder abduction with lateral rotation. There are a number of reasons why the clinician may choose to combine in this way and include:

- Further information of a movement dysfunction
- To mimic a functional activity
- To increase the stress of the underlying tissues, particularly the joint. This can be quickly veri-

fied by moving your index finger at the MCP joint into extension and end range rotation; you will feel your joint stretch, it may even click (!) The clinician may want to increase the stress in this way to help determine whether the joint is the source of the patient's symptoms.

To further verify whether the joint is a source of the patient's symptoms, accessory movements may be carried out (see later). The use of combined movements and accessory movements, together, form what is sometimes referred to as 'joint clearing tests'; this is an abbreviation. Normally, if strong end-of-range combined movements and accessory movements do not reproduce the patient's symptoms and reassessment asterisks remain the same, then the joint is not considered to be a source of the patient's symptoms; hence the joint is 'cleared'. If symptoms are produced or there is reduced range of movement, the joint cannot be considered 'normal' and may need further examination. Suggested combined movements to 'clear' each joint are given in Table 3.5 and generally are the more stressful physiological movements.

A movement can be added prior to another movement; for example, the glenohumeral joint can be medially rotated prior to flexion. Alternatively, a movement can be added at the end of another movement; for example, the hip can be moved into flexion and then adduction can be added. The effect of altering the sequence of these movements might be expected to alter the symptom response.

Combining spinal movements has been thoroughly explored by Edwards (1999). Similar to the examples above, the lumbar spine can be moved into flexion and then lateral flexion, or it can be moved into lateral flexion and then flexion. Once again, the signs and symptoms will vary according to the order of these movements. Recording of the findings of combined movements for the lumbar spine is illustrated in Figure 3.12, which demonstrates that left rotation, extension and left lateral flexion in extension are limited to half normal range, both symptoms being produced in the left posterior part of the body. Following examination of the active movements and various combined movements, the patient can be categorized into one of three patterns (Edwards 1999):

Table 3.5   Joint clearing tests

Joint	Physiological movement	Accessory movement
Cervical spine	Quadrants (flexion and extension)	All movements
Thoracic spine	Rotation and quadrants (flexion and extension)	All movements
Lumbar spine	Flexion and quadrants (flexion and extension)	All movements
Sacroiliac joint	Anterior and posterior gapping	
Shoulder girdle	Elevation, depression, protraction and retraction	
Shoulder joint	Flexion and hand behind back	
Acromioclavicular joint	All movements (particularly horizontal flexion)	
Sternoclavicular joint	All movements	
Elbow joint	All movements	
Wrist joint	Flexion/extension and radial/ulnar deviation	
Thumb	Extension carpometacarpal and thumb opposition	
Fingers	Flexion at interphalangeal joints and grip	
Hip joint	Squat and hip quadrant	
Knee joint	All movements	
Ankle joint	Plantarflexion/dorsiflexion and inversion/eversion	
Patellofemoral joint	Medial/lateral glide and cephalad/caudad glide	
Temporomandibular joint	Open/close jaw, side to side movement, protraction/retraction	All movements

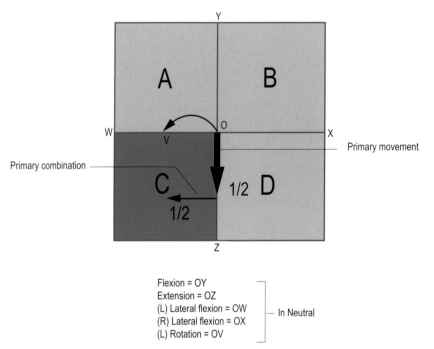

Flexion = OY
Extension = OZ
(L) Lateral flexion = OW
(R) Lateral flexion = OX
(L) Rotation = OV

In Neutral

Figure 3.12   Recording combined movements. Movements can be quickly and easily recorded using this box. It assumes that the clinician is standing behind the patient so that A and B refer to anterior, and C and D to posterior parts of the body; A and C are left side and B and D are right side. The box depicts the following information: left rotation is limited to half range; extension and left lateral flexion in extension range are half normal range. The symptoms are in the left posterior part of the body (represented by the cross-hatching). (From Edwards 1992, with permission.)

- *Regular stretch pattern*. This occurs when the symptoms are produced on the opposite side from that to which movement is directed. An example of this would be if left-sided cervical spine pain is reproduced on flexion, lateral flexion to the right and rotation to the right, and all other movements are full and pain-free. In this case, the patient is said to have a regular stretch pattern. The term stretch is used to describe the general stretch of spinal structures, in this example on the left-hand side of the cervical spine.
- *Regular compression pattern*. This occurs when the symptoms are reproduced on the side to which the movement is directed. If left-sided cervical spine pain is reproduced on extension, left lateral flexion and left rotation and all other movements are full and pain-free, the patient is said to have a regular compression pattern. The term compression is used to describe the general compression of spinal structures, in this example on the left-hand side of the cervical spine.
- *Irregular pattern*. Patients who do not clearly fit into a regular stretch or compression pattern are categorized as having an irregular pattern. In this case, symptoms are provoked by a mixture of stretching and compressing movements.

This information, along with the severity, irritability and nature (SIN) factors, can help to direct treatment. The clinician can position the patient in such a way as to increase or decrease the stretching or compression effect during palpation techniques. For example, accessory movements can be carried out with the spine at the limit of a physiological movement or in a position of maximum comfort.

Compression or distraction. Compression or distraction of the joint articular surfaces can be added during the movement. For example, compression or distraction of the shoulder joint can be applied with passive shoulder flexion. If the lesion is intra-articular then the symptoms are often made worse by compression and eased by distraction (Maitland 1985; Maitland et al 2001).

Sustained movements. A movement is held at end range or at a point in range and the effects on symptoms are noted. In this position, tissue creep will occur, whereby the soft tissue structures that are being stretched lengthen (Kazarian 1972). Range of movement would therefore increase in normal tissue.

Injuring movement. The movement carried out at the time of injury can be tested. This may be necessary when symptoms have not been reproduced by the previous movements described above or if the patient has momentary symptoms.

Differentiation tests. These tests are useful to distinguish between two structures suspected to be a source of the symptoms (Maitland et al 2001, Maitland 1991). A position that provokes symptoms is held constant and then a movement that increases or decreases the stress on one of the structures is added and the effect on symptoms is noted. For example, in the straight leg raise test, hip flexion with knee extension is held constant, which stretches the sciatic nerve and the hip extensor muscles (particularly hamstrings), and dorsiflexion of the ankle is then added. This increases the stretch of the sciatic nerve without altering the length of the hip extensors. Increased or reduced symptoms on dorsiflexion or plantarflexion would implicate the sciatic nerve.

Another example is the addition of cervical flexion and extension when the patient is in lumbar spine flexion and feels pain over the posterior thigh. Increased thigh pain on cervical flexion, reduced on cervical extension, can help to differentiate symptoms originating from neural tissue and those from other structures around the lumbar spine.

Functional ability. Some functional ability may be tested in the observation section, but further testing may be carried out at this stage, to examine gait analysis, stair climbing, lifting, etc. There are a number of functional rating scales available for the different joints, which will be briefly explored in relevant chapters. Assessment of general function using standardized tests is recommended, as it facilitates objectivity and evaluation of the treatment (Harding et al 1994).

Capsular pattern. In arthritic joint conditions affecting the capsule of the joint, the range of movement can become restricted in various directions and to different degrees. Each joint has a typical pattern of restricted movement (Table 3.6) and, because the joint capsule is involved, the phenomenon is known as a capsular pattern (Cyriax 1982). Where the capsular pattern involves a number of movements, these are listed in descending order of limitation; for instance, lateral rotation is the most limited range in the shoulder capsular pattern, followed by abduction and then medial rotation.

Passive physiological movements

A comparison of the response of symptoms to the active and passive movements can help to determine whether the structure at fault is non-contractile (articular) or contractile (extra-articular) (Cyriax 1982). If the lesion is of non-contractile tissue, such as ligamentous tissue, then active and passive movements will be painful and/or restricted in the same direction. For instance, if the anterior joint capsule of the proximal interphalangeal joint of the index finger is shortened, there will be pain and/or restriction of finger extension, whether this movement is carried out actively or passively. If the lesion is in a contractile tissue (i.e. muscle) then active and passive movements are painful and/or restricted in opposite directions. For example, a muscle lesion in the anterior fibres of deltoid will be painful on active flexion of the shoulder joint and on passive extension of the shoulder.

The range of active physiological movements of the spine is the accumulated movement at a number of vertebral segments and is thus a rather crude measure of range that does not in any way localize which segment is affected. For this reason, passive physiological intervertebral movements (PPIVMs) are carried out to determine the range of movement at each intervertebral level. To do this, the clinician feels the movement of adjacent spinous processes, articular pillars or transverse

Table 3.6 Capsular patterns (Cyriax 1982). Movements are listed in descending order of limitation

Joint	Movement restriction
Temporomandibular joint	Opening mouth
Cervical spine	Side flexion and rotation are equally limited; flexion is full but painful, and extension is limited
Thoracic and lumbar spine	Difficult to detect capsular pattern
Sacroiliac, pubic symphysis and sacrococcygeal joints	Pain when the joint is stressed
Sternoclavicular and acromioclavicular joints	Pain at extremes of range
Shoulder joint	Lateral rotation then abduction then medial rotation
Elbow joint	More limitation of flexion than extension
Inferior radioulnar joint	Full range but pain at extremes of range
Wrist joint	Flexion and extension equally limited
Carpometacarpal joint of the thumb	Full flexion, limited abduction and extension
Thumb and finger joints	More limitation of flexion than extension
Hip joint	Medial rotation, extension, abduction, flexion, then lateral rotation
Knee joint	Gross limitation of flexion with slight limitation of extension Rotation full and painless in early stages
Tibiofibular joints	Pain when the joint is stressed
Ankle joint	More limitation of plantarflexion than dorsiflexion
Talocalcaneal joint	Limitation of inversion
Midtarsal joint	Limitation of dorsiflexion, plantarflexion, adduction and medial rotation; abduction and lateral rotation are full range
Metatarsophalangeal joint of the big toe	More limitation of extension than flexion
Metatarsophalangeal joint of the other four toes	Variable; tend to fix in extension with interphalangeal joints flexed

processes during physiological movements. A brief reminder of how to perform the technique is given in each relevant chapter and a full description can be found in Maitland et al (2001). A quick and easy method of recording PPIVMs is shown in Figure 3.13. This method can also be used for a range of active movements.

Muscle tests

In the last 15 years or so, there has been considerable interest in muscle examination, assessment and treatment (Hides 1995, Hides et al 1996, Hodges 1995, Hodges & Richardson 1996, Janda 1986, Jull & Janda 1987, Jull & Richardson 1994, Richardson et al 2004, Sahrmann 2002, White & Sahrmann 1994).

Muscle function was classified by Bergmark (1989), in relation to the lumbar spine, into local and global systems. This classification system was further refined by Comerford & Kinetic Control (2000) which expanded the system to include all muscles and increased muscle function into three broad headings: local stabilizer, global stabilizer and global mobilizer. Generally speaking, the local stabilizer muscles maintain a low, continuous activation in all joint positions regardless of the direction of joint motion, which tend to become inhibited when dysfunctional; examples include vastus medialis oblique, the deep neck flexors and

transversus abdominis. The global stabilizers become activated on specific directions of joint movement, particularly eccentric control and rotation movement, and when dysfunctional tend to become long and weak; examples include gluteus medius, superficial multifidus and internal and external obliques. The global mobilizers are activated to produce specific directions of joint movement, particularly concentric movement, and when dysfunctional tend to become short and overactive; examples include rectus abdominis, hamstrings and levator scapula. Further characteristics of each classification are given in Table 3.7. It should be noted that a muscle may be allocated into more that one category; for example, serratus anterior and longus colli could be considered local stabilizers and subscapularis could fall into local or global stabilizer; middle and lower trapezius, the deep cervical flexors and latissimus dorsi could be considered to be global stabilizer muscles. In addition, sternocleidomastoid and pectoralis major and minor are considered to be global mobilizers. Normal muscle function requires normal muscle strength, length and coordination. A muscle does not function in isolation – it is also dependent on the normality of its antagonist muscle as well as other local and distant muscle groups. The effect of muscle dysfunction can therefore be widespread throughout the musculoskeletal system.

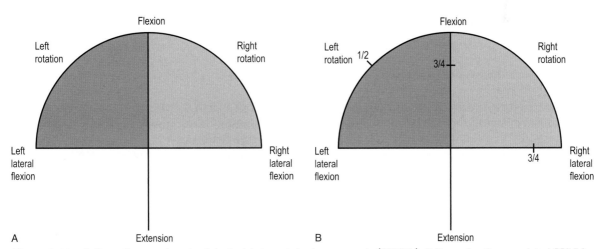

Figure 3.13 **A** Recording passive physiological intervertebral movements (PPIVMs). **B** Example of a completed PPIVM recording for a segmental level. Interpretation: there is $^3/_4$ range of flexion and right lateral flexion and $^1/_2$ range of left rotation. There is no restriction of extension.

Table 3.7   Classification of muscle function (Comerford & Kinetic Control 2000)

Local stabilizer	Global stabilizer	Global mobilizer
Examples:		
Transversus abdominis	Internal & external obliques	Rectus abdominis
Deep lumbar multifidus	Superficial multifidus	Iliocostalis
Psoas major (posterior fasciculi)	Spinalis	Hamstrings
Vastus medialis oblique	Gluteus medius	Latissimus dorsi
Middle & lower trapezius	Serratus anterior	Levator scapulae
Deep cervical flexors	Longus colli (oblique fibres)	Scalenus anterior, medius & posterior
Function and characteristics:		
Increase muscle stiffness to control segmental movement	Generates force to control range of movement	Generates torque to produce movement
Controls the neutral joint position. Contraction does not produce change in length and so does not produce movement. Proprioceptive function: information on joint position, range and rate of movement	Controls particularly the inner and outer ranges of movement. Tends to contract eccentrically for low load deceleration of momentum and for rotational control	Produces joint movement, especially movements in the sagittal plane. Tends to contract concentrically. Absorbs shock
Activity is independent of direction of movement	Activity is direction dependent	Activity is direction dependent
Continuous activation throughout movement	Non-continuous activity	Non-continuous activity
Dysfunction:		
Reduced muscle stiffness, loss of joint neutral position (segmental control). Delayed timing and recruitment	Poor control of inner and outer ranges of movement, poor eccentric control and rotation dissociation. Inner and outer range weakness of muscle	Muscle spasm. Loss of muscle length (shortened), limiting accessory and/or physiological range of movement
Becomes inhibited	Reduced low threshold tonic recruitment	Overactive low threshold, low load recruitment
Local inhibition	**Global imbalance**	**Global imbalance**
Loss of segmental control	Increased length and inhibited stabilizing muscles result in underpull at a motion segment	Shortened and overactive mobilizing muscles result in overpull at a motion segment

There is a close functional relationship between agonist and antagonist muscles. Muscle activation is associated with inhibition of its antagonist so that overactivation of a muscle group, as occurs in muscle spasm, will be associated with inhibition of the antagonist group, which may then become weak. This situation produces what is known as muscle imbalance, i.e. a disruption of the coordinated interplay of muscles. Muscle imbalance can occur where a muscle becomes shortened and alters the position of the joint in such a way that the antagonist muscle is elongated and then becomes weak. Another example is where there is reflex inhibition of muscle and weakness in the presence of pain and/or injury, such as is seen with patellofemoral joint pain (Mariani & Caruso 1979, Voight & Wieder 1991) and low back pain (Hides 1995, Hodges 1995). Muscle testing therefore involves examination of the strength and length of both agonist and antagonist muscle groups.

The following tests are commonly used to assess muscle function: muscle strength, muscle control, muscle length, isometric muscle testing and some other muscle tests.

Muscle strength

This is usually tested manually with an isotonic contraction through the available range of movement and graded according to the Medical Research Council (MRC) scale (Medical Research Council 1976) shown in Table 3.8. Groups of muscles are tested, as well as more specific testing of individual muscles. The strength of a muscle contraction will depend on the age, gender, build and usual level of physical activity of the patient. Details of these tests can be found in various texts, including Cole et al (1988), Hislop & Montgomery (1995) and Kendall et al (1999).

Some muscles are thought to be prone to inhibition and weakness and are shown in Table 3.2 (Comerford & Kinetic Control 2000, Janda 1994, 2002, Jull & Janda 1987). They are characterized by hypotonia, decreased strength and delayed activation with atrophy over a prolonged period of time (Janda 1993). While the mechanism behind this process is still unclear, it seems reasonable to suggest that the strength of these muscles in particular needs to be examined. White & Sahrmann (1994) suggest that the postural muscles tend to lengthen as a result of poor posture and that this occurs because the muscle rests in an elongated position. The muscles then appear weak when tested in a shortened position, although their peak tension in outer range is actually larger than the peak tension generated by a 'normal length' muscle (Fig. 3.14) (Gossman et al 1982). Crawford (1973) found that the peak tension of the lengthened muscle in outer range may be 35% greater than normal muscle. In addition, muscles that lose their length will, over a period of time, become weak. Methods of testing the strength of individual muscles are outlined in Figure 3.15. The patient is asked to move against the resistance applied by the clinician.

Muscle control

Muscle control is tested by observing the recruitment and coordination of muscles during active movements. Some of these movements will have already been carried out (under joint tests) but there are other specific tests, which will be carried out here. The relative strength, endurance and control of muscles are considered to be more important than the overall strength of a muscle or muscle group (Janda 1994, 2002, Jull & Janda 1987, Jull & Richardson 1994, Sahrmann 2002, White & Sahrmann 1994). Relative strength is assessed by observing the pattern of muscle recruitment and the quality of movement and by palpating muscle activity in various positions. It should be noted that this relies on the observational skills of the clinician. A common term within the concept of muscle control is recruitment (or activation), which refers to timed onset of muscle activity; an aspect of motor control by the central nervous system.

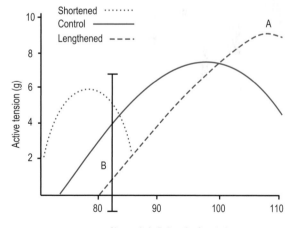

Figure 3.14   Effects of muscle length on muscle strength. The normal length–tension curve (control) moves to the right for a lengthened muscle, giving it a peak tension some 35% greater than the control (point A). When tested in an inner range position, however (point B), the muscle tests weaker than normal. (From Norris 1995, with permission.)

Table 3.8   Grades of muscle strength (Medical Research Council 1976)

Grade	Muscle activity
0	No contraction
1	Flicker or trace of contraction
2	Active movement, with gravity eliminated
3	Active movement against gravity
4	Active movement against gravity and resistance
5	Normal strength

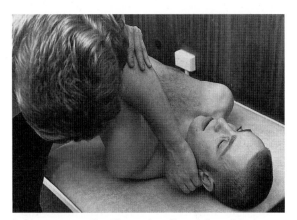

A Serratus anterior. The patient lies supine with the shoulder flexed to 90° and the elbow in full flexion. Resistance is applied to shoulder girdle protraction.

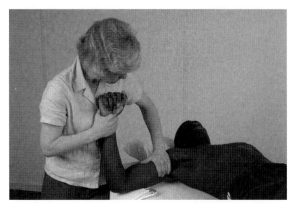

B Subscapularis. In supine with the shoulder in 90° abduction and the elbow flexed to 90°. A towel is placed underneath the upper arm so that the humerus is in the scapular plane. The clinician gently resists medial rotation of the upper arm. The subscapularis tendon can be palpated in the axilla, just anterior to the posterior border. There should be no scapular movement or alteration in the abduction position.

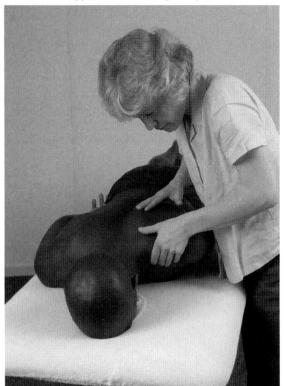

C Lower fibres of trapezius. In prone lie with the arm by the side and the glenohumeral joint placed in medial rotation, the clinician passively moves the coracoid process away from the plinth such that the head of the humerus and body of scapula lie horizontal. Poor recruitment of lower fibres of trapezius would be suspected from an inability to hold this position without substitution by other muscles such as levator scapulae, rhomboid major and minor or latissimus dorsi.

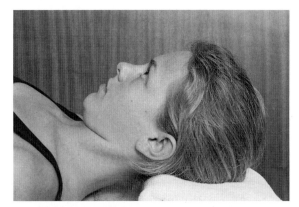

D Deep cervical flexors. The patient lies supine and is asked to tuck the chin in. If there is poor recruitment the sternocleidomastoid initiates the movement.

Figure 3.15(A–J) Testing the strength of individual muscles prone to become weak (Cole et al 1988, Janda 1994, Jull & Janda 1987).

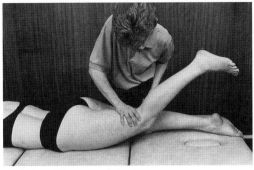

E Gluteus maximus. The clinician resists hip extension. A normal pattern would be hamstring and gluteus maximus acting as prime movers and the erector spinae stabilizing the lumbar spine and pelvis. Contraction of gluteus maximus is delayed when it is weak.
Alternatively, the therapist can passively extend the hip into an inner range position and ask the patient to hold this position isometrically (Jull & Richardson 1994).

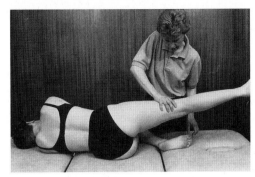

F Posterior gluteus medius. The patient is asked to actively abduct the uppermost leg. Resistance can be added by the clinician. Lateral rotation of the hip may indicate excessive activity of tensor fasciae latae, and using hip flexors to produce the movement may indicate a weakness in the lateral pelvic muscles. Other substitution movements include lateral flexion of the trunk or backward rotation of the pelvis. Inner range weakness is tested by passively abducting the hip; if the range is greater than the active abduction movement, this indicates inner range weakness.

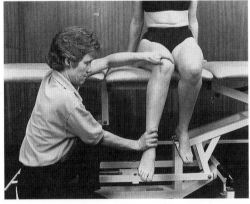

G Gluteus minimus. The clinician resists medial rotation of the hip.

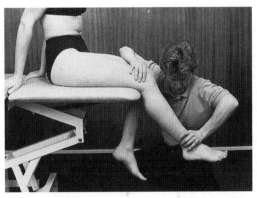

H Vastus lateralis, medialis and intermedius. The clinician resists knee extension.

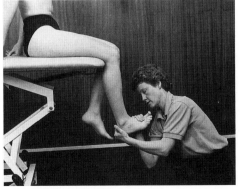

I Tibialis anterior. The clinician resists ankle dorsiflexion and inversion.

Figure 3.15 *Continued*

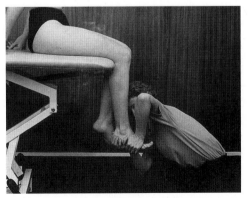

J Peroneus longus and brevis. The clinician resists ankle eversion.

Muscle length

Muscle length may be tested, in particular for those muscles that tend to become tight and thus lose their extensibility (Comerford & Kinetic Control 2000, Janda 1994, 2002, Jull & Janda 1987) (Table 3.2). These muscles are characterized by hypertonia, increased strength and quickened activation time (Janda 1993). Methods of testing the length of individual muscles are outlined in Figure 3.16.

There are two important comments to make regarding muscle length tests. Firstly, while these tests are described according to individual muscles, it is clear that a number of muscles will be lengthened (as well as underlying joints and nerves). This awareness is important when interpreting a test; it cannot be assumed that when testing 'upper trapezius' muscle that it is this muscle and no other muscle that is reduced in length; levator scapula and scalene muscles, for example, may also be contributing to the reduced movement. Secondly, the photographs show minimum muscle length test; further testing may often be required for patients. For example, to fully test the length of the hamstring muscles, the clinician may investigate hip flexion with some adduction/abduction and/or with some medial/lateral rotation. Similarly, for levator scapula, the clinician may examine varying degrees of cervical flexion, contralateral lateral flexion and contralateral rotation as well as varying the order of the movements. Testing muscle length in this way, outside of pure planes of movement, brings to muscle length tests what Brian Edwards brought to physiological movement with the addition of combined movements. For further information on fully investigating muscle length tests, see Hunter (1998).

Muscle length is tested by the clinician stabilizing one end of the muscle and slowly and smoothly moving the body part to stretch the muscle. The following information is noted:

- The quality of movement
- The range of movement
- The presence of resistance through the range of movement and at the end of the range of movement; the quality of the resistance may identify whether muscle, joint or neural tissues are limiting the movement
- Pain behaviour (local and referred) through the range.

Reduced muscle length, i.e. muscle shortness or tightness, occurs when the muscle cannot be stretched to its normal length. This state may occur with overuse, which causes the muscle initially to become short and strong but later, over a period of time, to become weak (because of reduced nutrition). This state is known as stretch weakness (Janda 1993).

Isometric muscle testing

This may help to differentiate symptoms arising from inert from that of contractile tissues. The joint is put into a resting position (so that the inert structures are relaxed) and the patient is asked to hold this position against the resistance of the clinician. If symptoms are reproduced on contraction, this suggests that symptoms are coming from the muscle. It must be appreciated that there will be some shearing and compression of the inert structures, so the test is not always conclusive. In addition, the clinician observes the quality of the muscle contraction to hold this position (this can be done with the patient's eyes shut). The patient may, for example, be unable to prevent the joint from moving or may hold with excessive muscle activity; either of these circumstances would suggest a neuromuscular dysfunction. For a more thorough examination of muscle function the patient is asked to hold position in various parts of the physiological range.

Cyriax (1982) describes six possible responses to isometric muscle testing:

- Strong and painless – normal
- Strong and painful – suggests minor lesion of muscle or tendon, e.g. tennis elbow
- Weak and painless – complete rupture of muscle or tendon or disorder of the nervous system
- Weak and painful – suggests gross lesion, e.g. fracture of patella
- All movements painful – suggests emotional hypersensitivity
- Painful on repetition – suggests intermittent claudication.

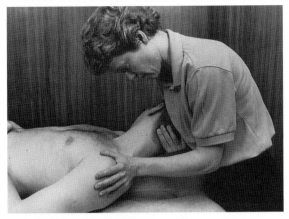

A Levator scapulae. A passive stretch is applied by contralateral lateral flexion and rotation with flexion of the neck and shoulder girdle depression. Restricted range of movement and tenderness on palpation over the insertion of levator scapula indicates tightness of the muscle.

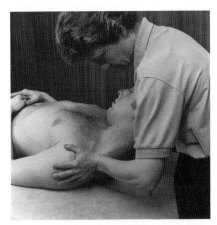

B Upper trapezius. A passive stretch is applied by passive contralateral lateral flexion, ipsilateral rotation and flexion of the neck with shoulder girdle depression. Restricted range of movement indicates tightness of the muscle.

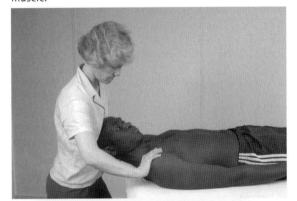

C Sternocleidomastoid. The clinician tucks the chin in and then laterally flexes the head away and rotates towards the side of testing. The clavicle is stabilized with the other hand.

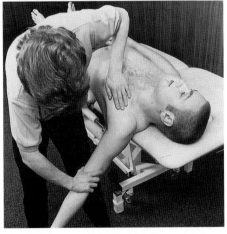

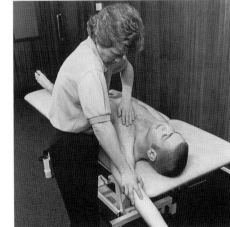

i   ii

D Pectoralis major. (i) Clavicular fibres – the clinician stabilizes the trunk and abducts the shoulder to 90°. Passive overpressure of horizontal extension will be limited in range and the tendon becomes taut if there is tightness of this muscle. (ii) Sternocostal fibres – the clinician elevates the shoulder fully. Restricted range of movement and the tendon becoming taut indicates tightness of this muscle.

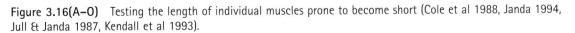

Figure 3.16(A–O)   Testing the length of individual muscles prone to become short (Cole et al 1988, Janda 1994, Jull & Janda 1987, Kendall et al 1993).

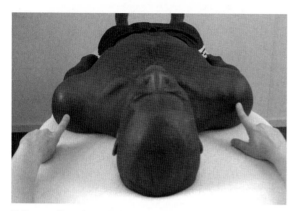

E Pectoralis minor. With the patient in supine and arm by side, the coracoid is found to be pulled anteriorly and inferiorly if there is a contracture of this muscle. In addition, the posterior edge of the acromion may rest further from the plinth on the affected side.

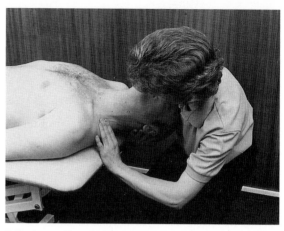

F Scalenes. The clinician extends the head and laterally flexes away and rotates towards the side of testing for anterior scalene; neutral rotation tests the middle fibres and contralateral rotation tests the posterior scalene muscle.

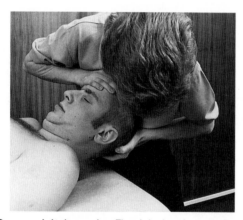

G Deep occipital muscles. The right hand passively flexes the upper cervical spine while palpating the deep occipital muscles with the left hand. Tightness on palpation indicates tightness of these muscles.

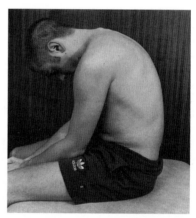

H Erector spinae. The patient slumps the shoulders towards the groin. Lack of flattening of the lumbar lordosis may indicate tightness (Lewit 1991).

Figure 3.16 *Continued*

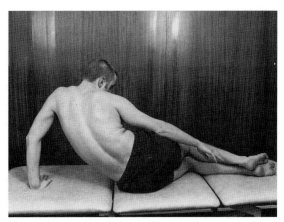

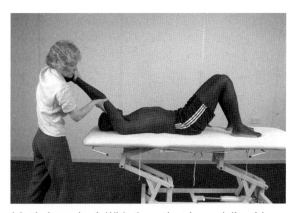

I Quadratus lumborum. The patient pushes up sideways as far as possible without movement of the pelvis. Limited range of movement, lack of curvature in the lumbar spine and/or abnormal tension on palpation (just above the iliac crest and lateral to erector spinae) indicate tightness of the muscle.

J Latissimus dorsi. With the patient in crook lie with the lumbar spine flat against the plinth and the glenohumeral joints laterally rotated, the patient is asked to elevate the arms through flexion. Shortness of latissimus dorsi is evidenced by an inability to maintain the lumbar spine in against the plinth and/or inability to fully elevate the arms.

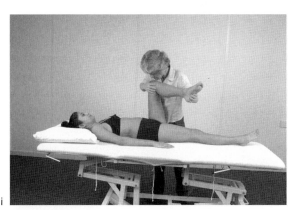

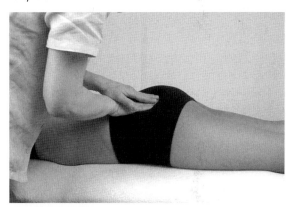

i

ii

K Piriformis. (i) The clinician passively flexes the hip to 90°, adducts it and then adds lateral rotation to the hip feeling the resistance to the limit of the movement. There should be around 45° of lateral rotation. (ii) Piriformis can be palpated if it is tight by applying deep pressure at the point at which an imaginary line between the iliac crest and ischial tuberosity crosses a line between the posterior superior iliac spine and the greater trochanter.

Figure 3.16 *Continued*

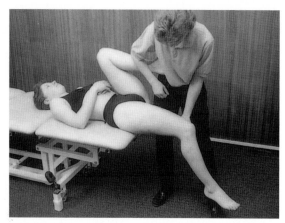

L Iliopsoas, rectus femoris and tensor fasciae latae. The left leg is stabilized against the clinician's side. The free leg will be flexed at the hip if there is tightness of iliopsoas. An extended knee indicates tight rectus femoris. Abduction of the hip, lateral deviation of the patella and a well-defined groove on the lateral aspect of the thigh indicate tight tensor fasciae latae and iliotibial band. Overpressure to each of these movements, including hip abduction for the short adductors, will confirm any tightness of these muscles.

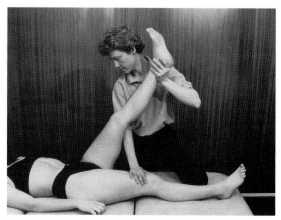

M Hamstrings. With the patient lying supine, the clinician passively flexes the hip while holding down the other leg.

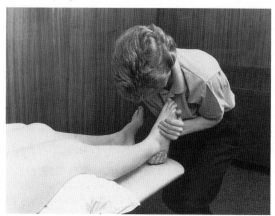

N Tibialis posterior. The clinician dorsiflexes the ankle joint and everts the forefoot. Limited range of movement indicates tightness of the muscle.

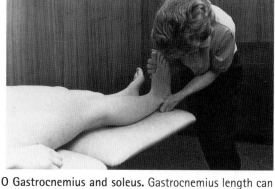

O Gastrocnemius and soleus. Gastrocnemius length can be tested by the range of ankle dorsiflexion with the knee extended and then flexed. If the range increases when the knee is flexed, this indicates tightness of gastrocnemius.

Figure 3.16 *Continued*

Other muscle tests

For years clinicians have measured, with a tape measure, the circumference of the muscle bulk at a measured distance from a bony point and compared left and right sides. This test attempts to measure the size of a muscle in order to measure its strength. There are a number of difficulties with this method. Firstly, it is not a pure measure of muscle size since it includes the subcutaneous fat (Stokes & Young 1986). Secondly, it assumes that the muscle fibres are running at right angles to the limb (so that the physiological cross-sectional area is being measured) but this is not the case for most muscles, which have a pennate structure (Newham 2001). Thirdly, there is no relationship between limb girth and muscle girth: a 22–33% reduction in the cross-sectional area of the quadriceps (measured by ultrasound scanning) may cause only a 5% reduction in the circumference of the limb using a tape measure (Young et al 1982). The test is therefore of limited value, and is not discussed in subsequent chapters.

These are particular tests that attempt to diagnose a muscle dysfunction. Examples include Speed's test for bicipital tendinitis and the drop arm test for rotator cuff tear (Magee 1997).

Neurological tests

Neurological examination includes neurological integrity testing, neurodynamic tests and some other nerve tests.

Integrity of the nervous system

The effects of compression of the peripheral nervous system are:

- Reduced sensory input
- Reduced motor impulses along the nerve
- Reflex changes
- Pain usually in the myotome or dermatome distribution
- Autonomic disturbance such as hyperaesthesia, paraesthesia or altered vasomotor tone.

Reduced sensory input. Sensory changes are due to a lesion of the sensory nerves anywhere from the spinal nerve root to its terminal branches in the skin. Figure 3.17 serves to illustrate this. Knowledge of the cutaneous distribution of nerve roots (dermatomes) and peripheral nerves enables the clinician to distinguish the sensory loss due to a root lesion from that due to a peripheral nerve lesion. The cutaneous nerve distribution and dermatome areas are shown in Figures 3.18–3.21. It must be remembered, however, that there is a great deal of variability from person to person and an overlap between the cutaneous supply of peripheral nerves (Walton 1989) and dermatome areas (Hockaday & Whitty 1967). A sclerotome is the region of bone supplied by one nerve root; the areas are shown in Figure 3.22 (Grieve 1981, Inman & Saunders 1944).

Reduced motor impulses along the nerve. A loss of muscle strength is indicative of either a lesion of the motor nerve supply to the muscle(s) – located anywhere from the spinal cord to its terminal branches in the muscle – or a lesion of the muscle itself. If the lesion occurs at nerve root level then all the muscles supplied by the nerve root (the myotome) will be affected. If the lesion occurs in a peripheral nerve then the muscles that it supplies will be affected. A working knowledge of the muscular distribution of nerve roots (myotomes) and peripheral nerves enables the clinician to distinguish the motor loss due to a root lesion from that due to a peripheral nerve lesion. The peripheral nerve distribution and myotomes are shown in Table 3.9 and Figures 3.23–3.25. It should be noted that most muscles in the limbs are innervated by more than one nerve root (myotome) and that the predominant segmental origin is given.

Over a period of time of motor nerve impairment there will be muscle atrophy and weakness, as is seen for example in the thenar eminence in carpal tunnel syndrome.

Reflex changes. The deep tendon reflexes test the integrity of the spinal reflex arc consisting of an afferent or sensory neurone and an efferent or motor neurone. The reflexes test individual nerve roots as shown in Table 3.9. If there is sufficient compression of the nerve, the reflex will be absent; if there is only some compression, there will be a diminished reflex. An increased reflex response is

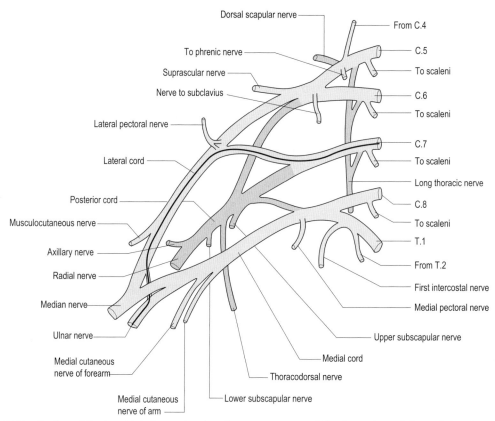

Figure 3.17 A plan of the brachial plexus showing the nerve roots and the formation of the peripheral nerves. (From Williams et al 1995, with permission.)

indicative of an upper motor neurone lesion and is confirmed by the plantar response; if this is positive, the clinician should refer the patient to an appropriate medical practitioner.

Procedure for examining the integrity of the nervous system. In order to examine the integrity of the peripheral nerves, three tests are carried out: skin sensation, muscle strength and deep tendon reflexes.

If a nerve root lesion is suspected, the tests carried out are referred to as dermatomal (area of skin supplied by one nerve root), myotomal (group of muscles supplied by one nerve root) and reflexal.

Testing skin sensation. It is important that any diminished skin sensation is identified accurately and sensitively by the clinician. Cotton wool is often used to test the ability to feel light touch. The clinician strokes an unaffected area of the skin first so that the patient knows what to expect. The clinician then lightly strokes across the skin and the patient is asked whether it feels the same or different to the other side. Alternatively, the cotton wool may be placed on the skin with the patient's eyes shut, and the patient is asked to say yes every time they feel they are being touched; if there is doubt the patient can be asked to say when and where they are being touched. Whichever of the above methods is used, the clinician needs to accurately identify and map out the area of diminished sensation using the cotton wool. The next step may be to further explore the area of diminished sensation, by testing pinprick (the ability to feel pain) and sometimes deep pressure, two-point discrimination, vibration sensation, hot/cold

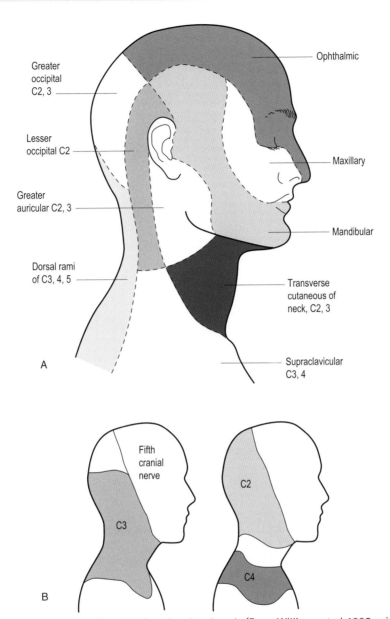

Greater
occipital
C2, 3

Lesser
occipital C2

Greater
auricular C2, 3

Dorsal rami
of C3, 4, 5

Ophthalmic

Maxillary

Mandibular

Transverse
cutaneous of
neck, C2, 3

Supraclavicular
C3, 4

A

Fifth
cranial
nerve

C3

C2

C4

B

Figure 3.18   A Cutaneous nerve supply to the face, head and neck. (From Williams et al 1995, with permission.)
B Dermatomes of the head and neck. (From Grieve 1981, with permission.)

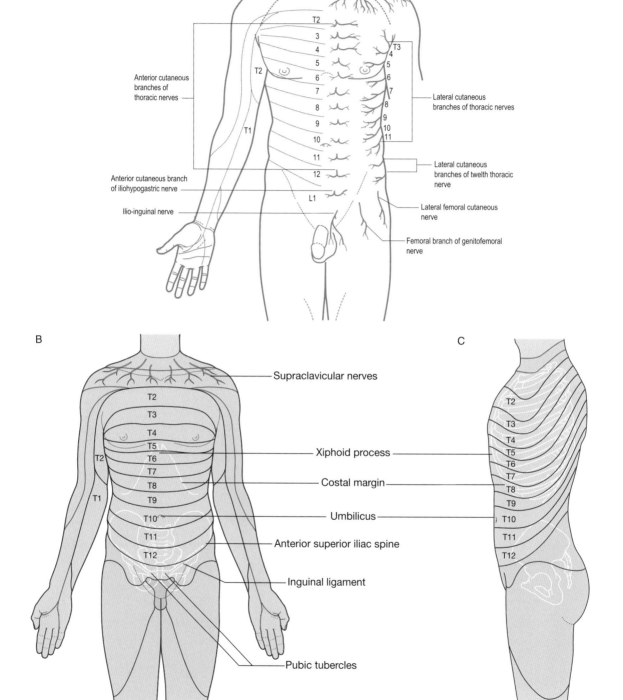

Figure 3.19 **A** Cutaneous nerve supply to the trunk. (From Williams et al 1995, with permission.) **B** Anterior view of thoracic dermatomes associated with thoracic spinal nerves. **C** Lateral view of dermatomes associated with thoracic spinal nerves. (From Drake et al 2005.)

A

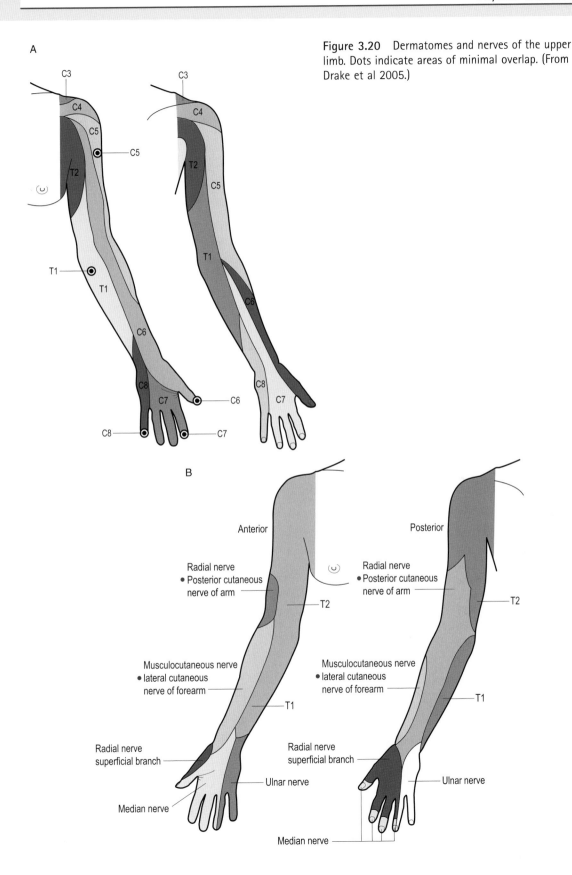

Figure 3.20   Dermatomes and nerves of the upper limb. Dots indicate areas of minimal overlap. (From Drake et al 2005.)

B

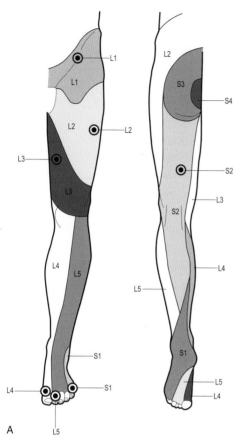

Figure 3.21   Dermatomes and major nerves of the lower limb. Dots indicate areas of minimal overlap. (From Drake et al 2005.)

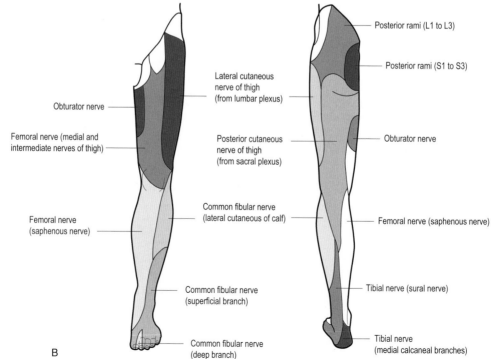

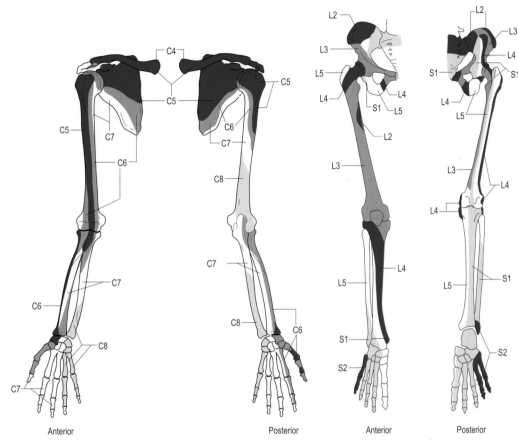

Figure 3.22 Sclerotomes of the upper and lower limbs. (From Grieve 1991, with permission.)

sensation, proprioception and stereognosis. Areas of sensory abnormality can be documented on the body chart. Mapping out an area needs to be accurate, as a change, particularly an increase in the area, indicates a worsening neurological state and may require the patient to be referred to a medical practitioner; for example, progressive signs due to a prolapsed intervertebral disc pressing on the spinal cord or cauda equina may require immediate surgery. For this reason, sensation is often reassessed at each appointment, until it is established that the diminished sensation is stable.

An alternative and more standardized method of assessment of light touch to deep pressure is to use monofilaments (Semmes-Weinstein or West). Each monofilament relates to a degree of pressure,

is repeatable and scales from loss of protective sensation through diminished light touch to normal sensation (Hunter 2002).

Testing muscle strength. Muscle strength testing consists of carrying out an isometric contraction of a muscle group over a few seconds. The muscle is placed in mid-position and the patient is asked to hold the position against the resistance of the clinician. The resistance is applied slowly and smoothly to enable the patient to give the necessary resistance, and the amount of force applied must be appropriate to the specific muscle group and to the patient. Myotome testing is shown in Figures 3.26 and 3.27. If a peripheral nerve lesion is suspected, the clinician may test the strength of individual muscles supplied by the nerve using the MRC scale, as mentioned earlier.

Table 3.9   Myotomes (Grieve 1991)

Root	Joint action	Reflex
V cranial (trigeminal N)	Clench teeth, note temporalis and masseter muscles	Jaw
VII cranial (facial N)	Wrinkle forehead, close eyes, purse lips, show teeth	
XI cranial (accessory N)	Shoulder girdle elevation and sternocleidomastoid	
C1	Upper cervical flexion	
C2	Upper cervical extension	
C3	Cervical lateral flexion	
C4	Shoulder girdle elevation	
C5	Shoulder abduction	Biceps jerk
C6	Elbow flexion	Biceps jerk
C7	Elbow extension	Triceps jerk and brachioradialis
C8	Thumb extension; finger flexion	
T1	Finger abduction and adduction	
T2–L1	No muscle tes or reflex	
L2	Hip flexion	
L3	Knee extension	Knee jerk
L4	Foot dorsiflexion	Knee jerk
L5	Extension of the big toe	
S1	Eversion of the foot	Ankle jerk
	Contract buttock	
	Knee flexion	
S2	Knee flexion	
	Toe standing	
S3–4	Muscles of pelvic floor, bladder and genital function	

Further details of peripheral nerve injuries are beyond the scope of this text, but they can be found in standard orthopaedic and neurological textbooks.

Reflex testing.   The deep tendon reflexes are elicited by tapping the tendon a number of times. The commonly-used deep tendon reflexes are the biceps brachii, triceps, patellar and tendocalcaneus (Fig. 3.28).

The reflex response may be graded as follows:

– or 0: absent
– or 1: diminished
+ or 2: average
++ or 3: exaggerated
+++ or 4: clonus.

Clonus is associated with exaggerated reflexes and is characterized by intermittent muscular contraction and relaxation produced by sustained stretching of a muscle. It is most commonly tested in the lower limb, where the clinician sharply dorsiflexes the patient's foot with the knee extended.

A diminished reflex response can occur if there is a lesion of the sensory or motor pathways. An exaggerated reflex response suggests an upper motor lesion and, if this is found, the plantar response should be tested. This involves stroking the lateral aspect of the foot and observing the movement of the toes. The normal response is for all the toes to plantarflex, while an abnormal response, confirming an upper motor neurone lesion, consists of dorsiflexion of the great toe and downward fanning out of the remaining toes (Walton 1989), which is known as the extensor or Babinski response.

Reflex changes alone, without sensory or motor changes, do not necessarily indicate nerve root involvement. Zygapophyseal joints injected with hypertonic saline can abolish ankle reflexes, which can then be restored by a steroid injection

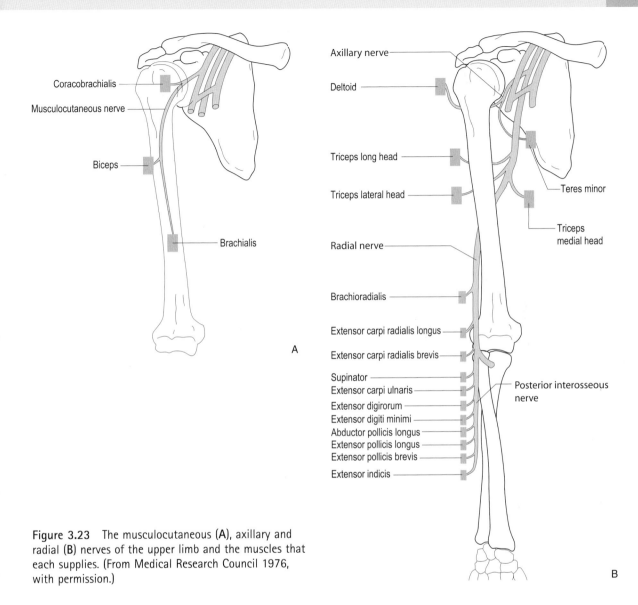

Coracobrachialis
Musculocutaneous nerve
Biceps
Brachialis

A

Axillary nerve
Deltoid
Triceps long head
Triceps lateral head
Teres minor
Triceps medial head
Radial nerve
Brachioradialis
Extensor carpi radialis longus
Extensor carpi radialis brevis
Supinator
Extensor carpi ulnaris
Posterior interosseous nerve
Extensor digirorum
Extensor digiti minimi
Abductor pollicis longus
Extensor pollicis longus
Extensor pollicis brevis
Extensor indicis

B

Figure 3.23 The musculocutaneous (**A**), axillary and radial (**B**) nerves of the upper limb and the muscles that each supplies. (From Medical Research Council 1976, with permission.)

(Mooney & Robertson 1976). For this reason, reflex changes alone may not be a relevant clinical finding. It should also be realized that all tendon reflexes can be exaggerated by tension and anxiety.

Neurodynamic tests

The mobility of the nervous system is examined by carrying out what are known as neurodynamic tests (Shacklock 1995). Some of these tests have been used by the medical profession for over 100 years (Dyck 1984), but they have been more fully developed by several therapists (Butler 1991, Elvey 1985, Maitland et al 2001). A summary of the tests is given here, but further details of the theoretical aspects of these tests and how the tests are performed can be found in Butler (1991). In addition to the length tests described below, the clinician can also palpate the nerve with and without the nerve under tension; details are given later in the section on palpation.

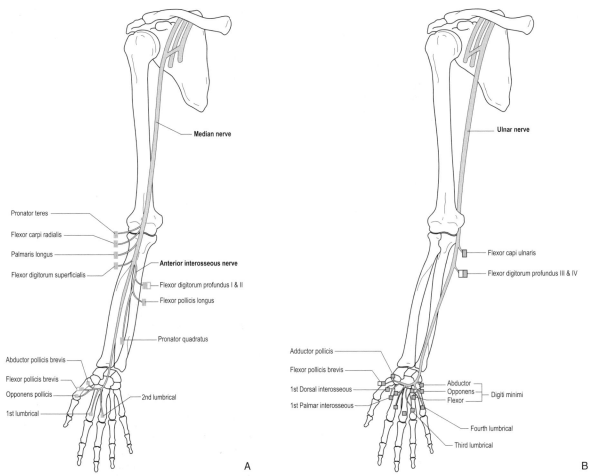

Figure 3.24 Diagram of the median (**A**) and ulnar (**B**) nerves of the upper limb and the muscles that each supplies. (From Medical Research Council 1976, with permission.)

The testing procedures follow the same format as that of joint movement. Thus, resting symptoms are established prior to any testing movement and then the following information is noted:

- The quality of movement
- The range of movement
- The resistance through the range and at the end of the range
- Pain behaviour (local and referred) through the range.

A test is considered positive if one or more of the following are found:

- All or part of the patient's symptoms have been reproduced

- Symptoms different from the 'normal' response are produced
- The range of movement in the symptomatic limb is different from that of the other limb.

The patient is first informed what the purpose of the test is and to tell the clinician if they feel any of their symptoms during the movement; single movements in one plane are then slowly added, gradually taking the upper or lower limb through a sequence of movements. The intention is to examine all of the possible movements for any given test (if possible) and to see if any of the patient's symptoms are produced. If this is achieved, then the clinician moves a part of the

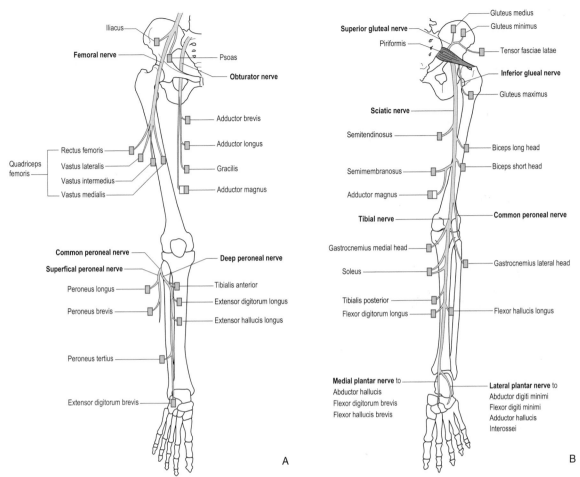

Figure 3.25 Diagram of the nerves on the anterior (**A**) and posterior (**B**) aspects of the lower limb and the muscles that they supply. (From Medical Research Council, with permission.)

spine, or limb that is far away from where the symptoms are, to either increase the overall length of the nervous system (sensitizing movement) or perhaps more preferable, to decrease the overall length of the nervous system. If all other body parts are kept still and the only movement is far away from the symptoms, then the clinician may assume a positive test if a desensitizing movement eases the patient's symptoms. For example, with the patient in supine with hip flexion with knee extension and this produces the patient's posterior thigh pain, the clinician may then add dorsiflexion: if the thigh pain is increased with dorsiflexion, this is a positive test and suggests a neurodynamic component to the thigh pain.

Neurodynamic tests include the following:

- Passive neck flexion (PNF)
- Straight leg raise
- Prone knee bend (PKB)
- Slump
- Upper limb tension tests (ULTT), also known as brachial plexus tension tests (BPTT).

Passive neck flexion. In the supine position, the head is flexed passively by the clinician (Fig. 3.29). The normal response would be pain-free full-range movement. Sensitizing tests include the straight leg raise (SLR) or one of the upper limb tension tests. Where symptoms are related to cervical extension, investigation of passive neck

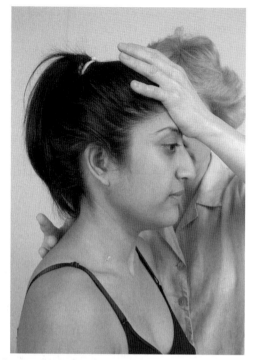

A C1, upper cervical flexion.

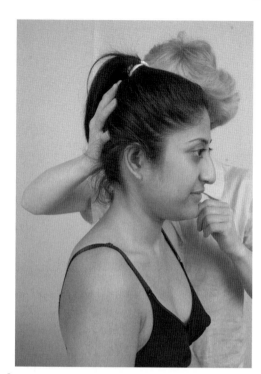

B C2, upper cervical extension.

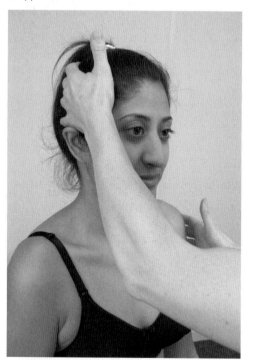

C C3, cervical lateral flexion.

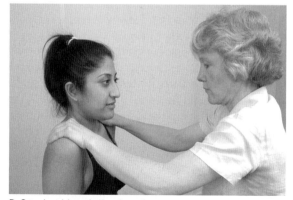

D C4, shoulder girdle elevation.

Figure 3.26(A–I) Myotome testing for the cervical and upper thoracic nerve roots. The patient is asked to hold the position against the force applied by the clinician.

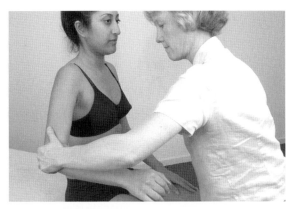

E C5, shoulder abduction.

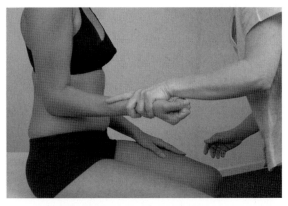

F C6, elbow flexion.

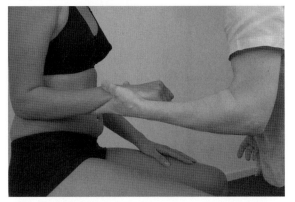

G C7, elbow extension.

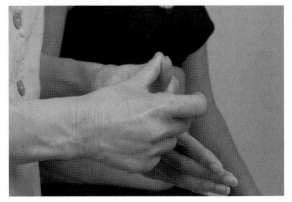

H C8, thumb extension.

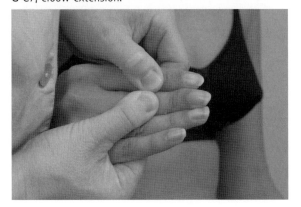

I T1, finger adduction.

Figure 3.26 *Continued*

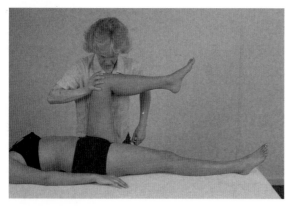

A L2, hip flexion.

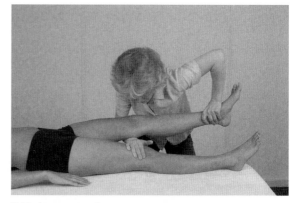

B L3, knee extension.

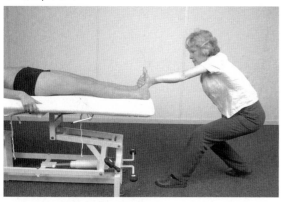

C L4, foot dorsiflexion.

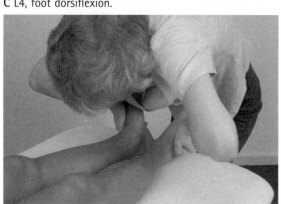

E S1, foot eversion.

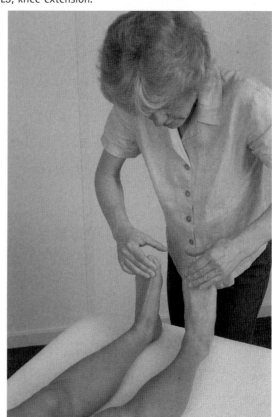

D L5, extension of the big toe.

Figure 3.27(A–H)   Myotome testing for the lumbar and sacral nerve roots.

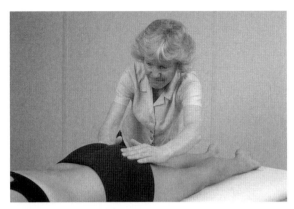

F S1, contract buttock.

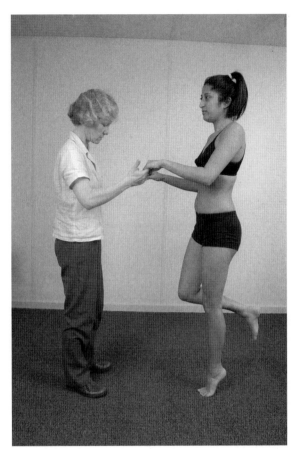

H S2, toe standing.

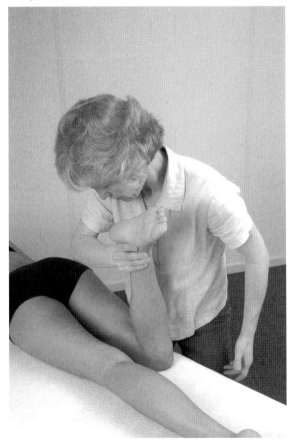

G S1 and S2, knee flexion.
Figure 3.27 *Continued*

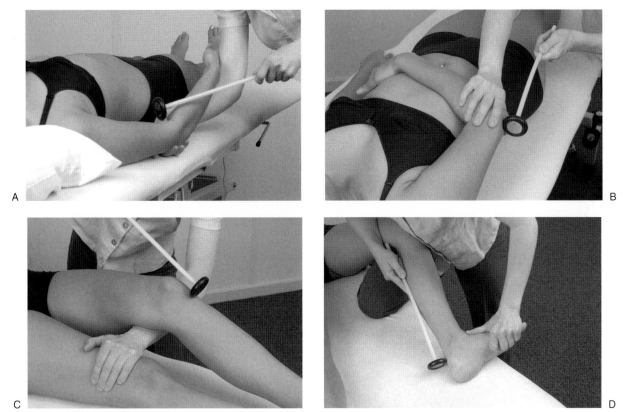

Figure 3.28   Reflex testing. **A** Biceps jerk (C5 and C6). **B** Triceps jerk (C7). **C** knee jerk (L3 and L4). **D** Ankle jerk (S1).

extension is necessary. Passively flexing the neck produces movement and tension of the spinal cord and meninges of the lumbar spine and of the sciatic nerve (Breig 1978, Tencer et al 1985).

Straight leg raise.   The patient lies supine. The way in which the SLR is carried out depends on where the patient's symptoms are. The basic component movements of the SLR are hip adduction, hip medial rotation, hip flexion and knee extension (affecting sciatic nerve); the foot can be moved into any position, but ankle dorsiflexion/forefoot eversion would alter tibial nerve and ankle plantarflexion/forefoot inversion, the common peroneal nerve. Other movements within the forefoot may be used to bias the medial and lateral plantar nerves; this may be useful if symptoms are in the foot. Neck flexion can be used to affect the spinal cord, meninges and sciatic

nerve, and/or trunk lateral flexion to lengthen the spinal cord and sympathetic trunk on the contralateral side.

The SLR moves and tensions the nervous system (including the sympathetic trunk) from the foot to the brain (Breig 1978). The normal response to hip flexion/adduction/medial rotation with knee extension and foot dorsiflexion would be a strong stretching feeling or tingling in the posterior thigh, posterior knee and posterior calf and foot (Miller 1987, Slater 1989).

Figure 3.30A demonstrates how the SLR could be carried out for a patient whose symptoms are in the posterior thigh. The clinician passively adducts, medially rotates and then flexes the hip to the onset of the patient's posterior thigh symptoms (assuming the symptoms are not severe or irritable); at this point the clinician then adds

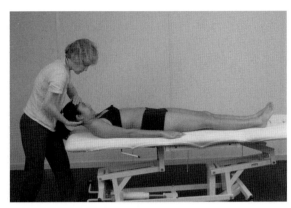

Figure 3.29 Passive neck flexion.

ankle dorsiflexion/forefoot eversion. If the posterior thigh symptoms are increased (or occasionally decreased) with dorsiflexion/eversion, this would be a positive test suggesting there is a neurodynamic component to the patient's posterior thigh symptoms. Figure 3.30B demonstrates how a SLR could be carried out for a patient whose symptoms are over the lateral calf. The clinician moves the foot to bring on the lateral calf symptoms, for example, with ankle plantarflexion and forefoot inversion. This position is then maintained while the clinician passively adducts and medially rotates the hip and then passively flexes the hip. If the lateral calf symptoms are increased (or occasionally decreased) with any of the additional hip movements, this is a positive test, indicating a neurodymamic component to the patient's lateral calf symptoms.

Prone knee bend. Traditionally, this test is carried out in the prone position, as the name suggests, with the test being considered positive if, on passive knee flexion, symptoms are reproduced. This does not, however, differentiate between nervous tissue (femoral nerve) and the hip flexor muscles, which are also being stretched. Carrying out the test in side lying with the head and trunk flexed allows cervical extension to be used as a desensitizing test (Fig. 3.31). The test movements are as follows:

- The clinician determines any resting symptoms and asks the patient to say immediately if any

of his/her symptoms are provoked during any of the movements

- The patient is placed in side lying with a pillow under the head (to avoid lateral flexion/rotation of the cervical spine). The patient is asked to hug both knees up on to the chest.
- The patient releases the uppermost knee to the clinician, flexes the knee and then passively extends the hip, making sure the pelvis and trunk remain still. The clinician may need to add hip medial or lateral rotation and/or hip abduction/adduction movement to produce the patient's symptoms.
- At the point at which symptoms occur the patient is then asked to extend the head and neck while the clinician maintains the trunk and leg position. A typical positive test would be for the cervical extension to ease the patient's anterior thigh pain and for the clinician to then be able to extend the hip further into range. However, if cervical extension increases the patient's anterior thigh pain, this is also a positive test.

A normal response would be full-range movement so that the heel approximates the buttock, accompanied by a feel of strong stretch over the anterior thigh.

Saphenous nerve length test. The patient lies prone and the hip is placed in extension and abduction with the knee flexed. The clinician then passively adds lateral rotation of the hip, foot dorsiflexion and eversion and then knee extension (Fig 3.32). The clinician can sensitize the test by, for example, moving the foot into plantarflexion if symptoms are above the knee (Fig. 3.32B) or by moving the hip into medial rotation if symptoms are below the knee.

Slump. This test is fully described by Maitland et al (2001) and Butler (1991) and is shown in Figure 3.33. The slump test can be carried out as follows:

- The clinician establishes the patient's resting symptoms and asks the patient to say immediately if any of his/her symptoms are provoked
- The patient sits with thighs fully supported at the edge of the plinth with hands behind his/her back

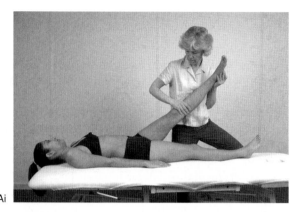
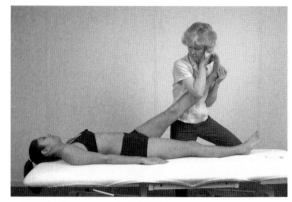

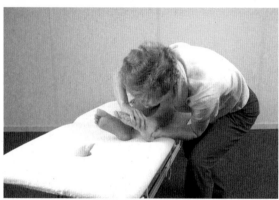
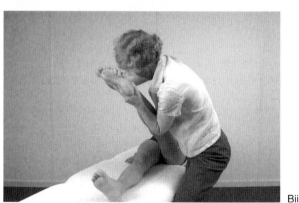

Figure 3.30 **A** Straight leg raise (SLR) if, for example, symptoms are in the posterior thigh. (i) Hip adduction, medial rotation and then flexion to the onset of patient's posterior thigh symptoms. (ii) The clinician then adds ankle dorsiflexion and forefoot eversion. If the posterior thigh symptoms are increased (or decreased) with the dorsiflexion/eversion, this would be a positive test. **B** Straight leg raise (SLR) if, for example, symptoms are over lateral calf brought on with ankle plantarflexion and forefoot inversion. (i) Passive ankle plantarflexion and forefoot inversion to the onset of the patient's lateral calf symptoms. (ii) The clinician then adds hip adduction, medial rotation and flexion. If the lateral calf symptoms are increased (or decreased) with the addition of hip movements, this would be a positive test.

- The patient is asked to flex the trunk by 'slumping the shoulders towards the groin'
- The clinician monitors or applies overpressure to the trunk flexion
- Active cervical flexion
- The clinician applies overpressure to the cervical flexion
- Active foot dorsiflexion on asymptomatic side
- Active knee extension on asymptomatic side
- Return the foot and knee back to neutral
- Active foot dorsiflexion on symptomatic side
- Active knee extension on symptomatic side
- Return the foot and knee back to neutral
- Active bilateral foot dorsiflexion

- Active bilateral knee extension
- Return the foot and knee back to neutral.

Now that all the combinations of lower limb movements have been explored, the clinician chooses the most appropriate movement to which to add a sensitizing movement. This would commonly be as follows:

- Active foot dorsiflexion on symptomatic side
- Active knee extension on symptomatic side
- The patient is asked to extend the head to look upwards and report on any change in the symptoms. It is vital that there is *no* change in position of the trunk and lower limbs when the

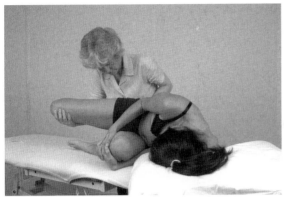
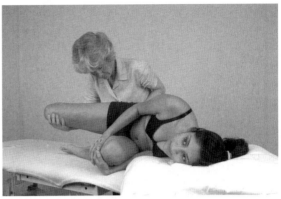

A   B

Figure 3.31   Prone knee bend if symptoms are in the anterior thigh. **A** With knee flexion, the clinician passively extends the hip to the point of onset of the patient's anterior thigh symptoms. **B** Patient extends their cervical spine. If the anterior thigh symptoms are reduced (or increased) with the neck movement, this would be a positive test.

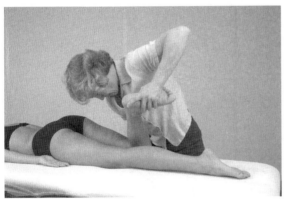
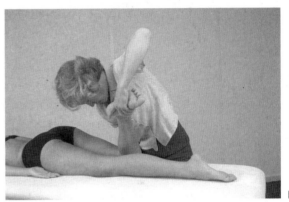

A   B

Figure 3.32   Saphenous nerve length test. **A** With the hip in extension and abduction, the clinician moves the foot into dorsiflexion and eversion, laterally rotates the hip and then extends the knee. **B** If symptoms are above the knee the clinician can then move the foot into plantarflexion and inversion. If the symptoms are reduced (or increased) with foot movement, this would be a positive test.

cervical spine is extended. A reduction in symptoms on cervical extension would be a typical positive test indicating a neurodynamic component to the patient's symptoms; but an increase in symptoms would also indicate a neurodynamic component.

The normal response might be:

- Pain or discomfort in the mid-thoracic area on trunk and neck flexion
- Pain or discomfort behind the knees or in the hamstrings in the trunk and neck flexion and knee extension position; symptoms are increased with ankle dorsiflexion

- Some restriction of knee extension in the trunk and neck flexion position
- Some restriction of ankle dorsiflexion in the trunk and neck flexion and knee extension position; this restriction should be symmetrical
- A decrease in pain in one or more areas with the release of the neck flexion
- An increase in the range of knee extension and/or ankle dorsiflexion with the release of the neck flexion.

The desensitizing test is cervical extension. Sensitizing tests can include cervical rotation, cervical lateral flexion, hip flexion, hip adduction, hip medial rotation, thoracic lateral flexion, altering

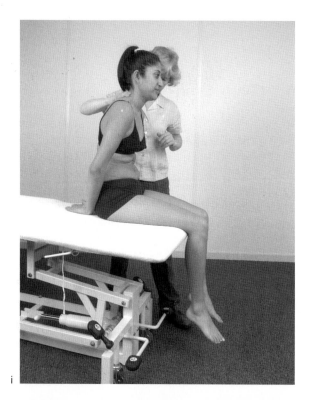

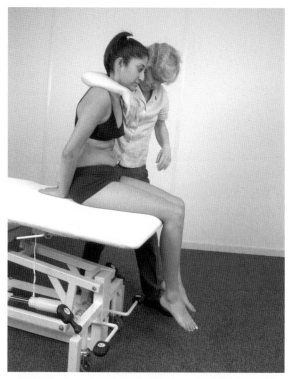

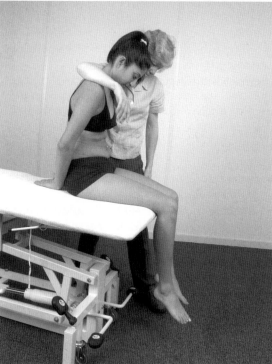

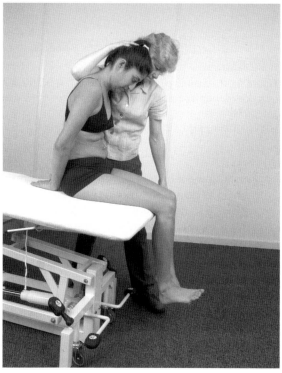

Figure 3.33(i–xii) Slump test. Demonstrated for a patient with left posterior thigh pain. (i) Active trunk flexion. (ii) Overpressure to trunk flexion. (iii) Active cervical flexion. (iv) Overpressure to cervical flexion.

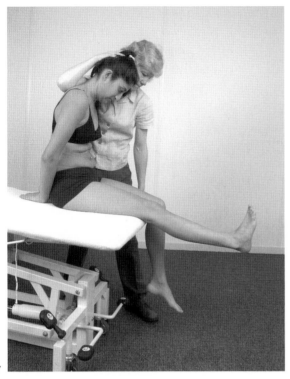

v

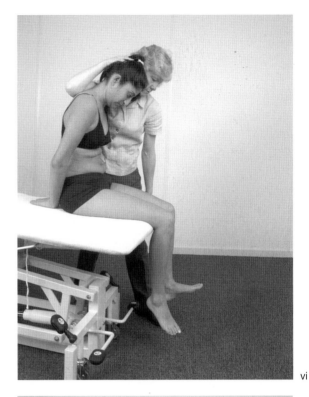

vi

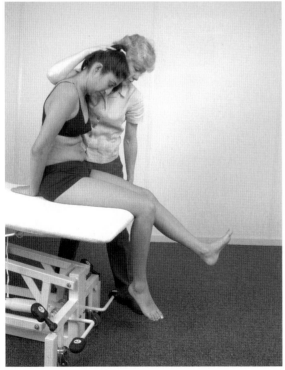

vii

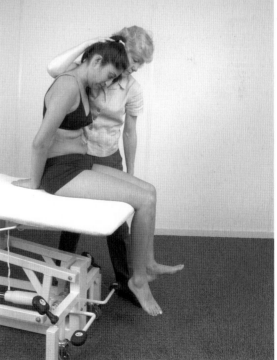

viii

Figure 3.33 *Continued*   (v) Right leg: dorsiflexion then knee extension. (vi) Return right knee. Left leg: dorsiflexion (vii) then knee extension (reduced range due to onset of left thigh pain). (viii) Return left leg.

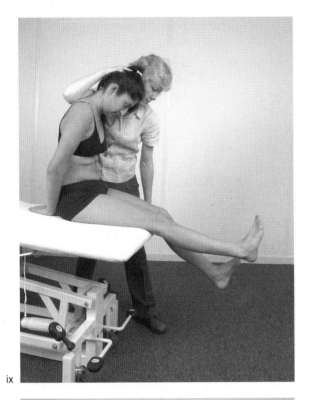

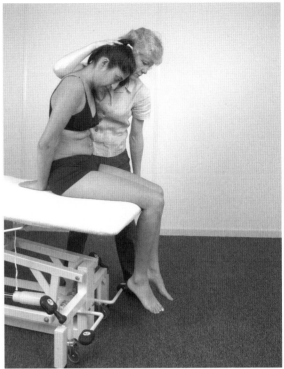

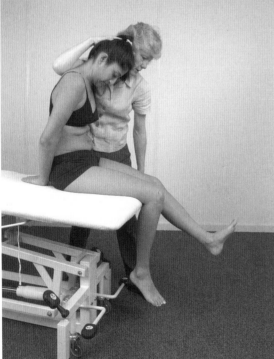

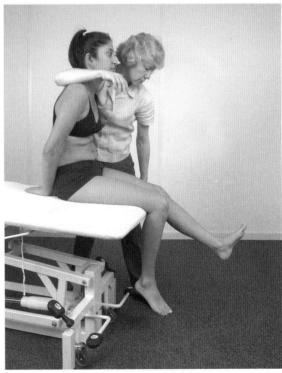

Figure 3.33 *Continued* (ix) Left and right leg: dorsiflexion and knee extension (same reduction in left knee extension). (x) Return to neutral. (xi) Clinician chooses to test position vii: left leg dorsiflexion and knee extension. (xii) Active cervical extension. If cervical extension reduces (or increases) the patient's left posterior thigh pain, this would be a positive test.

foot and ankle movements as for the SLR test, or one of the upper limb tension tests. Differentiation of groin strain due to muscle or nerve dysfunction can be carried out by positioning the patient in sitting and abducting the hip to the onset of symptoms. Slump and neck flexion are then added and if symptoms are increased this may suggest obturator nerve involvement; if there is no change in symptoms this may suggest a local groin strain. Greater emphasis on the sympathetic chain can be tested by adding cervical extension and thoracic lateral flexion.

Upper limb tension (brachial plexus tension) tests. There are four tests, each of which is biased towards a particular nerve:

- ULTT 1 – median nerve
- ULTT 2a – median nerve
- ULTT 2b – radial nerve
- ULTT 3 – ulnar nerve.

The test movements are outlined below. The order of the test movements is relatively unimportant; what matters is consistency in sequencing at each time of testing. The following tests are described with the assumption that the symptoms are in the upper limb. The order of the movements has been chosen so that the last movement is the easiest for the clinician to measure by eye. Each movement is added on slowly and carefully and the clinician monitors the patient's symptoms. The area of the patient's symptoms will help the clinician to decide which is the most appropriate ULTT; where symptoms are mainly in the distribution of the radial nerve, ULTT 2b would be carried out.

ULTT 1: median nerve bias (Fig. 3.34). The following sequence of movements would be appropriate, if, for example the patient has symptoms in the upper arm or below (in the forearm and hand):

1. Neutral position of body on couch
2. Contralateral lateral flexion of the cervical spine
3. Shoulder girdle depression
4. Shoulder abduction
5. Wrist and finger extension
6. Forearm supination
7. Lateral rotation of the shoulder
8. Elbow extension
9. Ipsilateral lateral flexion of the cervical spine

If symptoms are over the upper fibres of trapezius then:

10. Wrist flexion would be used, instead of ipsilateral lateral flexion of the cervical spine.

The movement of ipsilateral lateral flexion of the cervical spine is used to test whether or not there is a neurodynamic component to the patient's symptoms. If there were a neurodynamic component, it would be expected for the patient's symptoms to be produced at some stage during the arm movements from 2 to 8, and that these symptoms would be reduced (or increased) by ipsilateral lateral flexion of the cervical spine. This principle will occur with each of the ULTT below.

ULTT 2a: median nerve bias (Fig. 3.35). The following sequence of movements would be appropriate, if, for example, the patient has symptoms in the upper arm or below (in the forearm and hand):

1. Neutral position of body on couch, but with shoulder girdle overhanging the edge
2. Contralateral lateral flexion of the cervical spine
3. Shoulder girdle depression
4. Wrist, finger and thumb extension
5. Forearm supination
6. Elbow extension
7. Shoulder lateral rotation
8. Shoulder abduction
9. Desensitizing movement of ipsilateral lateral flexion of the cervical spine.

If symptoms were near the cervical spine, for example, over the upper fibres of trapezius, then the movement of wrist flexion, for example, could be used as the desensitizing movement.

ULTT 2b: radial nerve bias (Fig. 3.36). The following sequence of movements would be appropriate, if, for example, the patient has symptoms in the upper arm or below (in the forearm and hand):

1. Neutral position of body on couch, but with shoulder girdle overhanging the edge
2. Contralateral lateral flexion of the cervical spine
3. Shoulder girdle depression
4. Wrist finger and thumb flexion
5. Shoulder medial rotation
6. Elbow extension
7. Desensitizing movement of ipsilateral lateral flexion of the cervical spine.

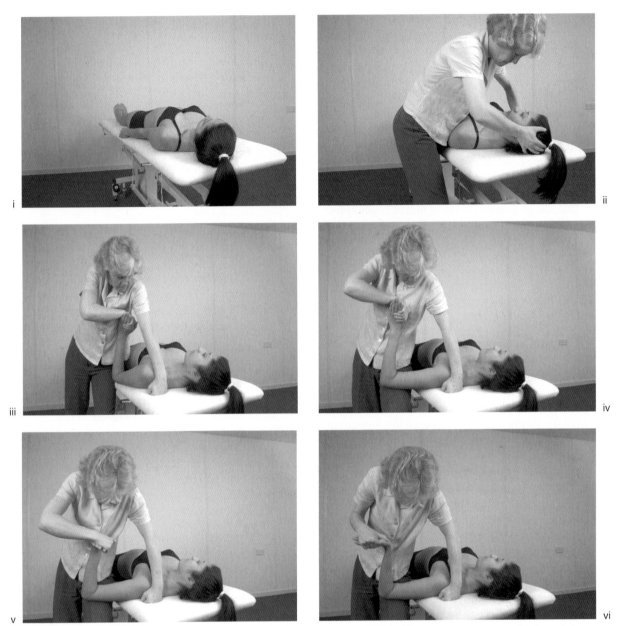

Figure 3.34(i–x) Upper limb tension test (ULTT) 1. (i) Neutral start position. (ii) Contralateral lateral flexion of the cervical spine. (iii) Shoulder girdle depression. (iv) Shoulder abduction. (v) Wrist and finger extension. (vi) Forearm supination.

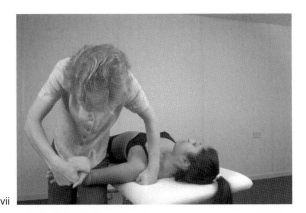
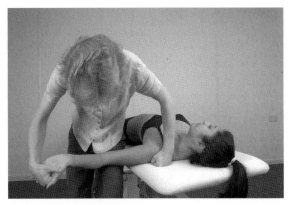

vii

viii

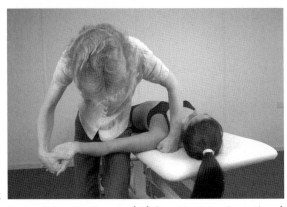
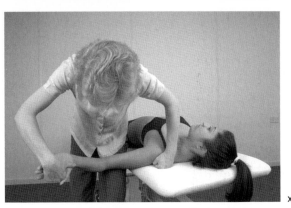

ix

x

Figure 3.34 *Continued* (vii) Shoulder lateral rotation. (viii) Elbow extension. (ix) Ipsilateral lateral flexion of the cervical spine if symptoms are in the arm. If ipsilateral lateral flexion reduces (or increases) the patient's symptoms, this would be a positive test. (x) Wrist flexion may be used to desensitize the movement, if the patient's symptoms are close to the cervical spine such as over the upper fibres of trapezius. If wrist flexion reduces (or increases) the patient's neck symptoms this would be a positive test.

Or

8. Wrist extension if symptoms are near the cervical spine, for example, over the upper fibres of trapezius.

   ULTT 3: ulnar nerve bias (Fig. 3.37). The following sequence of movements would be appropriate if, for example, the patient has symptoms in the upper arm or below (in the forearm and hand):

1. Neutral position of body on couch
2. Contralateral lateral flexion of the cervical spine
3. Shoulder girdle depression
4. Forearm pronation
5. Wrist and finger extension
6. Elbow flexion
7. Some shoulder abduction
8. Shoulder lateral rotation
9. Shoulder abduction
10. Desensitizing movement of ipsilateral lateral flexion of the cervical spine.

    Or

11. Wrist flexion if symptoms are near the cervical spine, for example, over the upper fibres of trapezius.

    Normal responses to ULTT 1 (Kenneally et al 1988) found a deep ache or stretch in the cubital fossa extending to the anterior and radial aspects of the forearm and hand, tingling in the thumb and first three fingers, a stretch feeling over the anterior aspect of the shoulder. Contralateral

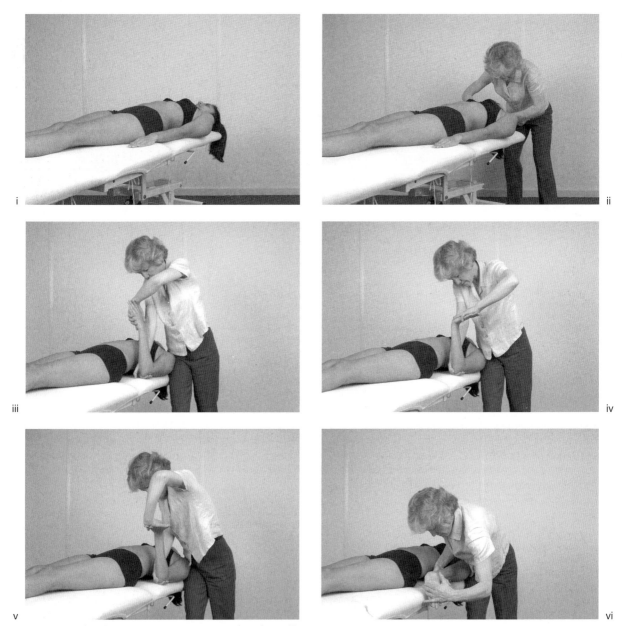

Figure 3.35(i–ix) Upper limb tension test (ULTT) 2a. (i) Neutral position of body on couch, but with shoulder girdle overhanging the edge. (ii) Contralateral lateral flexion of the cervical spine. (iii) Shoulder girdle depression. (iv) Wrist, finger and thumb extension. (v) Forearm supination. (vi) Elbow extension.

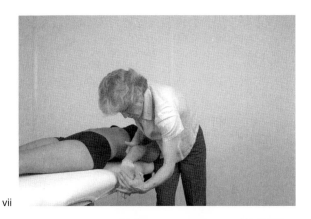
vii

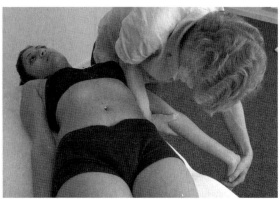
viii

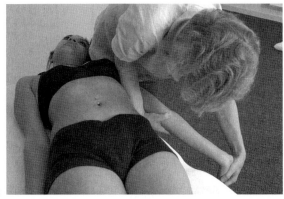
ix

Figure 3.35 *Continued*   (vii) Shoulder lateral rotation. (viii) Shoulder abduction. (ix) Desensitizing movement of ipsilateral lateral flexion of the cervical spine.

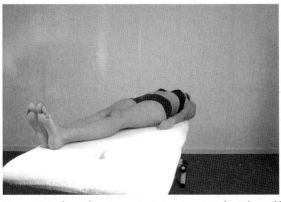
i

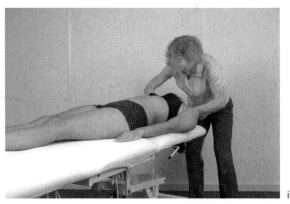
ii

Figure 3.36(i–viii)   Upper limb tension test (ULTT) 2b. (i) Neutral position of body on couch, but with shoulder girdle overhanging the edge. (ii) Contralateral lateral flexion of the cervical spine.

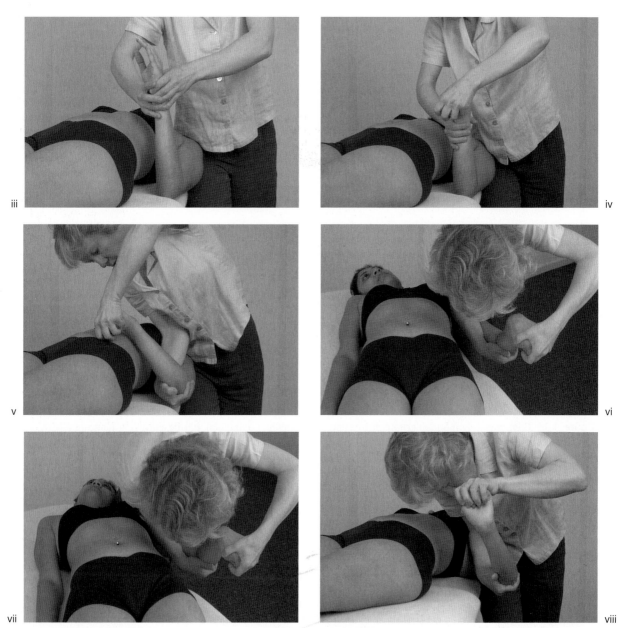

Figure 3.36 *Continued* (iii) Shoulder girdle depression. (iv) Wrist, finger and thumb flexion. (v) Shoulder medial rotation. (vi) Elbow extension. (vii) Desensitizing movement of ipsilateral lateral flexion of the cervical spine, or (viii) wrist extension would be used as a desensitizing movement if symptoms are near the cervical spine, for example, over the upper fibres of trapezius.

cervical lateral flexion increased symptoms while ipsilateral cervical lateral flexion reduced the symptoms.

Normal responses to ULTT 2b (Yaxley & Jull 1993) on asymptomatic subjects felt a stretching pain over the radial aspect of the proximal forearm; these symptoms were usually increased with the addition of contralateral cervical lateral flexion.

Additional tests for the upper limb tension test include placing the other arm in a ULTT position

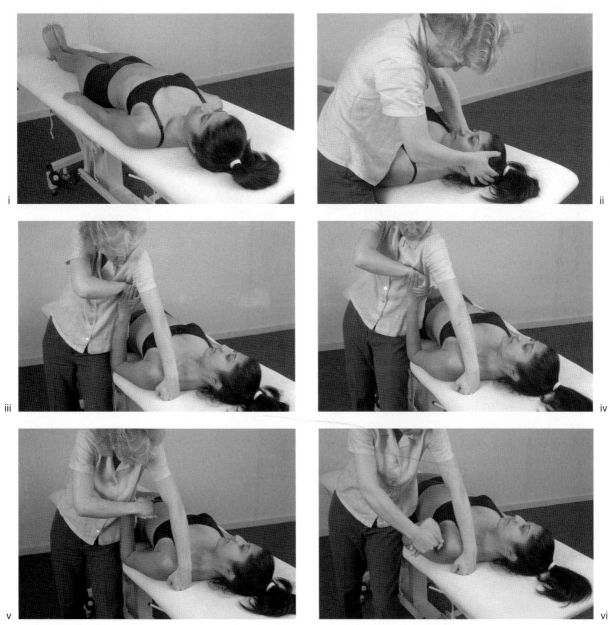

Figure 3.37(i–xi)   Upper limb tension test (ULTT) 3 (ulnar nerve bias). (i) Neutral position of body on couch. (ii) Contralateral lateral flexion of the cervical spine. (iii) Shoulder girdle depression. (iv) Wrist and finger extension. (v) Pronation of forearm. (vi) Elbow flexion.

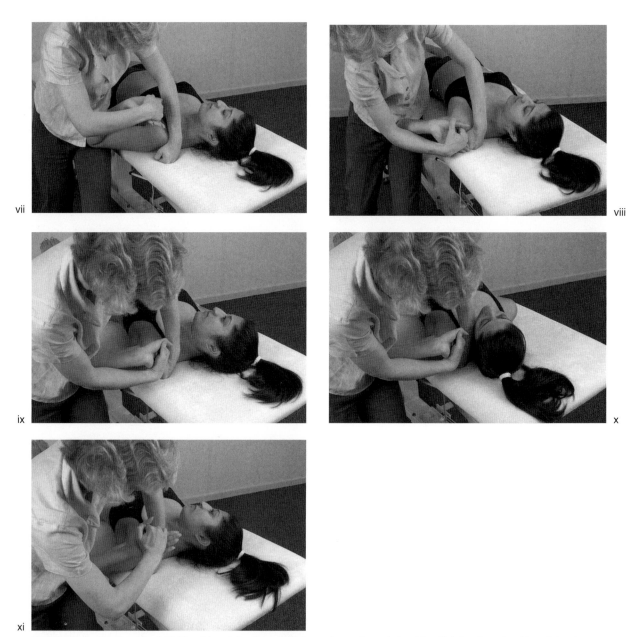

Figure 3.37 *Continued* (vii) Shoulder abduction. (viii) Lateral rotation of shoulder. (ix) Further shoulder abduction. (x) Desensitizing movement of ipsilateral lateral flexion of the cervical spine (if symptoms are in the forearm or hand), or (xi) Wrist flexion if symptoms are near the cervical spine or shoulder.

and adding in either the SLR or the slump test. The tests can also be carried out with the subject in other starting positions; for instance, the ULTT can be performed with the patient prone, which allows accessory movements to be carried out at the same time. Other upper limb movements can be carried out in addition to those suggested, for instance, pronation/supination or radial/ulnar deviation can be added to ULTT 1.

Other neurological tests

These tests include various tests for spinal cord and peripheral nerve damage and are discussed in the relevant chapters.

Miscellaneous tests

These can include vascular tests, respiratory tests and tests of soft tissues (such as meniscal tears in the knee). These tests are all discussed in detail in the relevant chapters.

Palpation

It is useful to record palpation findings on a body chart (see Fig. 2.3) and/or palpation chart for the vertebral column (Fig. 3.38).

During the palpation of soft tissues and skeletal tissues, the following should be noted:

- The temperature of the area (increase is indicative of local inflammation)
- Localized increased skin moisture (indicative of autonomic disturbance)
- The presence of oedema and effusion
- Mobility and feel of superficial tissues, e.g. ganglions, nodules
- The presence or elicitation of muscle spasm
- Tenderness of bone, ligament, muscle, tendon, tendon sheath, trigger point and nerve
- Increased or decreased prominence of bones
- Joint effusion or swelling of a limb can be measured using a tape measure, and comparing left and right sides
- Pain provoked or reduced on palpation.

Hints on the method of palpation are given in Box 3.2. Further guidance on palpation of the soft tissues can be found in Hunter (1998).

Trigger points

A trigger point is 'a focus of hyperirritability in a tissue that, when compressed, is locally tender and, if sufficiently hypersensitive, gives rise to referred pain and tenderness, and sometimes to referred autonomic phenomena and distortion of proprioception. Types include myofascial, cutaneous, fascial, ligamentous, and periosteal trigger points' (Travell & Simons 1983).

Trigger points can be divided into latent and active: a latent trigger point is where the tenderness is found on examination yet the person has no symptoms, while an active trigger point is one

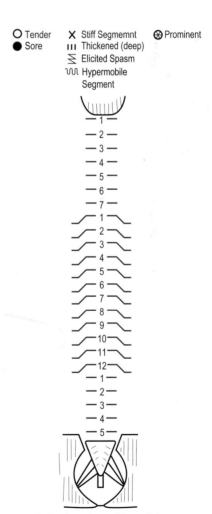

Figure 3.38 Palpation chart. (From Grieve 1991, with permission.)

where symptoms are produced locally and/or in an area of referral. Active trigger points lead to shortening and weakening of the muscle and are thought to be caused by trauma to the muscle (Baldry 1993). Commonly-found myofascial trigger points and their characteristic area of referral can be seen in Figure 3.39. In order to examine for a trigger point, the muscle is put on a slight stretch and the clinician searches for trigger points by firm pressure with the fingers over the muscle.

Palpable nerves in the upper limb are as follows:

- The brachial plexus can be palpated in the posterior triangle of the neck; it emerges at the lower third of sternocleidomastoid
- The suprascapular nerve can be palpated along the superior border of the scapula in the suprascapular notch
- The dorsal scapular nerve can be palpated medial to the medial border of the scapula
- The median nerve can be palpated over the anterior elbow joint crease, medial to the biceps tendon, also at the wrist between palmaris longus and flexor carpi radialis
- The radial nerve can be palpated around the spiral groove of the humerus, between brachioradialis and flexor carpi radialis, in the forearm and also at the wrist in the snuffbox.

Palpable nerves in the lower limb are as follows:

- The sciatic nerve can be palpated two-thirds of the way along an imaginary line between the greater trochanter and the ischial tuberosity with the patient in the prone position

- The common peroneal nerve can be palpated medial to the tendon of biceps femoris and also around the head of the fibula
- The tibial nerve can be palpated centrally over the posterior knee crease medial to the popliteal artery; it can also be felt behind the medial malleolus, which is more noticeable with the foot in dorsiflexion and eversion
- The superficial peroneal nerve can be palpated on the dorsum of the foot along an imaginary line over the fourth metatarsal; it is more noticeable with the foot in plantar flexion and inversion
- The deep peroneal nerve can be palpated between the first and second metatarsals, lateral to the extensor hallucis tendon
- The sural nerve can be palpated on the lateral aspect of the foot behind the lateral malleolus, lateral to the tendocalcaneus.

Accessory movements

Accessory movements are defined as those movements which a person cannot perform actively but which can be performed on that person by an external force (Maitland et al 2001). They take the form of gliding (sometimes referred to as translation or sliding) of the joint surfaces (medially, laterally, anteriorly or posteriorly), distraction and compression of the joint surfaces and, in some joints, rotation movements where this movement cannot be performed actively – e.g. rotation at the metacarpal and interphalangeal joints of the fingers. These movements are possible because all joints have a certain amount of play or 'slack' in the capsule and surrounding ligaments (Kaltenborn 2002).

Accessory movements are important to examine because they occur during all physiological movements and, very often, if there is a limitation of the accessory range of movement this will affect the range of physiological movement available. For example, during knee flexion in a non-weight-bearing position, the tibia rolls backwards and slides backwards on the femoral condyles; and during shoulder elevation through abduction, the head of the humerus rolls upwards and translates inferiorly on the glenoid cavity. The direction in which the bone glides during

---

Box 3.2   Hints on palpation

- Palpate the unaffected side first and compare this with the affected side
- Palpate from superficial to deep
- Use just enough force to feel – excessive force can reduce feel
- Never assume that a relevant area does not need palpating

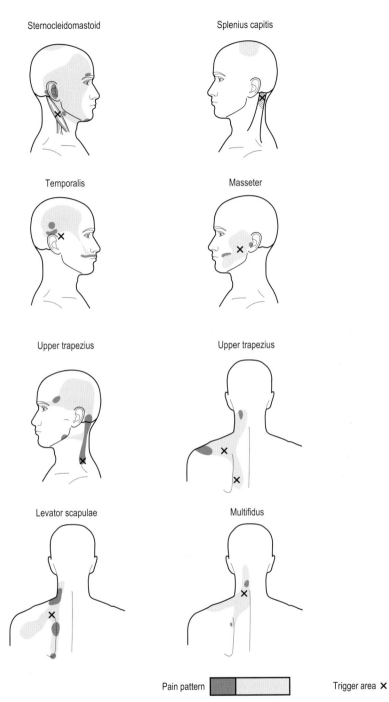

Figure 3.39 Myofascial trigger points.

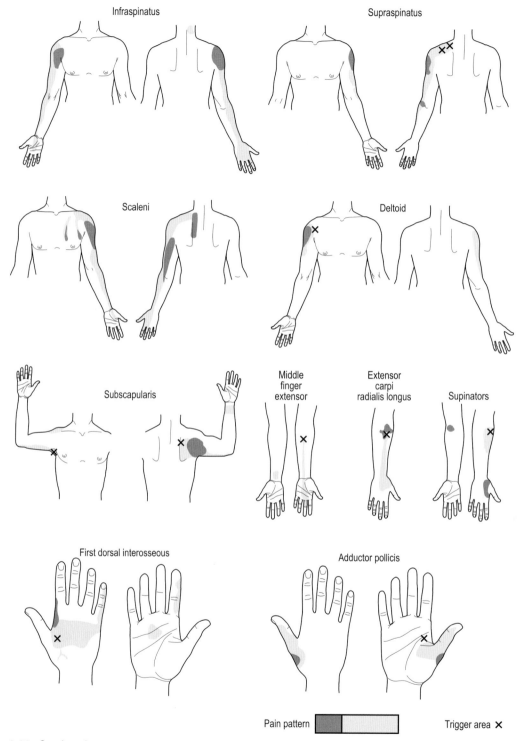

Figure 3.39 *Continued*

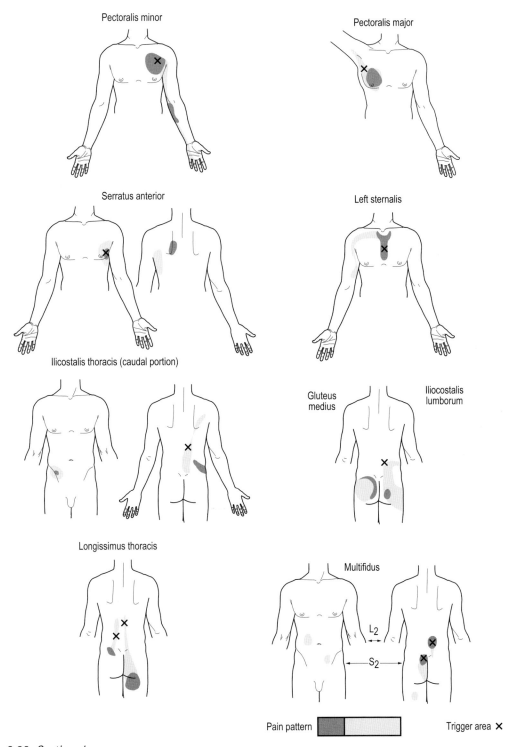

Pectoralis minor

Pectoralis major

Serratus anterior

Left sternalis

Ilicostalis thoracis (caudal portion)

Gluteus medius

Iliocostalis lumborum

Longissimus thoracis

Multifidus

L₂

S₂

Pain pattern   Trigger area ✕

Figure 3.39 *Continued*

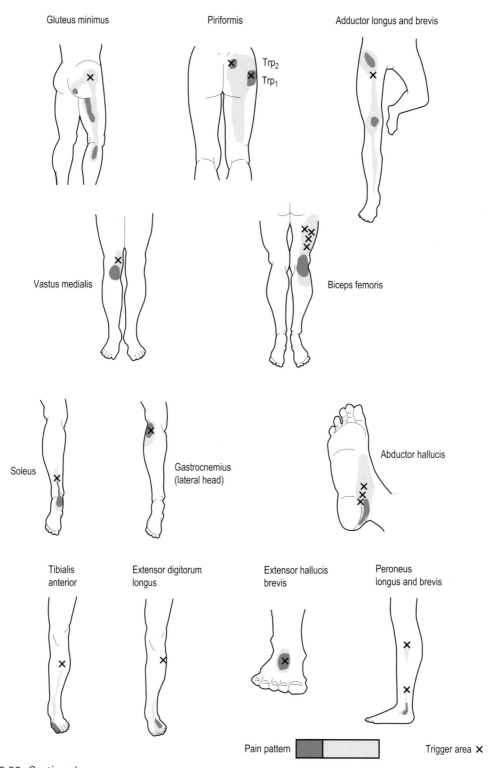

Gluteus minimus

Piriformis

Trp₂
Trp₁

Adductor longus and brevis

Vastus medialis

Biceps femoris

Soleus

Gastrocnemius (lateral head)

Abductor hallucis

Tibialis anterior

Extensor digitorum longus

Extensor hallucis brevis

Peroneus longus and brevis

Pain pattern

Trigger area ✗

Figure 3.39 *Continued*

physiological movements depends upon the shape of the moving articular surface (Fig. 3.40). When the joint surface of the moving bone is concave, the glide occurs in the same direction as the bone is moving, so that with flexion of the knee joint (in non-weight-bearing), posterior glide of the tibia occurs on the femur; when the joint surface is convex, the glide is in the opposite direction to the bone movement, so that with shoulder abduction there is an inferior glide of the head of the humerus on the glenoid cavity.

Examination of the accessory movement is important as it can (adapted from Jull 1994):

- Identify and localize a symptomatic joint
- Define the nature of a joint motion abnormality
- Identify associated areas of joint motion abnormality
- Alter local muscle and nerve tissues and identify either source of the patient's symptoms or a contributing factor to the patient's condition.
- Provide a basis for the selection of treatment techniques.

Pressure is applied to a bone close to the joint line and the clinician increases movement progressively through the range and notes the:

- Quality of the movement
- Range of the movement
- Pain behaviour (local and referred) through the range, which may be provoked or reduced

- Resistance through range and at the end of the range
- Muscle spasm elicitation.

Hints on performing an accessory movement are given in Box 3.3. Findings can include the following:

- Undue skeletal prominence
- Undue tenderness
- Thickening of soft tissues
- Decreased mobility of soft tissues, such as periarticular tissues, muscles and nerves
- A point in the range of the accessory movement where symptoms are increased or reduced
- An indication as to the irritability of a problem (see Ch. 2)
- Evidence of joint hypermobility
- Evidence of joint hypomobility
- Elicitation of muscle spasm
- Joints that are not affected by the present problem
- The location(s) of the problem(s)
- The relationship of the problems to each other
- The possible nature of structures involved
- What is limiting the movement and the relationship of pain, resistance or muscle spasm within the available range of movement. A movement diagram (or joint picture) depicts this information.

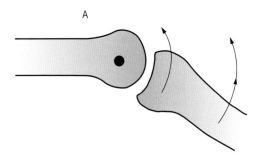
A

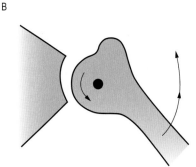
B

Figure 3.40 Movement of articular surfaces during physiological movements. The single arrow depicts the direction of movement of the articular surface and the double arrow depicts the physiological movement. A With knee extension (non-weight-bearing), the concave articular surface of the tibia slides superiorly on the convex femoral condyles. B With shoulder elevation through abduction, the convex articular surface of the humerus slides inferiorly on the concave glenoid cavity. (From Kaltenborn 2002, with permission.)

Movement diagrams

The movement diagram is useful for a student who is learning how to examine joint movement and is also a quick and easy way of recording information on joint movements. It was initially described by Maitland (1977) and then later refined by Margarey (1985) and Maitland et al (2001).

A movement diagram is a graph that describes the behaviour of pain, resistance and muscle spasm, showing the intensity and position in range at which each is felt during a passive accessory or passive physiological movement of a joint (Fig. 3.41).

The baseline AB is the range of movement of any joint. Point A is the beginning of range and

point B is the end of the passive movement. The exact position of B will vary with the strength and boldness of the clinician. It is thus depicted on the diagram as a thick line.

The vertical axis AC depicts the intensity of pain, resistance or muscle spasm. Point A is the absence of any pain, resistance or spasm and point C is the maximum intensity that the clinician is prepared to provoke.

Procedure for drawing a movement diagram. *To draw resistance* (Fig. 3.42). The clinician moves the joint and the first point at which resistance is felt is called R_1 and is marked on the baseline AB. A normal joint, when moved passively, has the feel of being well-oiled and friction-free until near the end of range, when some resistance is felt that increases to limit the range of movement. As mentioned previously, the resistance to further movement is due to bony apposition, increased tension in the surrounding ligaments and muscles or soft tissue apposition.

The joint is then taken to the limit of range and the point of limitation is marked by L on the baseline AB. If resistance limits the range, the point of limitation is marked by R_2 vertically above L on the CD line to indicate that it is resistance that limits the range. R_2 is the point beyond which the clinician is not prepared to push. The behaviour of the resistance between R_1 and R_2 is then drawn.

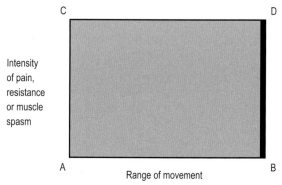

Figure 3.41 A movement diagram. The baseline AB is the range of movement of any joint and the vertical axis AC depicts the intensity of pain, resistance or muscle spasm.

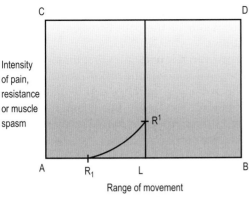

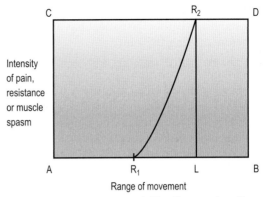

Figure 3.42   Resistance depicted on a movement diagram for physiological movements. **A** The diagram describes a joint movement that is limited (L) to $^1/_2$ range. Resistance is first felt at around $^1/_4$ of full range (R_1) and increases a little at the end of the available range (R'). **B** The diagram describes a joint movement that is limited (L) to $^3/_4$ range. Resistance is first felt at around $^1/_2$ of full range (R_1) and gradually increases to the limit range of movement (R_2).

If, on the other hand, pain limits the range of movement, an estimate of the intensity of resistance is made at the end of the available range and is plotted vertically above L as R'. The behaviour of the resistance between R_1 and R' is then described by drawing a line between the two points.

The resistance curve of the movement diagram, during physiological movements, is essentially a part of the load-displacement curve of soft tissue (Lee & Evans 1994, Panjabi 1992) and is shown in Figure 3.43. In a normal joint, the initial range of movement has minimal resistance and this part is known as the toe region (Lee & Evans 1994) or neutral zone (Panjabi 1992). As the joint is moved further into range, resistance increases; this is known as the linear region (Lee & Evans 1994) or elastic zone (Panjabi 1992). R_1 is the point at which the therapist perceives an increase in the resistance and it will lie somewhere between the toe region/neutral zone and the linear region/elastic zone. The ease with which a therapist can feel this change in resistance might be expected to depend on the range of joint movement and the type of movement being examined. It seems reasonable to suggest that it would be easier to feel R_1 when the range of movement is large and where there is a relatively long toe region, such as elbow flexion.

By contrast, accessory movements may only have a few millimetres of movement and no clear

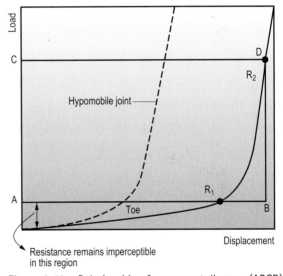

Figure 3.43   Relationship of movement diagram (ABCD) to a load – displacement curve. (From Lee & Evans 1994, with permission.)

toe region (Petty et al 2002); in this case R_1 may be perceived at the beginning of the range. For this reason, resistance occurs at the beginning of the range of movement for accessory movements, shown in Figure 3.44. A further complication in finding R_1 occurs with spinal accessory movements, because the movement is not localized to any one joint but produces a general movement of the spine (Lee & Svensson 1990).

To draw pain (Fig. 3.45). In this case, the clinician must establish whether the patient has any resting pain before moving the joint.

The joint is then moved passively through range, asking the patient to report any discomfort immediately. Several small oscillatory movements are carried out, gradually moving further into range up to the point where the pain is first felt, so that the exact position in the range at which the pain occurs can be recorded on the diagram. The point at which pain first occurs is called P_1 and is marked on the baseline AB.

The joint is then moved passively beyond P_1 to determine the behaviour of the pain through the available range of movement. If pain limits range, the point of limitation is marked as L on the baseline AB. Vertically above L, P_2 is marked on the CD

line to indicate that it is pain that limits the range. The behaviour of the pain between P_1 and P_2 is now drawn.

If, however, it is resistance that limits the range of movement, an estimate of the intensity of pain is made at the end of range and is plotted vertically above L as P′. The behaviour of the pain between P_1 and P′ is then described by drawing a line between the two points.

To draw muscle spasm (Fig. 3.46). The joint is taken through range and the point at which resistance due to muscle spasm is first felt is marked on the baseline AB as S_1.

The joint is then taken to the limit of range. If muscle spasm limits range, the point of limitation is marked as L on the baseline AB. Vertically above L, S_2 is marked on the CD line to indicate that it is muscle spasm that limits the range. The behaviour of spasm is then plotted between S_1 and S_2. When spasm limits range, it always reaches its maximum quickly and is more or less a straight line almost vertically upwards. The resistance from muscle spasm varies depending on the speed at which the joint is moved – as the speed increases, so the resistance increases.

Examples of movement diagrams are given in Figure 3.47.

Joint pictures. Grieve (1981) uses 'joint pictures' to describe essentially the same information as movement diagrams, i.e. the behaviour of pain,

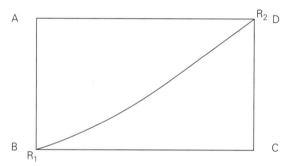

Figure 3.44   A movement diagram of an accessory movement, where R_1 starts at the beginning of range (at A).

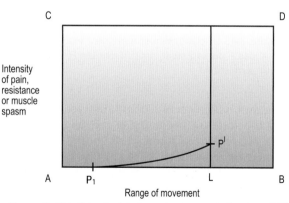

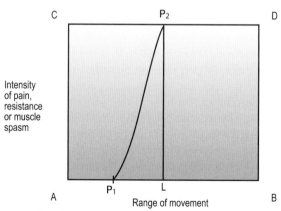

Figure 3.45   Pain depicted on a movement diagram. **A** The diagram describes a joint movement that is limited to $^3/_4$ range (L). Pain is first felt at around $^1/_4$ of full range (P_1) and increases a little at the end of available range (P′). **B** The diagram describes a joint movement that is limited to $^1/_2$ range (L). Pain is first felt at around $^1/_4$ of full range (P_1) and gradually increases to limit range of movement (P_2).

resistance and muscle spasm throughout the available range of movement (Fig. 3.48). A horizontal line depicts normal range, with the start of movement to the left. Pain is shown above the line, muscle spasm below, and resistance is shown as a number of vertical lines across the horizontal line. Limitation to movement is depicted by a vertical line from the dominant factor responsible for restricting the range of movement. A few examples of movement diagrams and joint pictures are shown for comparison in Figure 3.49.

Modifications to accessory movement examination

Accessory movements can be modified by altering the:

- Speed of applied force; pressure can be applied slowly or quickly and it may or may not be oscillated through the range
- Direction of the applied force
- Point of application of the applied force
- Resting position of the joint.

The joint can be placed in any number of resting positions; for example, accessory movements on the patella can be applied with the knee anywhere between full flexion and full extension, and accessory movements to any part of the spine can be

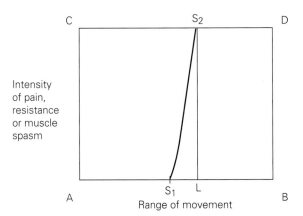

Figure 3.46 Muscle spasm depicted on a movement diagram. The diagram describes a joint movement that is limited to $^{3}/_{4}$ range (L). Muscle spasm is first felt just before $^{3}/_{4}$ of full range (S_1) and quickly increases to limit the range of movement (S_2).

performed with the spine in flexion, extension, lateral flexion or rotation, or indeed any combination of these positions. The effect of this positioning alters the effect of the accessory movement. For example, central posteroanterior pressure on C5 causes the superior articular facets of C5 to slide upwards on the inferior articular facets of C4, a movement similar to cervical extension; this upward movement can be enhanced with the cervical spine positioned in extension. Specific techniques have been described by Maitland et al (2001), Maitland (1991) and Edwards (1999) and readers are referred to these authors for further information.

Accessory movements are carried out on each joint suspected to be a source of the symptoms. After each joint is examined in this way, all relevant asterisks are reassessed to determine the effect of the accessory movements on the signs and symptoms. For example, in a patient with cervical spine, shoulder and elbow pain, it may be found that, following accessory movements to the cervical spine, there is an increase in range and reduction in pain in both the cervical spine and the shoulder joint but that there is no change in elbow movement. Accessory movements to the elbow joint, however, may be found to improve the elbow range of movements. Such a scenario suggests that the cervical spine is giving rise to the pain in the cervical spine and the shoulder, and the local tissues around the elbow are responsible for producing the pain at the elbow. This process had been termed the 'analytical assessment' by Maitland et al (2001) and is shown in Figure 3.50.

Accessory movements have been described by various authors (Cyriax 1982, Grieve 1991, Kaltenborn 2002, 2003, Maitland 1991, Maitland et al 2001, Mulligan 1999). This text will deal mainly with those described by Maitland, Kaltenborn and Mulligan and they will be covered in the relevant chapters.

Natural apophyseal glides (NAGs), sustained natural apophyseal glides (SNAGs) and mobilization with movement (MWM). These are a development from Kaltenborn's work and have been devised and fully described by Mulligan (1999). As mentioned earlier, during normal physiological movements there is a combination of

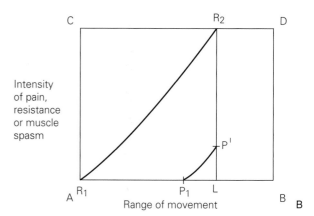

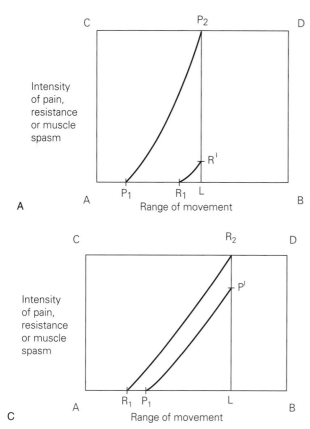

Figure 3.47 Examples of completed movement diagrams. **A** Shoulder joint flexion. Interpretation: Shoulder joint flexion is limited to just over half range (L). Pain first comes on at about $^1/_4$ of full range (P$_1$) and increases to limit the range of movement (P$_2$). Resistance is first felt just before the end of the available range (R$_1$) and increases a little (R'). The movement is therefore predominantly limited by pain. **B** Central posteroanterior (PA) pressure on L3. Interpretation: The PA movement is limited to $^3/_4$ range (L). Resistance is felt immediately, at the beginning of range (R$_1$) and increases to limit the range of movement (R$_2$). Pain is first felt just before the limit of the available range (P$_1$) and increases slightly (P'). The movement is therefore predominantly limited by resistance. **C** Left cervical rotation. Interpretation: Left cervical rotation is limited to $^3/_4$ range (L). Resistance is first felt at $^1/_4$ of full range (R$_1$) and increases to limit range of movement (R$_2$). Pain is felt very soon after resistance (P$_1$) and increases (P') to an intensity of about $^8/_{10}$ (where 0 represents no pain and 10 represents the maximum pain ever felt by the patient). Cervical rotation is therefore limited by resistance but pain is a significant factor.

(i) The horizontal line represents normal range and movement is from left to right

(ii) Pain is depicted above it

(iii) Spasm is depicted below it

(iv) Movement limitation is represented by a vertical line from the dominant factor responsible

(v) Resistance (other than spasm) is represented by a number of vertical lines which always cross the range line

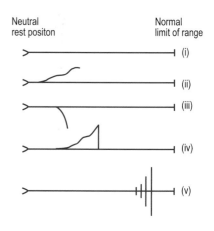

Figure 3.48 Joint pictures. (From Grieve 1991, with permission.)

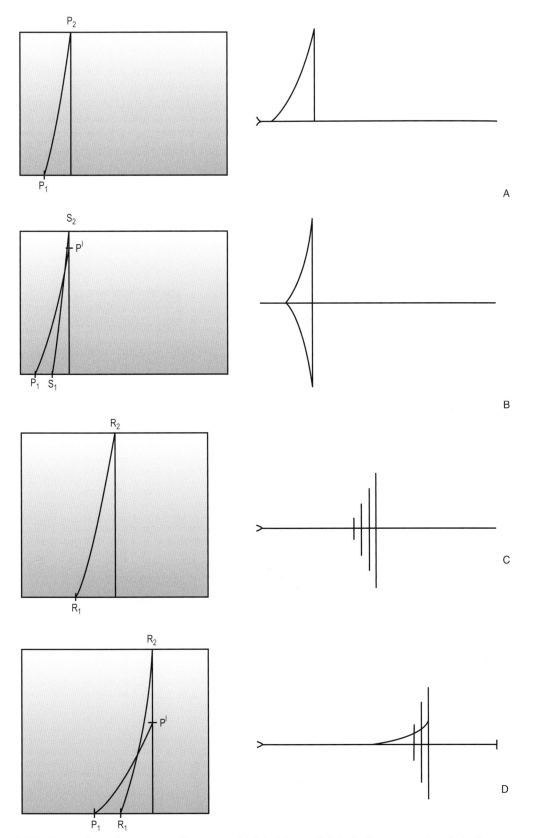

Figure 3.49 Comparison of movement diagrams and joint pictures. **A** Pain limits movement early in the range. **B** Spasm and pain limit movement early in range. **C** Resistance limits movement halfway through range. **D** Limitation of movement to $^3/_4$ range because of resistance, with some pain provoked from halfway through range.

rolling and gliding of bony surfaces at the joint. Examination (and treatment) aims to restore the glide component of the movement and thus enable full pain-free movement at the joint. During examination (and later treatment), the clinician moves the bone parallel (translation) or at right angles (distraction/separation) to the treatment plane. The treatment plane passes through the joint and lies 'in' the concave articular surface (Fig. 3.51). During examination with these accessory movements, it is the relief of symptoms that implicates the joint as the source of symptoms, since the technique aims to facilitate movement (compare accessory movements used by Maitland et al 2001 and Maitland 1991). The examination tests can be used as a treatment technique but details of these are outside the scope of this book.

Natural apophyseal glides (NAGs). These are mid-range rhythmic or sustained mobilizations applied centrally or unilaterally in the cervical and upper thoracic spine (between C2 and T3). They

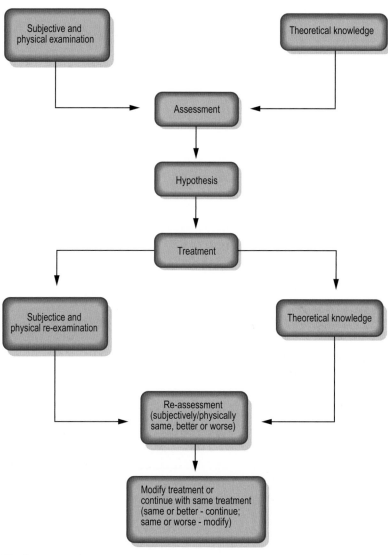

Figure 3.50 Analytical assessment.

are carried out in a weight-bearing position and the direction of the force is along the facet treatment plane (anterosuperiorly). They should eliminate the pain provoked during the movement. Further description of this examination procedure can be found in relevant chapters.

Sustained natural apophyseal glides (SNAGs). These are end-range sustained mobilizations, which are combined with active movements and can be used for all areas of the spine. They are, like NAGs, carried out in a weight-bearing position with the direction of the force along the facet treatment plane. They should eliminate the pain provoked during the movement. Further description can be found in relevant chapters.

Mobilizations with movement (MWM). These are sustained mobilizations carried out with active or passive movements or resisted muscle contraction and are used for the peripheral joints. They are generally applied close to the joint at right angles to the plane of the movement taking place. They should eliminate the pain provoked during the movement. It is proposed that the mobilization affects and corrects a bony positional fault, which produces abnormal tracking of the articular surfaces during movement (Exelby 1996, Mulligan

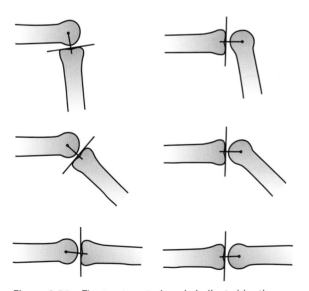

Figure 3.51 The treatment plane is indicated by the line and passes through the joint and lies 'in' the concave articular surface. (From Kaltenborn 1989, with permission.)

1993, 1999). Further description can be found in relevant chapters.

COMPLETION OF THE PHYSICAL EXAMINATION

Once all the above steps have been carried out, the physical examination is complete. It is vital at this stage to highlight with an asterisk (*) important findings from the examination. These findings must be reassessed at, and within, subsequent treatment sessions to evaluate the effects of treatment on the patient's condition. An outline examination chart that summarizes the physical examination is shown in Figure 3.52.

The physical testing procedures which specifically indicate joint, nerve or muscle tissues, as a source of the patient's symptoms, are summarized in Table 3.10. At one end of the scale the findings may provide strong evidence, and at the other end, may provide weak evidence. A variety of presentation between these two extremes, may, of course, be found.

The strongest evidence that a joint is the source of the patient's symptoms is that active and passive physiological movements, passive accessory movements, and joint palpation all reproduce the patient's symptoms, and that following a treatment dose, reassessment identifies an improvement in the patient's signs and symptoms. For example, let us assume a patient has lateral elbow pain caused by a radiohumeral joint dysfunction. In the physical examination, there is limited elbow flexion and extension movements due to reproduction of the patient's elbow pain, with some resistance. Active movement is very similar to passive movement in terms of range, resistance and pain reproduction. Accessory movement examination of the radiohumeral joint reveals limited posteroanterior and anteroposterior glide of the radius due to reproduction of the patient's elbow pain with some resistance. Following the examination of accessory movements, sufficient to be considered a treatment dose, reassessment of the elbow physiological movements are improved, in terms of range and pain. This scenario would indicate that there is a dysfunction at the radiohumeral joint, firstly because elbow movements, both active and passive

Observation	Isometric muscle testing
Joint integrity tests	Other muscle tests
Active and passive physiological movements	Neurological integrity tests
	Neurodynamic tests
	Other nerve tests
Capsular pattern yes/no	Miscellaneous tests
Muscle strength	
	Palpation
Muscle control	
	Accessory movements and reassessment of each relevant region
Muscle length	

Figure 3.52   Physical examination chart.

Table 3.10 Physical tests which, if positive, indicate joint, nerve and muscle as a source of the patient's symptoms

Test	Strong evidence	Weak evidence
Joint		
Active physiological movements	Reproduces patient's symptoms	Dysfunctional movement: reduced range, excessive range, altered quality of movement, increased resistance, decreased resistance
Passive physiological movements	Reproduces patient's symptoms; this test same as for active physiological movements	Dysfunctional movement: reduced range, excessive range, increased resistance, decreased resistance, altered quality of movement
Accessory movements	Reproduces patient's symptoms	Dysfunctional movement: reduced range, excessive range, increased resistance, decreased resistance, altered quality of movement
Palpation of joint	Reproduces patient's symptoms	Tenderness
Reassessment following therapeutic dose of accessory movement	Improvement in tests which reproduce patient's symptoms	No change in physical tests which reproduce patient's symptoms
Muscle		
Active movement	Reproduces patient's symptoms	Reduced strength Poor quality
Passive physiological movements	Do not reproduce patient's symptoms	
Isometric contraction	Reproduces patient's symptoms	Reduced strength Poor quality
Passive lengthening of muscle	Reproduces patient's symptoms	Reduced range Increased resistance Decreased resistance
Palpation of muscle	Reproduces patient's symptoms	Tenderness
Reassessment following therapeutic dose of muscle treatment	Improvement in tests which reproduce patient's symptoms	No change in physical tests which reproduce patient's symptoms
Nerve		
Passive lengthening and sensitizing movement, i.e. altering length of nerve by a movement at a distance from patient's symptoms	Reproduces patient's symptoms and sensitizing movement alters patient's symptoms	Reduced length Increased resistance
Palpation of nerve	Reproduces patient's symptoms	Tenderness

physiological, and accessory movements, reproduce the patient's symptoms, and secondly, because following accessory movements, the active elbow movements are improved. Even if the active movements are made worse, this would still suggest a joint dysfunction, since it is likely that the accessory movements would predominantly affect the joint, with much less effect on nerve and muscle tissues around the area. Collectively, this evidence would suggest there is a joint dysfunction, as long as this is accompanied by negative muscle and nerve tests.

Weaker evidence includes an alteration in range, resistance or quality of physiological and/or accessory movements and tenderness over the joint, with no alteration in signs and symptoms after treatment. One or more of these findings may indicate a dysfunction of a joint which may or may not be contributing to the patient's condition.

The strongest evidence that a muscle is the source of a patient's symptoms is if active movements, an isometric contraction, passive lengthening and palpation of a muscle all reproduce the patient's symptoms, and that following a treatment dose, reassessment identifies an improvement in the patient's signs and symptoms. For example, let us assume that a patient has lateral elbow pain caused by lateral epicondylalgia, a primary muscle problem. In this case reproduction of the lateral elbow pain is found on active wrist and finger extension, isometric contraction of the wrist extensors and/or finger extensors, and passive lengthening of the extensor muscles to the wrist and hand. These signs and symptoms are found to improve following soft tissue mobilization examination, sufficient to be considered a treatment dose. Collectively, this evidence would suggest there is a muscle dysfunction, as long as this is accompanied by negative joint and nerve tests.

Further evidence of muscle dysfunction may be suggested by reduced strength or poor quality during the active physiological movement and the isometric contraction, reduced range, and/or increased/decreased resistance, during the passive lengthening of the muscle, and tenderness on palpation, with no alteration in signs and symptoms after treatment. One or more of these findings may indicate a dysfunction of a muscle which may or may not be contributing to the patient's condition.

The strongest evidence that a nerve is the source of the patient's symptoms is when active and/or passive physiological movements reproduce the symptoms, which are then increased or decreased with an additional sensitizing movement, at a distance from the patient's symptoms. In addition, there is reproduction of the patient's symptoms on palpation of the nerve and neurodynamic testing, sufficient to be considered a treatment dose, results in an improvement in the above signs and symptoms. For example, let us assume this time that the lateral elbow pain is caused by a neurodynamic dysfunction of the radial nerve supplying this region. The patient's lateral elbow pain is reproduced during the component movements of

ULTT 2b and is eased with ipsilateral cervical lateral flexion sensitizing movement. There is tenderness over the radial groove in the upper arm and testing of ULTT 2b, sufficient to be considered a treatment dose, results in an improvement in the patient's signs and symptoms. Collectively, this evidence would suggest there is a neurodynamic dysfunction, as long as this is accompanied by negative joint and muscle tests. Further evidence of nerve dysfunction may be suggested by reduced range (compared to the asymptomatic side) and/or increased resistance to the various arm movements, and tenderness on nerve palpation.

It can be seen that the common factor for identifying joint, nerve and muscle dysfunction as a source of the patient's symptoms, is the reproduction of the patient's symptoms, the alteration in the patient's signs and symptoms following a treatment dose and the lack of evidence from other potential sources of symptoms. It is assumed that if a test reproduces a patient's symptoms, then it is somehow stressing the structure at fault. As mentioned earlier, each test is not purely a test of one structure; every test, to a greater or lesser degree, involves all structures. For this reason, it is imperative that the treatment given proves its value by altering the patient's signs and symptoms. The other factor common in identifying joint, nerve or muscle dysfunction is the lack of positive findings in the other possible tissues; for example, a joint dysfunction is considered when joint tests are positive and muscle and nerve tests are negative. Thus the clinician collects evidence to implicate tissues and evidence to negate tissues; both being equally important.

Inexperienced clinicians may find the treatment and management planning form shown in Figure 3.53 helpful in guiding them through what is often a complex clinical reasoning process. Figure 3.54 is a more advanced clinical reasoning form for more experienced clinicians.

On completion of the physical examination the clinician:

● Warns the patient of possible exacerbation up to 24–48 hours following the examination. With severe and/or irritable conditions, the patient may have increased symptoms following examination.

- Requests the patient to report details on the behaviour of the symptoms following examination at the next attendance.

- Explains the findings of the physical examination and how these findings relate to the sub-

jective assessment. An attempt should be made to clear up any misconceptions patients may have regarding their illness or injury.

- Evaluates the findings, formulates a clinical hypothesis and writes up a problem list, i.e. a concise numbered list of the patient's problems at the time of the examination. Problems for a

What subjective and physical reassessment asterisks will you use?	
Subjective	Physical
What is your treatment plan for the:	
Source of symptoms	Contributing factors
What are your goals for discharge?	

Figure 3.53   Management planning form (to be completed after the physical examination). (After Maitland 1986.)

1.1 Source of symptoms

Symptomatic area	Structures under area	Structures which can refer to area	Supporting evidence

1.2 What is the mechanism of each symptom? Explain from information from the subjective and *physical examination findings*

	Symptom:	Symptom:	Symptom:	Symptom:
Subjective				
Physical				

Figure 3.54   Clinical reasoning form.

1.3 Following the physical examination what is your clinical diagnosis?

2. Contributing factors

2.1   What factors need to be examined/explored in the physical examination?

2.2   How will you address each contributing factor?

3. Precautions and contraindications

3.1 Are any symptoms severe? Which symptoms, and explain why	Yes	No
3.2 Are any symptoms irritable? Which symptoms, and explain why	Yes	No

Figure 3.54 *Continued*

3.3   How much of each symptom are you prepared to provoke in the physical examination?

Symptom	Short of P1	Point of onset or increase in resting symptoms	Partial reproduction	Total reproduction

3.4   Will a neurological examination be necesssary in the physical?

yes   no   Explain why

3.5   Following the subjective examination are there any precautions or contraindications?

yes   no   Explain why

4   Management

4.1   What tests will you do in the physical and what are the expected findings?

Physical tests	Expected findings

Figure 3.54 *Continued*

4.2   *Were there any unexpected findings from the physical? Explain*

4.3   *What will be your subjective and physical reassessment asterisks?*

4.4   *What is your first choice of treatment (be exact) and explain why?*

4.5   *What do you expect the response to be over the next 24 hours following the first visit? Explain*

4.6   *How do you think you will treat and manage the patient at the second visit, if the patient returns:*

Same

Better

Worse

4.7   *What advice and education will you give the patient?*

Figure 3.54 *Continued*

4.8 What needs to be examined on the second and third visits?

Second visit	Third visit

5 Prognosis

5.1 List the positive and negative factors (from both the subjective *and physical examination findings*) in considering the patient's prognosis?

	Positive	Negative
Subjective		
Physical		

5.2 Overall, is the patient's condition:
      improving   *worsening*   *static*

5.3 What is your overall prognosis for this patient? Be specific

Figure 3.54 *Continued*

6. After third attendance

6.1 Has your understanding of the patient's problem changed from your interpretations made following the initial subjective and physical examination? If so explain

6.2 On reflection, were there any clues that you initially missed, misinterpreted, under- or over-weighted? If so explain

7. After discharge

7.1 Has your understanding of the patient's problem changed from your interpretations made following the third attendance? If so explain how

7.2 What have you learnt from the management of this patient which will be helpful to you in the future?

Figure 3.54 *Continued*

patellofemoral problem, for example, could include pain over the knee and difficulty ascending and descending stairs, inhibition of vastus medialis oblique (VMO), tightness of the iliotibial band and hamstring muscle group, and lateral tilt and external rotation of the patella. More general problems, such as lack of general fitness or coping behaviour should be also be included.

- Determines the long- and short-term objectives for each problem in consultation with the patient. Short-term objectives for the above example might be relief of some of the knee pain, increased contraction of VMO, increased extensibility of the iliotibial band and hamstrings, and correction of patellar malalignment by the end of the third treatment session. The long-term objective might be complete resolution of the patient's problem after six treatment sessions.

- Devises an initial treatment plan in order to achieve the short- and long-term objectives. This includes the modalities and frequency of treatment and any patient education required. In the example above, this might be treatment twice a week to consist of passive stretches to the iliotibial band and hamstrings; passive accessory movements to the patella; taping to correct the patellar malalignment; and exercises with biofeedback to alter the timing and intensity of VMO contraction in squat standing, pro-gressing to steps and specific functional exercises and activities.

By the end of the physical examination the clinician will have further developed the hypotheses categories initiated in the subjective examination (adapted from Jones & Rivett 2004):

- Function: abilities and restrictions.
- Patient's perspectives on the experience.
- Source of symptoms. This includes the structure or tissue that is thought to be producing the patient's symptoms, the nature of the structure or tissues in relation to the healing process, and the pain mechanisms.
- Contributing factors to the development and maintenance of the problem. There may be environmental, psychosocial, behavioural, physical or heredity factors.
- Precautions/contraindications to treatment and management. This includes the severity and irritability of the patient's symptoms and the nature of the patient's condition.
- Management strategy and treatment plan.
- Prognosis – this can be affected by factors such as the stage and extent of the injury as well as the patient's expectation, personality and lifestyle.

For further information on treatment and management of patients with neuromusculoskeletal dysfunction, please see the companion to this text: *Principles of Neuromusculoskeletal Treatment and Management* (Petty 2004).

References

American Academy of Orthopaedic Surgeons 1990 Joint motion. Method of measuring and recording, 3rd edn. Churchill Livingstone, New York

Amevo B, Aprill C, Bogduk N 1992 Abnormal instantaneous axes of rotation in patients with neck pain. Spine 17(7): 748–756

Baldry P E (1993) Acupuncture, trigger points and musculoskeletal pain. Churchill Livingstone, Edinburgh

Bergmark A 1989 Stability of the lumbar spine. A study in mechanical engineering. Acta Orthopaedica Scandinavica 230(suppl): 20–24

Breig A 1978 Adverse mechanical tension in the central nervous system. Almqvist & Wiksell, Stockholm

Butler D S 1991 Mobilisation of the nervous system. Churchill Livingstone, Melbourne

Chaitow L 1996 Muscle energy techniques. Churchill Livingstone, New York

Cole J H, Furness A L, Twomey L T 1988 Muscles in action, an approach to manual muscle testing. Churchill Livingstone, Edinburgh

Comerford M & Kinetic Control 2000 Movement dysfunction focus on dynamic stability and muscle balance. Kinetic Control course notes

Crawford G N C 1973 The growth of striated muscle immobilized in extension. Journal of Anatomy 114: 165–183

Cyriax J 1982 Textbook of orthopaedic medicine – diagnosis of soft tissue lesions, 8th edn. Baillière Tindall, London

Drake R L, Vogl W, Mitchell A W M 2005 Gray's anatomy for students. Churchill Livingstone, Philadelphia

Dyck P 1984 Lumbar nerve root: the enigmatic eponyms. Spine 9(1): 3–6

Edwards B C 1992 Manual of combined movements: their use in the examination and treatment of mechanical vertebral column disorders. Churchill Livingstone, Edinburgh

Edwards B C 1999 Manual of combined movements: their use in the examination and treatment of mechanical vertebral column disorders, 2nd edn. Butterworth-Heinemann, Oxford

Elvey R L 1985 Brachial plexus tension tests and the pathoanatomical origin of arm pain. In: Glasgow E F, Twomey L T, Scull E R, Kleynhans A M, Idczak R M (eds) Aspects of manipulative therapy, 2nd edn. Churchill Livingstone, Melbourne, ch 17, p 116

Exelby L 1996 Peripheral mobilisations with movement. Manual Therapy 1(3): 118–126

Frankel V H, Burstein A H, Brooks D B 1971 Biomechanics of internal derangement of the knee. Pathomechanics as determined by analysis of the instant centres of motion. Journal of Bone and Joint Surgery 53A(5): 945–962

Gerhardt J J 1992 Documentation of joint motion, 3rd edn. Isomed, Oregon

Gilmore K L 1986 Biomechanics of the lumbar motion segment. In: Grieve G P (ed) Modern manual therapy of the vertebral column. Churchill Livingstone, Edinburgh, ch 9, p 103

Gossman M R, Sahrmann S A, Rose S J 1982 Review of length-associated changes in muscle. Physical Therapy 62(12): 1799–1808

Grieve G P 1981 Common vertebral joint problems. Churchill Livingstone, Edinburgh

Grieve G P 1991 Mobilisation of the spine, 5th edn. Churchill Livingstone, Edinburgh

Harding V, Williams A C de C, Richardson P, Nicholas M K, Jackson J L, Richardson I H, Pither C E. 1994 The development of a battery of measures for assessing physical functioning in chronic pain patients. Pain 58: 367–375

Hides J 1995 Multifidus inhibition in acute low back pain: recovery is not spontaneous. In: Proceedings of the Manipulative Physiotherapists Association of Australia, 9th biennial conference, Gold Coast, pp 57–60

Hides J A, Richardson C A, Jull G A 1996 Multifidus muscle recovery is not automatic after resolution of acute, first-episode low back pain. Spine 21(23): 2763–2769

Hislop H, Montgomery J 1995 Daniels and Worthingham's muscle testing, techniques of manual examination, 7th edn. W B Saunders, Philadelphia

Hockaday J M, Whitty C W M 1967 Patterns of referred pain in the normal subject. Brain 90: 481–496

Hodges P 1995 Dysfunction of transversus abdominis associated with chronic low back pain. In: Proceedings of the Manipulative Physiotherapists Association of Australia, 9th biennial conference, Gold Coast, pp 61–62

Hodges P W, Richardson C A 1996 Inefficient muscular stabilization of the lumbar spine associated with low back pain, a motor control evaluation of transversus abdominis. Spine 21(22): 2640–2650

Hunter G 1998 Specific soft tissue mobilization in the management of soft tissue dysfunction. Manual Therapy 3(1): 2–11

Hunter J M (ed) 2002 Rehabilitation of the hand and upper extremity, 5th edn. Mosby, St Louis

Inman V T, Saunders J B de C M 1944 Referred pain from skeletal structures. Journal of Nervous and Mental Disease 90: 660–667

Janda V 1986 Muscle weakness and inhibition (pseudoparesis) in back pain syndromes. In: Grieve G P (ed) Modern manual therapy of the vertebral column. Churchill Livingstone, Edinburgh, ch 19, p 197

Janda V 1993 Muscle strength in relation to muscle length, pain and muscle imbalance. In: Harms-Ringdahl K (ed) Muscle strength. Churchill Livingstone, Edinburgh, ch 6, p 83

Janda V 1994 Muscles and motor control in cervicogenic disorders: assessment and management. In: Grant R (ed) Physical therapy of the cervical and thoracic spine, 2nd edn. Churchill Livingstone, Edinburgh, ch 10, p 195

Janda V 2002 Muscles and motor control in cervicogenic disorders. In: Grant R (ed) Physical therapy of the cervical and thoracic spine, 3rd edn. Churchill Livingstone, New York, ch 10, p 182

Jones M A, Jones H M 1994 Principles of the physical examination. In: Boyling J D, Palastanga N (eds) Grieve's modern manual therapy, 2nd edn. Churchill Livingstone, Edinburgh, ch 35, p 491

Jones M A, Rivett D A 2004 Clinical reasoning for manual therapists. Butterworth-Heinemann, Edinburgh

Jull G A 1994 Examination of the articular system. In: Boyling J D, Palastanga N (eds) Grieve's modern manual therapy, 2nd edn. Churchill Livingstone, Edinburgh, ch 37, p 511

Jull G A, Janda V 1987 Muscles and motor control in low back pain: assessment and management. In: Twomey L T, Taylor J R (eds) Physical therapy of the low back. Churchill Livingstone, Edinburgh, ch 10, p 253

Jull G A, Richardson C A 1994 Rehabilitation of active stabilization of the lumbar spine. In: Twomey L T, Taylor J R (eds) Physical therapy of the low back, 2nd edn. Churchill Livingstone, Edinburgh, ch 9, p 251

Kaltenborn F M 2002 Manual mobilization of the joints, vol I, The extremities, 6th edn. Olaf Norli, Oslo

Kaltenborn F M 2003 Manual mobilization of the joints, vol II, The spine, 4th edn. Olaf Norli, Oslo

Kazarian L 1972 Dynamic response characteristics of the human vertebral column. Acta Orthopaedica Scandinavica 146: 54–117

Kendall F P, McCreary E K, Provance P G 1993 Muscles: testing and function, 4th edn. Lippincott, Williams & Wilkins, Baltimore

Kenneally M, Rubenach H, Elvey R 1988 The upper limb tension test: the SLR test of the arm. In: Grant R (ed) Physical therapy of the cervical and thoracic spine. Churchill Livingstone, Edinburgh, ch 10, p 167

Lee R, Evans J 1994 Towards a better understanding of spinal posteroanterior mobilisation. Physiotherapy 80(2): 68–73

Lee M, Svensson N L 1990 Measurement of stiffness during simulated spinal physiotherapy. Clinical Physics and Physiological Measurement 11(3): 201–207

Lewit K 1991 Manipulative therapy in rehabilitation of the locomotor system, 2nd edn. Butterworth-Heinemann, Oxford

McKenzie R A 1981 The lumbar spine mechanical diagnosis and therapy. Spinal Publications, New Zealand

McKenzie R A 1990 The cervical and thoracic spine mechanical diagnosis and therapy. Spinal Publications, New Zealand

Magee D J 1997 Orthopedic physical assessment, 3rd edn. W B Saunders, Philadelphia

Maitland G D 1977 Vertebral manipulation, 4th edn. Butterworths, London

Maitland G D 1985 Passive movement techniques for intra-articular and periarticular disorders. Australian Journal of Physiotherapy 31(1): 3–8

Maitland G D 1991 Peripheral manipulation, 3rd edn. Butterworths, London

Maitland G D, Hengeveld E, Banks K, English K 2001 Maitland's vertebral manipulation, 6th edn. Butterworth-Heinemann, Oxford

Margarey M 1985 Selection of passive treatment techniques. In: Proceedings of the Manipulative Therapists Association of Australia, 4th biennial conference, Brisbane, pp 298–320

Mariani P P, Caruso I 1979 An electromyographic investigation of subluxation of the patella. Journal of Bone and Joint Surgery 61B(2): 169–171

Medical Research Council 1976 Aids to the investigation of peripheral nerve injuries. HMSO, London

Mercer S R, Jull G A 1996 Morphology of the cervical intervertebral disc: implications for McKenzie's model of the disc derangement syndrome. Manual Therapy 1(2): 76–81

Miller A M 1987 Neuro-meningeal limitation of straight leg raising. In: Dalziel B A, Snowsill J C (eds) Manipulative Therapists Association of Australia, 5th biennial conference proceedings, Melbourne, pp 70–78

Mooney V, Robertson J 1976 The facet syndrome. Clinical Orthopaedics and Related Research 115: 149–156

Mulligan B R 1993 Mobilisations with movement (MWMs). Journal of Manual and Manipulative Therapy 1(4): 154–156

Mulligan B R 1999 Manual therapy 'NAGs', 'SNAGs', 'MWMs' etc., 4th edn. Plane View Services, New Zealand

Newham D J 2001 Strength, power and endurance. In: Trew M, Everett T (eds) Human movement, 4th edn. Churchill Livingstone, Edinburgh, ch 6, p 105

Norris C M 1995 Spinal stabilisation, muscle imbalance and the low back. Physiotherapy 81(3): 127–138

Noyes F R, Delucas J L, Torvik P J 1974 Biomechanics of anterior cruciate ligament failure: an analysis of strain-rate sensitivity and mechanisms of failure in primates. Journal of Bone and Joint Surgery 56A(2): 236–253

Panjabi M M 1992 The stabilising system of the spine: part II. Neutral zone and instability hypothesis. Journal of Spinal Disorders 5(4): 390–396

Pennal G F, Conn G S, McDonald G, Dale G, Garside H 1972 Motion studies of the lumbar spine, a preliminary report. Journal of Bone and Joint Surgery 54B(3): 442–452

Petty N J 2004 Principles of neuromusculoskeletal treatment and management, a guide for therapists. Churchill Livingstone, Edinburgh

Petty N J, Maher C, Latimer J, Lee M 2002 Manual examination of accessory movements – seeking R1. Manual Therapy 7(1): 39–43

Richardson C, Hodges P W, Hides J 2004 Therapeutic exercise for lumbopelvic stabilization. A motor control approach for the treatment and prevention of low back pain, 2nd edn. Churchill Livingstone, Edinburgh

Sahrmann S A 1993 Diagnosis and treatment of movement system imbalances associated with musculoskeletal pain. Lecture notes, Washington University School of Medicine, Washington, DC

Sahrmann S A 2002 Diagnosis and treatment of movement impairment syndromes. Mosby, St Louis

Shacklock M 1995 Neurodynamics. Physiotherapy 81(1): 9–16

Shah J S, Hampson W G J, Jayson M I V 1978 The distribution of surface strain in the cadaveric lumbar spine. Journal of Bone and Joint Surgery 60B(2): 246–251

Shorland S 1998 Management of chronic pain following whiplash injuries. In Gifford L (ed) Topical issues in pain. NOI, Falmouth, ch 8, p 115–134

Slater H 1989 The effect of foot and ankle position on the response to the SLR test. In: Jones H M, Jones M A, Milde M R (eds) Manipulative Therapists Association of Australia, 6th biennial conference proceedings, Adelaide, pp 183–190

Stokes M, Young A 1986 Measurement of quadriceps cross–sectional area by ultrasonography: a description of the technique and its application in physiotherapy. Physiotherapy Practice 2: 31–36

Tencer A F, Allen B L, Ferguson R L 1985 A biomechanical study of thoracolumbar spine fractures with bone in the canal: part III. Mechanical properties of the dura and its tethering ligaments. Spine 10(8): 741–747

Travell J G, Simons D G 1983 Myofascial pain and dysfunction: the trigger point manual. Williams & Wilkins, Baltimore, MD

Voight M L, Wieder D L 1991 Comparative reflex response times of vastus medialis obliquus and vastus lateralis in normal subjects and subjects with extensor mechanism dysfunction. The American Journal of Sports Medicine 19(2): 131–137

Walton J H 1989 Essentials of neurology, 6th edn. Churchill Livingstone, Edinburgh

White S G, Sahrmann S A 1994 A movement system balance approach to musculoskeletal pain. In: Grant R (ed) Physical therapy of the cervical and thoracic spine, 2nd edn. Churchill Livingstone, Edinburgh, ch 16, p 339

Williams P L, Bannister L H, Berry M M, Collins P, Dyson M, Dussek J E, Ferguson M W J (eds) 1995 Gray's anatomy, 38th edn. Churchill Livingstone, Edinburgh

Yaxley G A, Jull G A 1993 Adverse tension in the neural system. A preliminary study of tennis elbow. Australian Journal of Physiotherapy 39(1): 15–22

Young A, Hughes I, Round J M, Edwards R H T 1982 The effect of knee injury on the number of muscle fibres in the human quadriceps femoris. Clinical Science 62: 227–234

Zusman M 1998 Structure orientated beliefs and disability due to back pain. Australian Journal of Physiotherapy 44: 13–20

Chapter 4

Examination of the temporomandibular region

POSSIBLE CAUSES OF PAIN AND/OR LIMITATION OF MOVEMENT

- Deviation in form
- Articular disc displacement (acute or chronic) with or without reduction
- Hypermobility
- Dislocation
- Degenerative conditions: osteoarthrosis or polyarthritides
- Inflammatory conditions: synovitis or capsulitis
- Ankylosis: fibrous or bony ankylosis
- Masticatory muscle disorders
- Neoplasm: malignant or benign
- Cranial neuralgia
- Referral of symptoms from the upper cervical spine, cervical spine, cranium, eyes, ears, nose, sinuses, teeth, mouth or other facial structures.

Disorders of the temporomandibular joint (TMJ) and overlying muscles can often be associated with symptoms from the upper cervical spine (C0–C3). The upper cervical spine can refer pain to the same areas as the TMJ, i.e. the frontal, retro-orbital, temporal and occipital areas of the head (Feinstein et al 1954). For this reason, it is suggested that examination of the temporomandibular region is always accompanied by examination of the upper cervical spine. The TMJ may also refer pain into the preauricular area or along the mandible. Interested readers may like to read further and a textbook devoted to this region by von Piekartz & Bryden (2001) may prove useful.

Further details of the questions asked during the subjective examination and the tests carried out during the physical examination can be found in Chapters 2 and 3 respectively.

The order of the subjective questioning and the physical tests described below can be altered as appropriate for the patient being examined.

SUBJECTIVE EXAMINATION

Body chart

The following information concerning the area and type of current symptoms can be recorded on a body chart (see Fig. 2.3).

Area of current symptoms

Be exact when mapping out the area of the symptoms. Symptoms can include crepitus, clicking (on opening and/or closing), grating, thudding sounds and joint locking, limitation or difficulty in jaw movement, as well as pain around the joint, head and neck. Ascertain the worst symptom and record the patient's interpretation of where s/he feels the symptoms are coming from.

Areas relevant to the region being examined

All other relevant areas are checked for symptoms; it is important to ask about pain or even stiffness, as this may be relevant to the patient's main symptom. Mark unaffected areas with ticks (✓) on the body chart. There are anatomical (Ayub et al 1984, Darling et al 1987, Rocabado 1983) links between the temporomandibular joint and the cervical spine, particularly the upper cervical spine, and so the clinician should check carefully for any symptoms in the cervical spine. Symptoms in the thoracic spine, head, mouth and teeth should also be checked.

Ask whether the patient has ever experienced any dizziness. This is relevant for symptoms emanating from the cervical spine where vertebrobasilar insufficiency (VBI) may be provoked. If dizziness is a feature described by the patient, the clinician determines what factors aggravate and what factors ease the symptoms, the duration and severity of the dizziness and its relationship with other symptoms such as disturbance in vision, diplopia, nausea, ataxia, 'drop attacks', impairment of trigeminal sensation, sympathoplegia, dysarthria, hemianaesthesia and hemiplegia (Bogduk 1994).

Quality of pain

Establish the quality of the pain.

Intensity of pain

The intensity of pain can be measured using, for example, a visual analogue scale (VAS) as shown in Figure 2.8. A pain diary (see Ch. 2) may be useful for patients with chronic temporomandibular joint or cervical spine pain and/or headaches, to determine the pain patterns and triggering factors over a period of time.

Depth of pain

Establish the depth of the pain. Does the patient feel that it is on the surface or deep inside?

Abnormal sensation

Check for any altered sensation locally over the temporomandibular region and, if appropriate, over the face, cervical spine, upper thoracic spine or upper limbs.

Constant or intermittent symptoms

Ascertain the frequency of the symptoms; whether they are constant or intermittent. If symptoms are constant, check whether there is variation in the intensity of the symptoms, as constant unremitting pain is indicative of neoplastic disease.

Relationship of symptoms

Determine the relationship between the symptomatic areas – do they come together or separately? For example, the patient may have pain over the jaw without neck pain, or they may always be present together.

Behaviour of symptoms

Aggravating factors

For each symptomatic area, discover what movements and/or positions aggravate the patient's symptoms, i.e. what brings them on (or makes them worse), can this position or movement be maintained (severity), what happens to other symptom(s) when this symptom is produced (or is made worse), and how long does it take for symptoms to ease once the position or movement is stopped (irritability). These questions help to confirm the relationship between the symptoms.

The clinician also asks the patient about theoretically known aggravating factors for structures that could be a source of the symptoms. Common aggravating factors for the temporomandibular region are opening the mouth, yawning and chewing more challenging foods such as nuts, meat, raw fruit and vegetables. Aggravating factors for other regions, which may need to be queried if they are suspected to be a source of the symptoms, are shown in Table 2.3.

The clinician ascertains how the symptoms affect function, such as: static and active postures, e.g. sitting, reading, writing (the patient may lean the hand on the jaw to support the head when reading or writing), using the telephone (it may be held between the head and shoulder), eating, drinking, etc. The patient may have a habit of biting fingernails or chewing hair, pen or pencil tops, all of which may stress the temporomandibular region. Sports that might affect the TMJ could be shot putting and snooker. The clinician finds out if the patient is left- or right-handed as there may be increased stress on the dominant side.

Detailed information on each of the above activities is useful in order to help determine the structure(s) at fault and to identify functional restrictions. This information can be used to determine the aims of treatment and any advice that may be required. The most notable functional restrictions are highlighted with asterisks (*), explored in the physical examination, and reassessed at subsequent treatment sessions to evaluate treatment intervention.

Easing factors

For each symptomatic area, the clinician asks what movements and/or positions ease the patient's symptoms, how long it takes to ease them and what happens to other symptoms when this symptom is relieved. These questions help to confirm the relationship between the symptoms.

The clinician asks the patient about theoretically known easing factors for structures that could be a source of the symptoms. For example, symptoms from the TMJ may be eased by placing the joint in a particular position, whereas symptoms from the upper cervical spine may be eased by supporting the head or neck. The clinician can then analyse the position or movement that eases the symptoms, to help determine the structure at fault.

Twenty-four-hour behaviour

The clinician determines the 24-hour behaviour of symptoms by asking questions about night, morning and evening symptoms.

Night symptoms. The following questions may be asked:

- Do you have any difficulty getting to sleep?
- What position is most comfortable/uncomfortable?
- What is your normal sleeping position?
- What is your present sleeping position?
- Do you grind your teeth at night?
- Do your symptom(s) wake you at night? If so,
  - Which symptom(s)?
  - How many times in the past week?
  - How many times in a night?
  - How long does it take to get back to sleep?
- How many and what type of pillows are used?

Morning and evening symptoms. The clinician determines the pattern of the symptoms first thing in the morning, through the day and at the end of the day. Patients who grind their teeth at night may wake up with a headache, and/or facial, jaw or tooth symptoms (Kraus 1994).

Stage of the condition

In order to determine the stage of the condition, the clinician asks whether the symptoms are getting better, getting worse or remaining unchanged.

Special questions

Special questions must always be asked, as they may identify certain precautions or contraindications to the physical examination and/or treatment (see Table 2.4). As mentioned in Chapter 2, the clinician must differentiate between conditions that are suitable for conservative treatment and systemic, neoplastic and other non-neuromusculoskeletal conditions, which require referral to a medical practitioner. Readers are referred to Appendix 2.3 for details of various serious pathological processes that can mimic neuromusculoskeletal conditions (Grieve 1994).

The following information is routinely asked for all patients.

General health.   The clinician ascertains the state of the patient's general health – find out if the patient suffers any malaise, fatigue, fever, nausea or vomiting, stress, anxiety or depression.

Weight loss.   Has the patient noticed any recent unexplained weight loss?

Rheumatoid arthritis.   Has the patient (or a member of his/her family) been diagnosed as having rheumatoid arthritis?

Drug therapy.   Find out what drugs are being taken by the patient. Has the patient ever been prescribed long-term (6 months or more) medication or steroid therapy? Has the patient been taking anticoagulants recently?

X-rays and medical imaging.   Has the patient been X-rayed or had any other medical tests recently? Routine spinal X-rays are no longer considered necessary prior to conservative treatment as they only identify the normal age-related degenerative changes, which do not correlate with the patient's symptoms (Clinical Standards Advisory Report 1994). The medical tests may include blood tests, magnetic resonance imaging, myelography, discography or a bone scan.

Neurological symptoms.   Has the patient experienced symptoms of spinal cord compression, which are bilateral tingling in hands or feet and/or disturbance of gait?

Vertebrobasilar insufficiency (VBI).   For symptoms emanating from the cervical spine, the clinician should ask about symptoms that may be caused by vertebrobasilar insufficiency (VBI). Symptoms include: dizziness (most commonly), altered vision (including diplopia), nausea, ataxia, drop attacks, altered facial sensation, difficulty speaking, difficulty swallowing, sympathoplegia, hemianaesthesia and hemiplegia (Bogduk 1994). If present, the clinician determines in the usual way, the aggravating and easing factors. These symptoms can also be due to upper cervical instability and diseases of the inner ear.

History of the present condition (HPC)

For each symptomatic area, the clinician needs to discover how long the symptom has been present, whether there was a sudden or slow onset and whether there was a known cause that provoked the onset of the symptom, such as trauma, stress, surgery or occupation. If the onset was slow, the clinician should find out if there has been any change in the patient's lifestyle, e.g. a new diet, recent dental treatment or other factors contributing to increased stress felt by the patient. To confirm the relationship between symptoms, the clinician asks what happened to other symptoms when each symptom began.

Past medical history (PMH)

The following information is obtained from the patient and/or dental/medical notes:

- The details of any relevant dental/medical history, particularly involving the teeth, jaw, cranium or cervical spine.
- The history of any previous attacks: how many episodes, when were they, what was the cause, what was the duration of each episode and did the patient fully recover between episodes? If there have been no previous attacks, has the patient had any episodes of stiffness in the TMJ or cervical spine? Check for a history of trauma or recurrent minor trauma.
- Ascertain the results of any past treatment for the same or similar problem. Past treatment records may be obtained for further information.

Social and family history (SH, FH)

Social and family history that is relevant to the onset and progression of the patient's problem is recorded. This includes the patient's perspectives, experience and expectations, their age, employment, home situation, and details of any leisure activities. Factors from this information may indicate direct and/or indirect mechanical influences on the TMJ. In order to treat the patient appropriately, it is important that the condition is managed within the context of the patient's social and work environment. The clinician may ask the following types of questions to elucidate psychosocial factors:

- Have you had time off work in the past with your pain?
- What do you understand to be the cause of your pain?
- What are you expecting will help you?
- How is your employer/co-workers/family responding to your pain?
- What are you doing to cope with your pain?
- Do you think you will return to work? When?

While these questions are described in relation to psychosocial risk factors for poor outcomes for patients with low back pain (Waddell 2004), they may be relevant to other patients.

Plan of the physical examination

When all this information has been collected, the subjective examination is complete. It is useful at this stage to highlight with asterisks (*), for ease of reference, important findings and particularly one or more functional restrictions. These can then be re-examined at subsequent treatment sessions to evaluate treatment intervention.

In order to plan the physical examination, the following hypotheses need to be developed from the subjective examination:

- The regions and structures that need to be examined as a possible cause of the symptoms, e.g. temporomandibular region, upper cervical spine, cervical spine, thoracic spine, muscles and nerves. Often, it is not possible to examine fully at the first attendance and so examination of the structures must be prioritized over subsequent treatment sessions.

- Other factors that need to be examined, e.g. working and everyday postures, vertebral artery, muscle weakness.
- In what way should the physical tests be carried out? Will it be easy or hard to reproduce each symptom? Will combined movements, repetitive movements, etc. need to be used to reproduce the patient's symptoms? Are symptom(s) severe and/or irritable? If symptoms are severe, physical tests may be carried out to just before the onset of symptom production or just to the onset of symptom production; no overpressures should be carried out, as the patient would be unable to tolerate this. If symptoms are irritable, physical tests may be examined to just before symptom production or just to the onset of provocation, with less physical tests being examined to allow for rest periods between tests.
- Are there any precautions and/or contraindications to elements of the physical examination that need to be explored further, such as VBI, neurological involvement, recent fracture, trauma, steroid therapy or rheumatoid arthritis; there may also be certain contraindications to further examination and treatment, e.g. symptoms of cord compression.

A planning form can be useful for clinicians to help guide them through the often complex clinical reasoning process (see Fig. 2.10 and Appendix 2.1).

PHYSICAL EXAMINATION

The information from the subjective examination helps the clinician to plan an appropriate physical examination. The severity, irritability and nature of the condition are the major factors that will influence the choice and priority of physical testing procedures. The first and over-arching question the clinician might ask is: 'is this patient's condition suitable for me to manage as a therapist?' For example, a patient presenting with cauda equina compression symptoms may only need neurological integrity testing, prior to an urgent medical referral. The nature of the patient's condition has had a major impact on the physical examination. The second question the clinician might ask is:'does this patient have a neuromusculoskeletal dysfunction that I may be able to help?' To answer that, the clinician needs to carry out a full physical examination; however, this may not be possible if the symptoms are severe and/or irritable. If the patient's symptoms are severe and/or irritable, the clinician aims to explore movements as much as possible, within a symptom-free range. If the patient has constant and severe and/or irritable symptoms, then the clinician aims to find physical tests that ease the symptoms. If the patient's symptoms are non-severe and non-irritable, then the clinician aims to find physical tests that reproduce each of the patient's symptoms.

Each significant physical test that either provokes or eases the patient's symptoms is highlighted in the patient's notes by an asterisk (*) for easy reference. The highlighted tests are often referred to as 'asterisks' or 'markers'.

The order and detail of the physical tests described below should be appropriate to the patient being examined; some tests will be irrelevant, some tests will be carried out briefly, while others will need to be investigated fully. It is important that readers understand that the techniques shown in this chapter are some of many; the choice depends mainly on the relative sizes of the clinician and patient, as well as the clinician's preference. For this reason, novice clinicians may initially want to copy what is shown, but then quickly adapt to what is best for them.

Observation

Informal observation

The clinician needs to observe the patient in dynamic and static situations; the quality of movement is noted, as are the postural characteristics and facial expression. Informal observation will have begun from the moment the clinician begins the subjective examination and will continue to the end of the physical examination.

Formal observation

Observation of posture. The clinician checks the bony and soft tissue contours of the face and TMJ. The clinician observes the resting position of the mandible (RPM), also known as the upper postural position of the mandible (UPPM). In the

RPM the back teeth are slightly apart, the mandible is in a relaxed position and the tip of the tongue lies against the palate just posterior to the inner surface of the upper central incisors. The clinician checks the intercuspal position (ICP), in which the back teeth are closed together, and observes the patient's teeth for malocclusion such as crossbite (mandibular teeth anterior to maxillary teeth), overbite (maxillary teeth anterior to mandibular teeth) or deviation of the mandible to one side. Check whether bipupital, otic and occlusive lines of the face are parallel (Fig. 4.1). Note whether the distance between the outer corner of the eye and mouth, AB, is equal to the distance from nose to chin, CD (Fig. 4.2); reduction of the latter distance by more than 1 mm indicates loss of teeth, overbite or temporomandibular dysfunction (Magee 1997). Check the wear of any false teeth and the state of the patient's gums.

It is useful to be aware that pure postural dysfunction rarely influences one region of the body in isolation and it will be necessary to examine the patient's posture when sitting and standing, noting the posture of head and neck, thoracic spine and upper limbs. The clinician passively corrects any asymmetry to determine its relevance to the patient's problem.

Observation of muscle form. The muscles of mastication are the masseter, temporalis, medial pterygoid and lateral pterygoid. Only the masseter and temporalis are visible and may be enlarged or atrophied. If there is postural abnormality that is thought to be due to a muscle imbal-

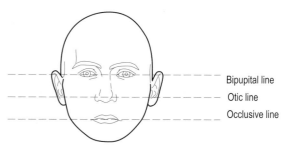

Figure 4.1   Symmetry of the face can be tested comparing the bipupital, otic and occlusive lines, which should be parallel. (From Magee 1997, with permission.)

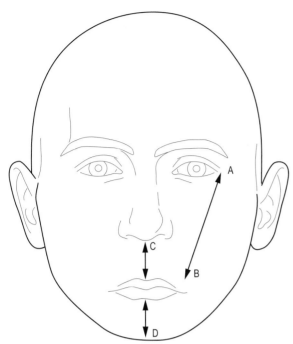

Figure 4.2 Measurement of the vertical dimension of face. Normally the distance AB is equal to CD. (From Trott 1986, with permission.)

ance, then the muscles around the cervical spine and shoulder girdle may need to be inspected. Some of these muscles are thought to shorten under stress, while other muscles weaken, producing muscle imbalance (see Table 3.2). Patterns of muscle imbalance are more fully dealt with in Chapter 3 and also more specifically in Table 6.1.

Observation of soft tissues. The clinician observes the colour of the patient's skin, any swelling over the TMJ, face or gums, and takes cues for further examination.

Observation of the patient's attitudes and feelings. The age, gender and ethnicity of patients and their cultural, occupational and social backgrounds will all affect their attitudes and feelings towards themselves, their condition and the clinician. The clinician needs to be aware of and sensitive to these attitudes, and empathize and communicate appropriately so as to develop a rapport with the patient and thereby enhance the patient's compliance with the treatment.

Active physiological movements

For active passive physiological movements, the clinician notes the following:

- The quality of movement: deviation, minor subluxation, crepitus or a click on opening and/or closing the mouth
- The range of movement; excessive range, particularly opening, may indicate hypermobility of the TMJ
- The behaviour of pain through the range
- The resistance through the range of movement and at the end of the range of movement
- Any provocation of muscle spasm.

A movement diagram can be used to depict this information. The active movements with overpressure listed below are shown in Figure 4.3 and can be tested with the patient sitting or lying supine. The clinician establishes the patient's symptoms at rest and prior to each movement, and corrects any movement deviation to determine its relevance to the patient's symptoms. Palpation of the movement of the condyles during active movements can be useful in feeling the quality of the movement. Excessive anterior movement of the lateral pole of the mandible may indicate TMJ hypermobility. During mouth opening, a small indent can normally be palpated posterior to the lateral pole. A large indentation may indicate hypermobility of the TMJ. If unilateral hypermobility is present, the mandible deviates towards the contralateral side of the hypermobile joint at the end of opening. Auscultation of the joint during jaw movements enables the clinician to listen to any joint sounds. The range of movement can be measured using a ruler.

Movements of the TMJ and the possible modifications are given in Table 4.1. Various differentiation tests (Maitland 1991) can be performed; the choice depends on the patient's signs and symptoms. For example, when cervical flexion reproduces the patient's TMJ pain in sitting, the addition of slump sitting (see Fig. 3.33) or knee extension may help to differentiate the structures at fault. Slump sitting or knee extension, for example, may increase symptoms if there is a neurodynamic component to the patient's symptoms.

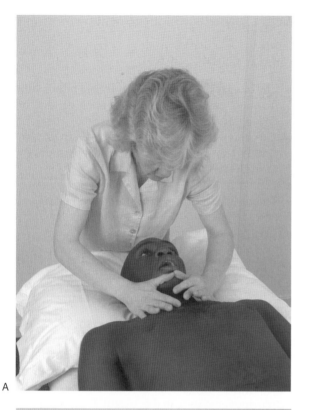

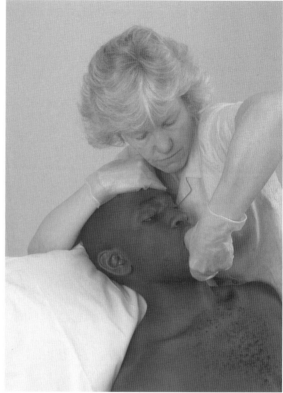

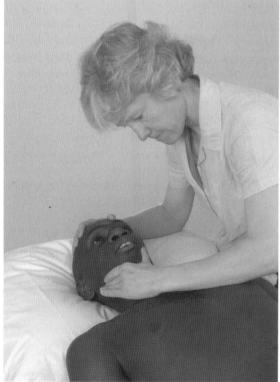

Figure 4.3 Overpressures to the TMJ. **A** Depression (opening) and elevation (closing). The fingers and thumbs of both hands gently grasp the mandible to depress and elevate the mandible. **B** Protraction and retraction. A gloved thumb is placed just inside the mouth on the posterior aspect of the bottom front teeth. Thumb pressure can then protract and retract the mandible. **C** Lateral deviation. The left hand stabilizes the head while the right hand cups around the mandible and moves the mandible to the left and right.

Table 4.1   Summary of active movements and their possible modification

Active movements	Modifications to active movements
TMJ	Repeated
Depression (opening)	Speed altered
Elevation (closing)	Combined, e.g.
Protraction	– opening then lateral
Retraction	deviation
Depression in retracted	– lateral deviation then
position	opening
Left lateral deviation	– protraction then opening
Right lateral deviation	– retraction then opening
?Upper cervical spine	Sustained
movements	Injuring movement
?Cervical spine movement	Differentiation tests
?Thoracic spine movements	Functional ability

Table 4.2   Joint clearing tests

Joint	Physiological movement	Accessory movement
Cervical spine	Quadrants (flexion and extension)	All movements
Thoracic spine	Rotation and quadrants (flexion and extension)	All movements
Temporomandibular joint	Open/close jaw, side to side movement, protraction/ retraction	All movements

Other regions may need to be examined to determine their relevance to the patient's symptoms; they may be the source of the symptoms, or they may be contributing to the symptoms. The regions most likely are the upper cervical spine, cervical spine and thoracic spine. The joints within these regions can be tested fully (see relevant chapter) or partially with the use of clearing tests (Table 4.2).

Some functional ability has already been tested by the general observation of jaw movement as the patient has talked during the subjective examination. Any further testing can be carried out at this point in the examination and may include sitting and sleeping postures, using the telephone, brushing teeth, etc. Clues for appropriate tests can be obtained from the subjective examination findings, particularly the aggravating factors.

Capsular pattern.   The capsular pattern for the TMJ is restriction in opening the mouth (Cyriax 1982).

Passive physiological movements

The clinician can move the TMJ passively with the patient in the supine position. A comparison of the response of symptoms to the active and passive movements can help to determine whether the structure at fault is non-contractile (articular) or contractile (extra-articular) (Cyriax 1982). If the lesion is non-contractile, such as ligament, then active and passive movements will be painful and/or restricted in the same direction. If the lesion is in a contractile tissue (i.e. muscle) then active and passive movements are painful and/or restricted in opposite directions.

Other regions may need to be examined to determine their relevance to the patient's symptoms; they may be the source of the symptoms, or they may be contributing to the symptoms. The regions most likely are the upper cervical spine, cervical spine and thoracic spine.

Muscle tests

Muscle tests include examining muscle strength, control and isometric contraction.

Muscle strength

The clinician may test muscle groups that depress, elevate, protract, retract and laterally deviate the mandible and, if applicable, the cervical flexors, extensors, lateral flexors and rotators. For details of these general tests, readers are directed to Cole et al (1988), Hislop & Montgomery (1995) or Kendall et al (1993). Kraus (1994), however, considers mandibular muscle weakness to be rare in TMJ disorders and difficult to determine manually. Janda (1994) considers that suprahyoid and mylohyoid muscles have a tendency to weaken.

Muscle control

Excessive masticatory muscle activity is thought to be a factor in TMJ conditions. Muscle hyperactivity alters the normal sequence of swallowing because of an altered position of the tongue, which is thrust forward in the mouth (tongue thrust). The clinician can determine muscle hyperactivity indirectly by palpating the hyoid bone and suboccipital muscles (Fig. 4.4) as the patient swallows some water (Kraus 1994). A slow and upward movement of the hyoid bone, as opposed to the normal quick up and down movement, and contraction of the suboccipital muscles, suggest a tongue thrust and indicate hyperactivity of the masticatory muscles.

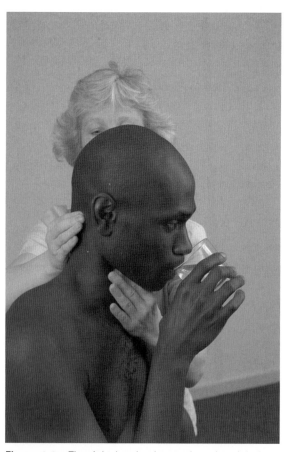

Figure 4.4   The right hand palpates the suboccipital muscles and the left hand palpates the hyoid bone as the patient swallows some water.

Testing the muscles of the cervical spine and shoulder girdle may be relevant for some patients and is described in Chapter 6.

Isometric muscle testing

Test the muscle groups that depress, elevate, protract, retract and laterally deviate the mandible in the resting position and, if indicated, in various parts of the physiological ranges. Also, if applicable, test the cervical flexors, extensors, lateral flexors and rotators. In addition the clinician observes the quality of the muscle contraction necessary to hold this position (this can be done with the patient's eyes shut). The patient may, for example, be unable to prevent the joint from moving or may hold with excessive muscle activity; either of these circumstances would suggest a neuromuscular dysfunction.

Neurological tests

Neurological examination includes neurological integrity testing, neurodynamic tests and some other nerve tests.

Integrity of nervous system

Generally, if symptoms are localized to the upper cervical spine and head, neurological examination can be limited to cranial nerves and C1–C4 nerve roots.

Dermatomes/peripheral nerves.   Light touch and pain sensation of the face, head and neck are tested using cotton wool and pinprick respectively, as described in Chapter 3. Knowledge of the cutaneous distribution of nerve roots (dermatomes) and peripheral nerves enables the clinician to distinguish the sensory loss due to a root lesion from that due to a peripheral nerve lesion. The cutaneous nerve distribution and dermatome areas are shown in Figure 3.18.

Myotomes/peripheral nerves.   The following myotomes are tested and are shown in Figure 3.26:

- Root–joint action
- V cranial (trigeminal N): clench teeth, note temporalis and masseter muscles

- VII cranial (facial N): wrinkle forehead, close eyes, purse lips, show teeth
- XI cranial (accessory N): sternocleidomastoid and shoulder girdle elevation
- C1–C2: upper cervical flexion
- C2: upper cervical extension
- C3: cervical lateral flexion
- C4 and XI cranial nerve: shoulder girdle elevation.

A working knowledge of the muscular distribution of nerve roots (myotomes) and peripheral nerves enables the clinician to distinguish the motor loss due to a root lesion from that due to a peripheral nerve lesion.

Reflex testing. There are no deep tendon reflexes for C1–C4 nerve roots. The jaw jerk (Vth cranial nerve) is elicited by applying a sharp downward tap on the chin with the mouth slightly open. A slight jerk is normal, excessive jerk suggests bilateral upper motor neurone lesion.

Neurodynamic tests

The following neurodynamic tests may be carried out in order to ascertain the degree to which neural tissue is responsible for the production of the patient's symptom(s):

- Passive neck flexion (PNF)
- Upper limb tension tests (ULTT)
- Straight leg raise (SLR)
- Slump.

These tests are described in detail in Chapter 3.

Other nerve tests

Chvostek test for facial nerve palsy. To carry out this test, the clinician taps the parotid gland over the masseter muscle; twitching of the facial muscles indicates facial nerve palsy (Magee 1997).

Plantar response to test for an upper motor neurone lesion (Walton 1989). Pressure applied from the heel along the lateral border of the plantar aspect of the foot produces flexion of the toes in the normal. Extension of the big toe with downward fanning of the other toes occurs with an upper motor neurone lesion.

Miscellaneous tests

In the case of the TMJ, these are vascular tests, as follows:

- Vertebral artery test (Sheehy et al 1990). This is described in detail in Chapter 5 on the examination of the upper cervical spine.
- If the circulation is suspected of being compromised, the clinician palpates the pulses of the carotid, facial and temporal arteries.

Palpation

The TMJ and the upper cervical spine (see Ch. 5 for details) are palpated. It is useful to record palpation findings on a body chart (see Fig. 2.3) and/or palpation chart (see Fig. 3.38).

The clinician should make a note of the following:

- The temperature of the area
- Localized increased skin moisture
- The presence of oedema or effusion
- Mobility and feel of superficial tissues, e.g. ganglions, nodules, thickening of deep suboccipital tissues
- Position and prominence of the mandible and TMJ
- The presence or elicitation of any muscle spasm
- Tenderness of bone, ligament, muscle (masseter, temporalis, medial and lateral pterygoids, splenius capitis, suboccipital muscles, trapezius, sternocleidomastoid, digastric), tendon, tendon sheath and nerve. Check for tenderness of the hyoid bone and thyroid cartilage. Test for the relevant trigger points shown in Figure 3.39
- Symptoms (often pain) provoked or reduced on palpation.

Accessory movements

It is useful to use the palpation chart and movement diagrams (or joint pictures) to record findings. These are explained in detail in Chapter 3.

The clinician should make a note of the following:

- Quality of movement
- Range of movement

- Resistance through the range and at the end of the range of movement
- Behaviour of pain through the range
- Provocation of any muscle spasm.

Temporomandibular joint

Dynamic loading and distraction. The clinician places a cotton roll between the upper and lower third molars on one side only and the patient is asked to bite on to the roll noting any pain produced. Pain may be felt on the left or right TMJ as there will be distraction of the TMJ on the side of the cotton roll and compression of the TMJ on the contralateral side (Hylander 1979). Pain on the side of the cotton roll is indicative of capsulitis (Kraus 1993).

Passive loading (retrusive overpressure). The patient is asked to hold the back teeth slightly apart. The clinician holds onto the chin with the thumb and index finger with one hand, and with the other hand supports the head to provide a counterforce. The clinician then applies a postero-superior force on the mandible centrally and then with some lateral inclination to the right and left. This test can be positive, reproducing the patient's pain, in both capsulitis and synovitis (Kraus 1993).

The temporomandibular joint accessory movements are shown in Figure 4.5 (Maitland 1991) and are listed with possible modifications in Table 4.3.

Following accessory movements to the TMJ, the clinician reassesses all the physical asterisks (movements or tests that have been found to reproduce the patient's symptoms) in order to establish the effect of the accessory movements on the patient's signs and symptoms. Accessory movements can then be tested for other regions suspected to be a source of the symptoms. Again, following accessory movements the clinician reassesses all the physical asterisks. Regions likely to be examined are the upper cervical spine, cervical spine and thoracic spine (Table 4.3).

COMPLETION OF THE EXAMINATION

Having carried out the above tests, the examination of the temporomandibular region is now complete. The subjective and physical examinations produce a large amount of information, which needs to be recorded accurately and quickly. An outline examination chart may be useful for some clinicians and one is suggested in Figure 4.6. It is important, however, that the clinician does not examine in a rigid manner, simply following the suggested sequence outlined in the chart. Each patient presents differently and this needs to be reflected in the examination process. It is vital at this stage to highlight with an asterisk (*) important findings from the examination. These findings must be reassessed at, and within, subsequent treatment sessions to evaluate the effects of treatment on the patient's condition.

Table 4.3 Accessory movements, choice of application and reassessment of the patient's asterisks

Accessory movements	Choice of application	Identify any effect of accessory movements on patient's signs and symptoms
TMJ: ↕ anteroposterior ↕ posteroanterior →• Med medial transverse →• Lat lateral transverse ←•→ Caud longitudinal caudad ←•→ Ceph longitudinal cephalad	Start position, e.g. with the mandible depressed, elevated, protracted, retracted, laterally deviated, or a combination of these positions • Speed of force application • Direction of the applied force • Point of application of applied force	Reassess all asterisks
?Upper cervical spine	As above	Reassess all asterisks
?Cervical spine	As above	Reassess all asterisks
?Thoracic spine		Reassess all asterisks

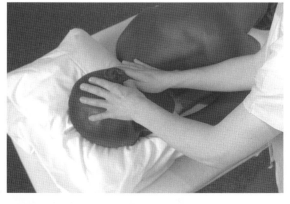

A

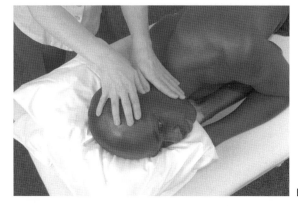

B

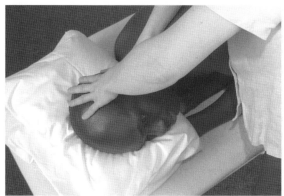

C

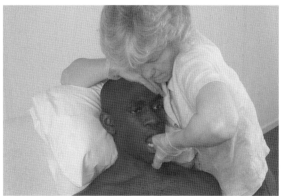

D

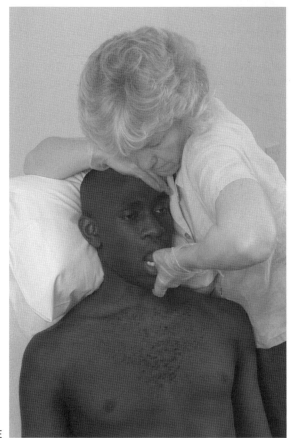

E

Figure 4.5 Accessory movements to the TMJ.
A Anteroposterior. With the patient in side lie, thumbs apply an anteroposterior pressure to the anterior aspect of the head of the mandible.
B Posteroanterior. With the patient in side lie, thumbs apply a posteroanterior pressure to the posterior aspect of the head of the mandible.
C Medial transverse. With the patient in side lie, thumbs apply a medial pressure to the lateral aspect of the head of the mandible.
D Lateral transverse. The patient is supported in sitting. The one hand supports the head while the gloved hand is placed inside the mouth so that the thumb rests along the medial surface of the mandible. Thumb pressure can then produce a lateral glide of the mandible.
E Longitudinal cephalad and caudad. With the patient sitting and the one hand supporting the head, the gloved hand is placed inside the mouth so that the thumb rests on the top of the lower back teeth. The thumb and outer fingers then grip the mandible and apply a downward pressure (longitudinal caudad) and an upward pressure (longitudinal cephalad).

Body chart	Name
	Age
	Date
	24-hour behaviour
	Improving static worsening
	Special questions General health Weight loss RA Drugs Steroids Anticoagulants X-ray Cord symptoms Cauda equina symptoms VBI symptoms
Relationship of symptoms	
Aggravating factors and function	HPC
	PMH
Severe Irritable	
Easing factors	SH & FH (Patient's perspective, experience, expectations. Yellow, blue, black flags)

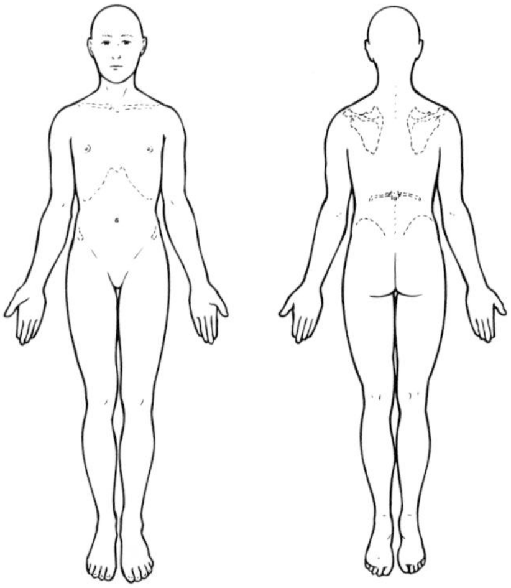

Figure 4.6   Temporomandibular joint examination chart.

| Physical examination

Observation	Isometric muscle testing
Active and passive physiological movements of TMJ and other relevant regions	Neurological integrity tests
	Neurodynamic tests
	Other nerve tests (Chvostek test)
	Miscellaneous tests (VBI testing, pulses)
Capsular pattern yes/no	
Muscle strength	Palpation
	Accessory movements and reassessment of each relevant region
Muscle control (swallowing)	

Figure 4.6 *Continued*

The physical testing procedures which specifically indicate joint, nerve or muscle tissues, as a source of the patient's symptoms, are summarized in Table 3.10. The strongest evidence that a joint is the source of the patient's symptoms is that active and passive physiological movements, passive accessory movements and joint palpation all reproduce the patient's symptoms, and that following a treatment dose, reassessment identifies an improvement in the patient's signs and symptoms. Weaker evidence includes an alteration in range, resistance or quality of physiological and/or accessory movements and tenderness over the joint, with no alteration in signs and symptoms after treatment. One or more of these findings may indicate a dysfunction of a joint which may or may not be contributing to the patient's condition.

The strongest evidence that a muscle is the source of a patient's symptoms is if active movements, an isometric contraction, passive lengthening and palpation of a muscle all reproduce the patient's symptoms, and that following a treatment dose, reassessment identifies an improvement in the patient's signs and symptoms. Further evidence of muscle dysfunction may be suggested by reduced strength or poor quality during the active physiological movement and the isometric contraction, reduced range, and/or increased/decreased resistance, during the passive lengthening of the muscle, and tenderness on palpation, with no alteration in signs and symptoms after treatment. One or more of these findings may indicate a dysfunction of a muscle which may, or may not, be contributing to the patient's condition.

The strongest evidence that a nerve is the source of the patient's symptoms is when active and/or passive physiological movements reproduce the patient's symptoms, which are then increased or decreased with an additional sensitizing movement, at a distance from the patient's symptoms. In addition, there is reproduction of the patient's symptoms on palpation of the nerve and following neurodynamic testing, sufficient to be considered a treatment dose, results in an improvement in the above signs and symptoms. Further evidence of nerve dysfunction may be suggested by reduced range (compared to the asymptomatic side) and/or increased resistance to the various arm movements, and tenderness on nerve palpation.

On completion of the physical examination the clinician:

- Warns the patient of possible exacerbation up to 24–48 hours following the examination.
- Requests the patient to report details on the behaviour of the symptoms following examination at the next attendance.
- Explains the findings of the physical examination and how these findings relate to the subjective assessment. It will be helpful to the patient, to clear up any misconceptions they may have regarding their illness or injury.
- Evaluates the findings, formulates a clinical diagnosis and writes up a problem list. Clinicians may find the management planning forms shown in Figures 3.53 and 3.54 helpful in guiding them through what is often a complex clinical reasoning process.
- Determines the objectives of treatment.
- Devises an initial treatment plan.

In this way, the clinician will have developed the following hypotheses categories (adapted from Jones & Rivett 2004):

- Function: abilities and restrictions.
- Patients' perspectives on their experience.
- Source of symptoms. This includes the structure or tissue that is thought to be producing the patients' symptoms, the nature of the structure or tissues in relation to the healing process, and the pain mechanisms.
- Contributing factors to the development and maintenance of the problem. There may be environmental, psychosocial, behavioural, physical or heredity factors.
- Precautions/contraindications to treatment and management. This includes the severity and irritability of the patient's symptoms and the nature of the patient's condition.
- Management strategy and treatment plan.
- Prognosis – this can be affected by factors such as the stage and extent of the injury as well as the patient's expectation, personality and lifestyle.

References

Ayub E, Glasheen-Wray M, Kraus S 1984 Head posture: a case study of the effects on the rest position of the mandible. Journal of Orthopaedic and Sports Physical Therapy 5(4): 179–183

Bogduk N 1994 Cervical causes of headache and dizziness. In: Boyling J D, Palastanga N (eds) Grieve's modern manual therapy, 2nd edn. Churchill Livingstone, Edinburgh, ch 22, p 317

Clinical Standards Advisory Report 1994 Report of a CSAG committee on back pain. HMSO, London

Cole J H, Furness A L, Twomey L T 1988 Muscles in action: an approach to manual muscle testing. Churchill Livingstone, Edinburgh

Cyriax J 1982 Textbook of orthopaedic medicine – diagnosis of soft tissue lesions, 8th edn. Baillière Tindall, London

Darling D W, Kraus S, Glasheen-Wray M B 1987 Relationship of head posture and the rest position of the mandible. Tenth International Congress of the World Confederation for Physical Therapy: 203–206

Feinstein B, Langton J N K, Jameson R M, Schiller F 1954 Experiments on pain referred from deep somatic tissues. Journal of Bone and Joint Surgery 36A(5): 981–997

Grieve G P 1994 Counterfeit clinical presentations. Manipulative Physiotherapist 26: 17–19

Hislop H, Montgomery J 1995 Daniels and Worthingham's muscle testing, techniques of manual examination, 7th edn. W B Saunders, Philadelphia

Hylander W L 1979 An experimental analysis of temporomandibular joint reaction forces in macaques. American Journal of Physical Anthropology 51: 433

Janda V 1994 Muscles and motor control in cervicogenic disorders: assessment and management. In: Grant R (ed) Physical therapy of the cervical and thoracic spine, 2nd edn. Churchill Livingstone, Edinburgh, ch 10, p 195

Jones M A, Rivett D A 2004 Clinical reasoning for manual therapists. Butterworth-Heinemann, Edinburgh

Kendall F P, McCreary E K, Provance P G 1993 Muscles testing and function, 4th edn. Williams & Wilkins, Baltimore, MD

Kraus S 1993 Evaluation and management of temporomandibular disorders. In: Saunders H D, Saunders R (eds) Evaluation, treatment and prevention of musculoskeletal disorders, vol 1. Saunders, Minneapolis, MN

Kraus S L 1994 Physical therapy management of TMD. In: Kraus S L (ed) Temporomandibular disorders, 2nd edn. Churchill Livingstone, Edinburgh

Magee D J 1997 Orthopedic physical assessment, 3rd edn. W B Saunders, Philadelphia

Maitland G D 1991 Peripheral manipulation, 3rd edn. Butterworths, London

Rocabado M 1983 Biomechanical relationship of the cranial, cervical and hyoid regions. Journal of Craniomandibular Practice 1(3): 62–66

Sheehy K, Middleditch A, Wickham S 1990 Vertebral artery testing in the cervical spine. Manipulative Physiotherapist 22(2): 15–18

Trott P H 1986 Examination of the temporomandibular joint. In: Grieve G P (ed) Modern manual therapy of the vertebral column. Churchill Livingstone, Edinburgh, ch 48, p 521

von Piekartz H, Bryden L 2001 Craniofacial dysfunction and pain, manual therapy, assessment and management. Butterworth-Heinemann, Oxford

Waddell G 2004 The back pain revolution, 2nd edn. Churchill Livingstone, Edinburgh

Walton J H 1989 Essentials of neurology, 6th edn. Churchill Livingstone, Edinburgh

Chapter 5

Examination of the upper cervical spine

POSSIBLE CAUSES OF PAIN AND/OR LIMITATION OF MOVEMENT

The upper cervical spine is defined here as the occiput and upper three cervical vertebrae (C1–C3) with their surrounding soft tissues.

- Trauma
  - Whiplash
  - Fracture of vertebral body, spinous or transverse process
  - Ligamentous sprain
  - Muscular strain
- Degenerative conditions
  - Spondylosis: degeneration of C2–C3 intervertebral disc
  - Arthrosis: degeneration of zygapophyseal joints
- Inflammatory conditions
  - Rheumatoid arthritis
  - Ankylosing spondylitis
- Neoplasm
- Infection
- Headache due to (Headache Classification Committee of the International Headache Society 1988)
  - Migraine
  - Tension-type headache
  - Cluster headache
  - Miscellaneous headaches unassociated with structural lesion, e.g. cold stimulus headache, cough or exertional headache
  - Headache associated with head trauma
  - Headache associated with vascular disorders, e.g. transient ischaemic attack, intracra-

nial haematoma, subarachnoid headache, arterial hypertension, carotid or vertebral artery pain
- Headache associated with non-vascular disorders, e.g. high or low cerebrospinal fluid pressure, intracranial infection or neoplasm
- Headache associated with substances or their withdrawal, e.g. monosodium glutamate, alcohol, analgesic abuse, caffeine, narcotics
- Headache associated with non-cephalic infection, e.g. bacterial or viral infection
- Headache associated with metabolic disorder, e.g. hypoxia, hypercapnia, sleep apnoea, hypoglycaemia
- Headache or facial pain associated with disorder of cranium, neck, eyes, ears, nose, sinuses, teeth, mouth or other facial or cranial structures, e.g. cervical spine, glaucoma of the eyes, acute sinus headache, temporomandibular joint disease. For further information on the physiotherapy management of headaches, readers are referred to a text by Edeling (1994)
- Cranial neuralgias, nerve trunk pain and deafferentation pain, e.g. diabetic neuritis, neck-tongue syndrome, herpes zoster, trigeminal neuralgia, occipital neuralgia
- Headache not classifiable.

Further details of the questions asked during the subjective examination and the tests carried out in the physical examination can be found in Chapters 2 and 3 respectively.

The order of the subjective questioning and the physical tests described below can be altered as appropriate for the patient being examined.

SUBJECTIVE EXAMINATION

Body chart

The following information concerning the area and type of current symptoms can be recorded on a body chart (see Fig. 2.3).

Area of current symptoms

Be exact when mapping out the area of the symptoms. Typically, patients with upper cervical spine disorders have neck pain high up around the occiput and pain over the head and/or face. Ascertain the worst symptom and record where the patient feels the symptoms are coming from.

Areas relevant to the region being examined

All other relevant areas are checked for symptoms; it is important to ask about pain or even stiffness, as this may be relevant to the patient's main symptom. Mark unaffected areas with ticks (✓) on the body chart. Check for symptoms in the lower cervical spine, thoracic spine, head and temporomandibular joint and if the patient has ever experienced any dizziness. This is relevant for symptoms emanating from the cervical spine where vertebrobasilar insufficiency (VBI) may be provoked. If dizziness is a feature described by the patient, the clinician determines what factors aggravate and what factors ease the symptoms, the duration and severity of the dizziness and its relationship with other symptoms such as disturbance in vision, diplopia, nausea, ataxia, 'drop attacks', impairment of trigeminal sensation, sympathoplegia, dysarthria, hemianaesthesia and hemiplegia (Bogduk 1994). In addition, the vertebral artery tests must be carried out in the physical examination (see below).

Quality of pain

Establish the quality of the pain. Headaches of cervical origin are often described as throbbing or as a pressure sensation. If the patient suffers from headaches, find out if there is any associated blurred vision, loss of balance, tinnitus, auditory disturbance, swelling and stiffness of the fingers, tendinitis and capsulitis, which could be due to irritation of the sympathetic plexus surrounding the vertebral artery or to irritation of the spinal nerve (Jackson 1966). Patients who have suffered a hyperextension injury to the cervical spine may complain of a sore throat, difficulty in swallowing and a feeling of something stuck in their throat resulting from an associated injury to the oesophagus (Dahlberg et al 1997).

Intensity of pain

The intensity of pain can also be measured using, for example, a visual analogue scale (VAS) as shown in Figure 2.8. A pain diary may be useful for patients with chronic neck pain or headaches, in order to determine the pain patterns and triggering factors, which may be unusual or complex.

Depth of pain

Establish the depth of the pain. Does the patient feel it is on the surface or deep inside?

Abnormal sensation

Check for any altered sensation locally over the cervical spine and head, as well as the face and upper limbs. Common abnormalities are paraesthesia and numbness.

Constant or intermittent symptoms

Ascertain the frequency of the symptoms, and whether they are constant or intermittent. If symptoms are constant, check whether there is variation in the intensity of the symptoms, as constant unremitting pain may be indicative of neoplastic disease. Headaches may change in frequency from one a month, to once a week, to daily (Edeling 1994).

Relationship of symptoms

Determine the relationship between the symptomatic areas – do they come together or separately? For example, the patient could have a headache without the cervical pain, or they may always be present together.

Behaviour of symptoms

Aggravating factors

For each symptomatic area, discover what movements and/or positions aggravate the patient's symptoms, i.e. what brings them on (or makes them worse), are they able to maintain this position or movement (severity), what happens to other symptom(s) when this symptom is produced (or is made worse), and how long does it take for symptoms to ease once the position or movement is stopped (irritability). These questions help to confirm the relationship between the symptoms.

The clinician also asks the patient about theoretically known aggravating factors for structures that could be a source of the symptoms. Common aggravating factors for the upper cervical spine are sustained cervical postures and movements. Headaches can be brought on with eye strain, noise, excessive eating, drinking, smoking, stress or inadequate ventilation. Aggravating factors for other regions, which may need to be queried if they are suspected to be a source of the symptoms, are shown in Table 2.3.

The clinician ascertains how the symptoms affect function, such as: static and active postures, e.g. sitting, standing, lying, washing, ironing, dusting, driving, reading, writing, work, sport and social activities. Note details of training regimen for any sports activities. The clinician finds out if the patient is left- or right-handed as there may be increased stress on the dominant side.

Detailed information on each of the above activities is useful in order to help determine the structure(s) at fault and identify functional restrictions. This information can be used to determine the aims of treatment and any advice that may be required. The most notable functional restrictions are highlighted with asterisks (*), explored in the physical examination, and reassessed at subsequent treatment sessions to evaluate treatment intervention.

Easing factors

For each symptomatic area, the clinician asks what movements and/or positions ease the patient's symptoms, how long it takes to ease them and what happens to other symptom(s) when this symptom is relieved. These questions help to confirm the relationship between the symptoms.

The clinician asks the patient about theoretically known easing factors for structures that could be a source of the symptoms. For example, symptoms from the upper cervical spine may be eased by supporting the head or neck. The clinician can analyse the position or movement that eases the symptoms, in order to help determine the structure at fault.

Twenty-four-hour behaviour of symptoms

The clinician determines the 24-hour behaviour of the symptoms by asking questions about night, morning and evening symptoms.

Night symptoms. The following questions may be asked:

- Do you have any difficulty getting to sleep?
- What position is most comfortable/uncomfortable?
- What is your normal sleeping position?
- What is your present sleeping position?
- Do your symptom(s) wake you at night? If so,
  - Which symptom(s)?
  - How many times in the past week?
  - How many times in a night?
  - How long does it take to get back to sleep?
- How many and what type of pillows are used? Is the mattress firm or soft?

Morning and evening symptoms. The clinician determines the pattern of the symptoms first thing in the morning, through the day and at the end of the day. Stiffness in the morning for the first few minutes might suggest cervical spondylosis; stiffness and pain for a few hours is suggestive of an inflammatory process such as rheumatoid arthritis.

Stage of the condition

In order to determine the stage of the condition, the clinician asks whether the symptoms are getting better, getting worse or remaining unchanged.

Special questions

Special questions must always be asked, as they may identify certain precautions or contraindications to the physical examination and/or treatment (see Table 2.4). As mentioned in Chapter 2, the clinician must differentiate between conditions that are suitable for conservative management and systemic, neoplastic and other non-neuromusculoskeletal conditions, which require referral to a medical practitioner. The reader is referred to Appendix 2.3 for details of various serious pathological processes that can mimic neuromusculoskeletal conditions (Grieve 1994).

The following information is routinely obtained from patients:

General health. The clinician ascertains the state of the patient's general health – find out if the patient suffers any malaise, fatigue, fever, epilepsy, diabetes, nausea or vomiting, stress, anxiety or depression.

Weight loss. Has the patient noticed any recent unexplained weight loss?

Rheumatoid arthritis. Has the patient (or a member of his/her family) been diagnosed as having rheumatoid arthritis?

Drug therapy. Find out what drugs are being taken by the patient. Has the patient ever been prescribed long-term (6 months or more) medication or steroid therapy? Has the patient been taking anticoagulants recently?

X-rays and medical imaging. Has the patient been X-rayed or had any other medical tests recently? Routine spinal X-rays are no longer considered necessary prior to conservative treatment as they only identify the normal age-related degenerative changes, which do not necessarily correlate with the patient's symptoms (Clinical Standards Advisory Report 1994). The medical tests may include blood tests, magnetic resonance imaging, myelography, discography or a bone scan.

Neurological symptoms. Has the patient experienced symptoms of spinal cord compression, which are bilateral tingling in the hands or feet and/or disturbance of gait?

Vertebrobasilar insufficiency (VBI). For symptoms emanating from the cervical spine, the clinician needs to ask about symptoms that may be caused by vertebrobasilar insufficiency. VBI symptoms include dizziness (most commonly), altered vision (including diplopia), nausea, ataxia, drop attacks, altered facial sensation, difficulty speaking, difficulty swallowing, sympathoplegia, hemianaesthesia and hemiplegia (Bogduk 1994). If present, the clinician determines in the usual way, the aggravating and easing factors. These symptoms can also be due to upper cervical instability and diseases of the inner ear. Risk factors associated with VBI are given in Box 5.1 (Barker et al

---

Box 5.1   Risk factors for symptoms related to vertebrobasilar insufficiency (Barker et al 2000)

- Drop attacks, blackouts, loss of consciousness
- Nausea, vomiting and general unwell feelings
- Dizziness or vertigo, particularly if associated with head positioning
- Disturbances of vision (e.g. decreased, blurred, diplopia)
- Unsteadiness of gait (ataxia) and general feeling of weakness
- Tingling or numbness (especially dysaesthesia, i.e. tingling around the lips, hemianaesthesia or any alteration in facial sensation)
- Difficulty in speaking (dysarthria) or swallowing
- Hearing disturbance (e.g. tinnitus, deafness)
- Headache
- Past history of trauma
- Cardiac disease, vascular disease, altered blood pressure, previous cerebrovascular accident or transient ischaemic attacks
- Blood clotting disorders
- Anticoagulant therapy
- Oral contraceptives
- Long-term use of steroids
- A history of smoking
- Immediately post partum

2000) and include some further screening questions that the clinician may need to ask some patients, particularly prior to treatment with a cervical manipulation.

History of the present condition (HPC)

For each symptomatic area the clinician needs to discover how long the symptom has been present, whether there was a sudden or slow onset and whether there was a known cause that provoked the onset of the symptom. If the patient complains of headaches, the clinician needs to find out whether there have been any factors that precipitated the onset, such as trauma, stress, surgery or occupation. If the onset was slow, the clinician finds out if there has been any change in the patient's lifestyle, e.g. a new job or hobby or a change in sporting activity. There may be an increased mechanical stress on the cervical spine or an increase in the patient's stress levels, which might explain the increase in the patient's symptoms. To confirm the relationship between the symptoms, the clinician asks what happened to other symptoms when each symptom began.

Past medical history (PMH)

The following information is obtained from the patient and/or medical notes:

- The details of any relevant medical history involving the cervical spine and related areas.
- The history of any previous attacks: how many episodes, when were they, what was the cause, what was the duration of each episode and did the patient fully recover between episodes? If there have been no previous attacks, has the patient had any episodes of stiffness in the cervical spine, thoracic spine or any other relevant region? Check for a history of trauma or recurrent minor trauma.
- Ascertain the results of any past treatment for the same or similar problem. Past treatment records may be obtained for further information.

Social and family history (SH, FH)

Social and family history that is relevant to the onset and progression of the patient's problem should be recorded. This includes the patient's perspectives, experience and expectations, their age, employment, home situation, and details of any leisure activities. Factors from this information may indicate direct and/or indirect mechanical influences on the cervical spine. In order to treat the patient appropriately, it is important that the condition is managed within the context of the patient's social and work environment.

The clinician may ask the following types of questions to elucidate psychosocial factors:

- Have you had time off work in the past with your pain?
- What do you understand to be the cause of your pain?
- What are you expecting will help you?

- How is your employer/co-workers/family responding to your pain?
- What are you doing to cope with your pain?
- Do you think you will return to work? When?

While these questions are described in relation to psychosocial risk factors for poor outcomes for patients with low back pain (Waddell 2004), they may be relevant to other patients.

Plan of the physical examination

When all this information has been collected, the subjective examination is complete. It is useful at this stage to highlight with asterisks (*), for ease of reference, important findings and particularly one or more functional restrictions. These can then be re-examined at subsequent treatment sessions to evaluate treatment intervention.

In order to plan the physical examination, the following hypotheses need to be developed from the subjective examination:

- The regions and structures that need to be examined as a possible cause of the symptoms, e.g. temporomandibular region, upper cervical spine, cervical spine, thoracic spine, muscles and nerves. Often it is not possible to examine fully at the first attendance and so examination of the structures must be prioritized over subsequent treatment sessions.
- Other factors that need to be examined, e.g. working and everyday postures, vertebral artery, muscle weakness.
- In what way should the physical tests be carried out? Will it be easy or hard to reproduce each symptom? Will combined movements, repetitive movements, etc. be necessary to reproduce the patient's symptoms? Are symptom(s) severe and/or irritable? If symptoms are severe, physical tests may be carried out to just before the onset of symptom production or just to the onset of symptom production; no overpressures will be carried out, as the patient would be unable to tolerate this. If symptoms are irritable, physical tests may be examined to just before symptom production or just to the onset of provocation with less physical tests being examined to allow for rest period between tests.

Are there any precautions and/or contraindications to elements of the physical examination that need to be explored further, such as vertebrobasilar insufficiency, neurological involvement, recent fracture, trauma, steroid therapy or rheumatoid arthritis? There may also be certain contraindications to further examination and treatment, e.g. symptoms of cord compression.

A physical examination planning form can be useful for clinicians to help guide them through the clinical reasoning process (see Fig. 2.10 and Appendix 2.1).

PHYSICAL EXAMINATION

The information from the subjective examination helps the clinician to plan an appropriate physical examination. The severity, irritability and nature of the condition are the major factors that will influence the choice and priority of physical testing procedures. The first and over-arching question the clinician might ask is: 'is this patient's condition suitable for me to manage as a therapist?' For example, a patient presenting with cauda equina compression symptoms may only need neurological integrity testing, prior to an urgent medical referral. The nature of the patient's condition has had a major impact on the physical examination. The second question the clinician might ask is: 'does this patient have a neuromusculoskeletal dysfunction that I may be able to help?' To answer that, the clinician must carry out a full physical examination; however, this may not be possible if the symptoms are severe and/or irritable. If the patient's symptoms are severe and/or irritable, the clinician aims to explore movements as much as possible, within a symptom-free range. If the patient has constant and severe and/or irritable symptoms, then the clinician aims to find physical tests that ease the symptoms. If the patient's symptoms are non-severe and non-irritable, then the clinician aims to find physical tests that reproduce each of the patient's symptoms.

Each significant physical test that either provokes or eases the patient's symptoms is highlighted in the patient's notes by an asterisk (*) for easy reference. The highlighted tests are often referred to as 'asterisks' or 'markers'.

The order and detail of the physical tests described below need to be appropriate to the patient being examined; some tests will be irrelevant, some tests will be carried out briefly, while others will need to be fully investigated. It is important that readers understand that the techniques shown in this chapter are some of many; the choice depends mainly on the relative size of the clinician and patient, as well as the clinician's preference. For this reason, novice clinicians may initially want to copy what is shown, but then quickly adapt to what is best for them.

Observation

Informal observation

The clinician needs to observe the patient in dynamic and static situations; the quality of movement is noted, as are the postural characteristics and facial expression. Informal observation will have begun from the moment the clinician begins the subjective examination and will continue to the end of the physical examination.

Formal observation

Observation of posture. The clinician examines spinal posture in sitting and standing, noting the posture of head and neck, thoracic spine and upper limbs. The clinician passively corrects any asymmetry to determine its relevance to the patient's problem.

A specific abnormal posture relevant to the upper cervical spine is the shoulder crossed syndrome (Janda 1994, 2002), which is described in Chapter 3. Patients who experience headaches may have a forward head posture (Watson 1994).

It is worth noting that pure postural dysfunction rarely influences one region of the body in isolation and it may be necessary to observe the patient more fully for a full postural examination.

Observation of muscle form. The clinician observes the muscle bulk and muscle tone of the patient, comparing left and right sides. It must be remembered that handedness and level and frequency of physical activity may well produce differences in muscle bulk between sides. Some muscles are thought to shorten under stress, while other muscles weaken, producing muscle imbalance (see Table 3.2). Patterns of muscle imbalance are thought to be the cause of the shoulder crossed syndrome mentioned above, as well as other abnormal postures outlined in Table 6.1.

Observation of soft tissues. The clinician observes the colour of the patient's skin and notes any swelling over the cervical spine or related areas, taking cues for further examination.

Observation of the patient's attitudes and feelings. The age, gender and ethnicity of patients and their cultural, occupational and social backgrounds will all affect their attitudes and feelings towards themselves, their condition and the clinician. The clinician needs to be aware of and sensitive to these attitudes, and to empathize and communicate appropriately so as to develop a rapport with the patient and thereby enhance the patient's compliance with the treatment.

Joint integrity tests (Pettman 1994)

These tests are applicable for patients who have suffered trauma to the spine, such as a whiplash, and who are suspected to have cervical spine instability. The tests described below are considered positive if the patient experiences one or more of the following symptoms: a loss of balance in relation to head movement, unilateral pain along the length of the tongue, facial lip paraesthesia, bilateral or quadrilateral limb paraesthesia, or nystagmus. The patient may require further diagnostic investigations of the upper cervical spine if the clinician finds instability during the tests below.

Distraction tests. With the head and neck in neutral position, the clinician gently distracts the head. If this is symptom-free then the test is repeated with the head flexed on the neck. Reproduction of symptoms suggests upper cervical ligamentous instability, particularly implicating the tectorial membrane (Pettman 1994).

Sagittal stress tests. The forces applied to test the stability of the spine are directed in the sagittal plane and are therefore known as sagittal stress tests. They include anterior and posterior stability tests for the atlanto-occipital joint and two anterior stability tests for the atlanto-axial joint.

Posterior stability test of the atlanto-occipital joint. With the patient supine, the clinician applies an anterior force bilaterally to the atlas and axis on the occiput (Fig. 5.1).

Anterior stability of the atlanto-occipital joint. With the patient supine, the clinician applies a posterior force bilaterally to the anterolateral aspect of the transverse processes of the atlas and axis on the occiput (Fig. 5.2).

Sharp–Perser test. With the patient sitting and the head and neck flexed, the clinician fixes the spinous process of C2 and gently pushes the head posteriorly through the forehead to translate the occiput and atlas posteriorly. The test is considered positive, indicating anterior instability of the atlanto-axial joint, if the patient's symptoms are provoked on head and neck flexion and relieved by the posterior pressure on the forehead (Fig. 5.3).

Anterior translation stress of the atlas on the axis. With the patient supine, the clinician fixes C2 (using thumb pressure over the anterior aspect of the transverse processes) and then lifts the head and atlas vertically (Fig. 5.4).

Coronal stress tests. The force applied to test the stability of the spine is directed in the coronal

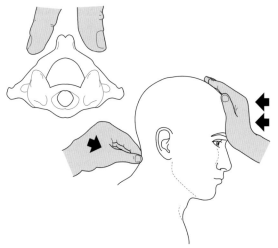

Figure 5.3 Sharp–Perser test of the atlanto-axial joint. (From Pettman 1994, with permission.)

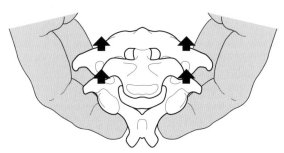

Figure 5.1 Posterior stability test of the atlanto-occipital joint. (From Pettman 1994, with permission.)

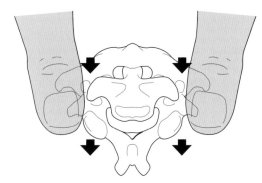

Figure 5.2 Anterior stability of the atlanto-occipital joint. (From Pettman 1994, with permission.)

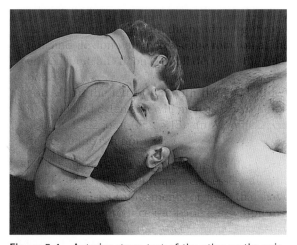

Figure 5.4 Anterior stress test of the atlas on the axis. The left hand grips around the anterior edge of the transverse processes of the axis while the right hand lifts the occiput upwards.

plane and is therefore known as a coronal stress test.

Lateral stability stress test for the atlanto-axial joint. With the patient supine, the clinician supports the occiput and the left side of the arch of the atlas, for example, with the other hand resting over the right side of the arch of the axis. A lateral shear of the atlas and occiput on the axis to the right is attempted. The test is then repeated to the other side. Excessive movement or reproduction of the patient's symptoms suggests lateral instability of this joint (Fig. 5.5).

Alar ligament stress tests. Two stress tests apply a lateral flexion and a rotation stress on the alar ligament (which attaches to the odontoid peg and foramen magnum). The alar ligaments limit contralateral lateral flexion and rotation movement of the occiput on the cervical spine.

Lateral flexion stress test for the alar ligaments. With the patient supine, the clinician fixes C2 along the neural arch and attempts to flex the craniovertebral joint laterally. No movement of the head is possible if the contralateral alar ligament is intact. The test is repeated with the upper cervical spine in flexion, neutral and extension. If motion is available in all three positions, the test is considered positive, suggesting an alar tear or arthrotic instability at the C0–C1 joint.

Rotational stress test for the alar ligament. This test is carried out if the previous lateral flexion stress test is positive, to determine whether the

instability is due to laxity of the alar ligament or due to instability at the C0–C1 joint. In sitting, the clinician fixes C2 by gripping the lamina and then rotates the head. More than 20–30° of rotation indicates a damaged contralateral alar ligament (Fig. 5.6). When the excessive rotational motion is in the same direction as the excessive lateral flexion (from the test above), this suggests damage to the alar ligament; when the excessive motions are in opposite directions, this suggests arthrotic instability (Pettman 1994).

Active physiological movements

For active physiological movements, the clinician notes the:

- Quality of movement (includes clicking or joint noises through the range)
- Range of movement
- Behaviour of pain through the range of movement
- Resistance through the range of movement and at the end of the range of movement
- Provocation of any muscle spasm.

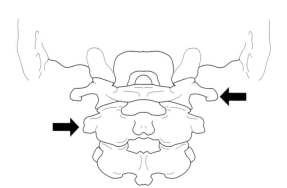

Figure 5.5 Lateral stability stress test for the atlanto-axial joint. (From Pettman 1994, with permission.)

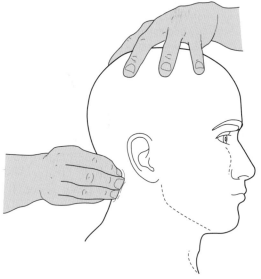

Figure 5.6 Rotational stress test for the alar ligament. (From Pettman 1994, with permission.)

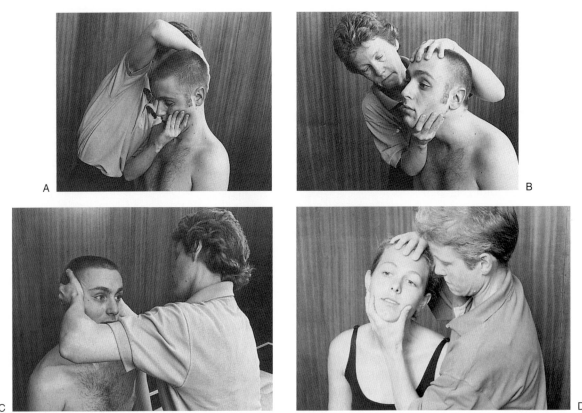

Figure 5.7 Overpressures to the upper cervical spine. **A** Flexion. The left hand cups around the anterior aspect of the mandible while the right hand grips over the occiput. Both hands then apply a force to cause the head to rotate forwards on the upper cervical spine. **B** Extension. The right hand holds underneath the mandible while the left hand and forearm lie over the head. The head and neck are displaced forwards and then both hands apply a force to cause the head to rotate backwards on the upper cervical spine. **C** Lateral flexion. The hands grasp around the head at the level of the ears and apply a force to tilt the head laterally on the upper cervical spine. **D** Left upper cervical quadrant. The hand position is the same as for upper cervical extension. The head is moved into upper cervical extension and then moved into left rotation and then left lateral flexion.

A movement diagram can be used to depict this information. The active movements with overpressure listed below and shown in Figure 5.7 for the upper cervical spine (and in Chapter 6 for the cervicothoracic spine) are often tested with the patient sitting. The clinician establishes the patient's symptom(s) at rest and prior to each movement and corrects any movement deviation to determine its relevance to the patient's symptoms.

Movements of the upper cervical spine and possible modifications are shown in Table 5.1. Numerous differentiation tests (Maitland et al

2001) can be performed; the choice depends on the patient's signs and symptoms. For example, when cervical flexion reproduces the patient's headache in sitting, the addition of slump sitting (see Fig. 3.33) or knee extension may help to differentiate the structures at fault. Slump sitting or knee extension may increase symptoms if there is a neurodynamic component to the patient's headache.

Other regions may need to be examined to determine their relevance to the patient's symptoms; they may be the source of the symptoms, or they may be contributing to the symptoms. The

Table 5.1   Active physiological movements and possible modifications

Active movement	Modification to active movements
Cervical spine	Repeated
Cervical flexion	Speed altered
Upper cervical flexion	Combined (Edwards 1994, 1999) e.g.
Cervical extension	– Upper cervical flexion then rotation
Upper cervical extension	– Upper cervical flexion, rotation and lateral flexion
L lateral flexion	– Upper cervical extension then rotation
R lateral flexion	– Rotation then flexion (shown in Fig. 5.8)
L rotation	– Rotation then extension
R rotation	Compression or distraction
Compression	Sustained
Distraction	Injuring movement
?Temporomandibular	Differentiation tests
?Lower cervical spine	Function
?Thoracic spine	

Table 5.2   Joint clearing tests

Joint	Physiological movement	Accessory movement
Cervical spine	Quadrants	All movements
Thoracic spine	Rotation and quadrants	All movements
Temporomandibular joint	Open/close jaw, side to side movement, protraction/ retraction	All movements

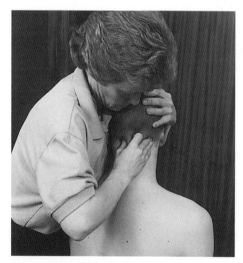

Figure 5.8 Combined movements to the upper cervical spine. The head is supported by the clinician's left hand and forearm and the right hand palpates the upper cervical spine. The left hand then rotates the patient's head and adds flexion while the right hand feels the movement.

regions most likely are the temporomandibular, lower cervical spine and thoracic spine. The joints within these regions can be tested fully (see relevant chapter) or partially with the use of clearing tests (Table 5.2).

Some functional ability has already been tested by the general observation of the patient during the subjective and physical examinations, e.g. the postures adopted during the subjective examination and the ease or difficulty of undressing prior to the examination. Any further functional testing can be carried out at this point in the examination and may include sitting postures or certain movements of the upper limb, etc. Clues for appropriate tests can be obtained from the subjective examination findings, particularly aggravating factors.

Passive physiological movements

This can take the form of passive physiological intervertebral movements (PPIVMs), which examine the movement at each segmental level of the spine. PPIVMs can be a useful adjunct to passive accessory intervertebral movements (PAIVMs) to identify segmental hypomobility and hypermobility. It can be performed with the patient supine or sitting. The clinician palpates between adjacent spinous processes or articular pillars to feel the range of intervertebral movement during the following physiological movements: upper cervical flexion and extension, lateral flexion and rotation. Figure 5.9 demonstrates upper cervical flexion PPIVM.

Other regions may need to be examined to determine their relevance to the patient's symptoms; they may be the source of the symptoms, or they may be contributing to the symptoms. The regions most likely are the temporomandibular region, lower cervical spine and thoracic spine.

Muscle tests

Muscle tests include examining muscle strength, control, length and isometric muscle testing.

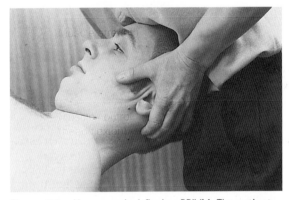

Figure 5.9 Upper cervical flexion PPIVM. The patient lies supine with the head over the end of the couch and supported on the clinician's stomach. The hands are placed so that the index and middle finger lie directly underneath the occiput and between the transverse process of C1 and the mastoid process. The head is then moved into upper cervical flexion and the palpating fingers feel the range of movement.

Muscle strength

The clinician may test the cervical flexors, extensors, lateral flexors and rotators. For details of these general tests, readers are directed to Cole et al (1988) , Hislop & Montgomery (1995) or Kendall et al (1993).

Greater detail may be required to test the strength of muscles, in particular those thought prone to become weak (Janda 1994, 2002, Sahrmann 2002), which include serratus anterior, middle and lower fibres of trapezius and the deep neck flexors. Testing the strength of these muscles is described in Chapter 3.

Muscle control

The relative strength of muscles is considered to be more important than the overall strength of a muscle group (Janda 1994, 2002, Sahrmann 2002). Relative strength is assessed indirectly by observing posture as already mentioned, by the quality of active movement, noting any changes in muscle recruitment patterns, and by palpating muscle activity in various positions.

In the neck, the deep neck flexors together with the muscles of the shoulder girdle are the important muscles that support and control the joints of the neck. Testing of the following muscles may be necessary: longus colli, longus capitis, upper, middle and lower fibres of trapezius and serratus anterior. These muscles stabilize the neck by supporting the weight of the head against gravity and allowing efficient functional activity of the upper limbs.

Weak deep neck flexors have been found to be associated with cervicogenic headaches (Watson 1994). These muscles are tested by the clinician observing the pattern of movement that occurs when the patient flexes the head from a supine position. When the deep neck flexors are weak, the sternocleidomastoid initiates the movement, causing the jaw to lead the movement and the upper cervical spine to hyperextend. After about 10° of head elevation, the cervical spine then curls up into flexion.

A pressure biofeedback unit (PBU; Chattanooga, Australia) can be used to measure the function of the deep neck flexors more objectively

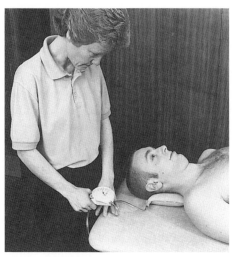

Figure 5.10 Testing the strength of the deep neck flexors.

(Jull 1994). The patient lies supine with a towel under the head to position the cervical spine in neutral, ensuring that the head is parallel to the ceiling. The PBU is placed under the cervical spine and inflated to fill the suboccipital space, to around 20 mmHg. The patient is then asked to carry out a gentle nod of the head, which will normally increase the pressure by 6–10 mmHg (Fig. 5.10). Normal function of the deep neck flexors is considered to be the ability to hold this contraction for 10 seconds and repeat the contraction 10 times (Jull, personal communication, 1999). The emphasis is on low load endurance and the patient should be able to sustain a pressure not exceeding 30 mmHg. Inability to hold an even pressure may indicate poor endurance of the deep neck flexors. Nodding of the head should occur without any activity in the superficial muscles of the neck. The clinician may be able to palpate sternocleidomastoid to feel for unwanted muscle activity.

Muscle length

The clinician tests the length of muscles, in particular those thought prone to shorten (Janda 1994); that is: levator scapula, upper trapezius, sterno-cleidomastoid, pectoralis major and minor, scalenes and the deep occipital muscles. Testing the length of these muscles is described in Chapter 3.

Isometric muscle testing

Test the cervical spine flexors, extensors, lateral flexors and rotators in resting position and, if indicated, in different parts of the physiological range. This is usually carried out with the patient sitting but may be done supine. In addition the clinician observes the quality of the muscle contraction to hold this position (this can be done with the patient's eyes shut). The patient may, for example, be unable to prevent the joint from moving or may hold with excessive muscle activity; either of these circumstances would suggest a neuromuscular dysfunction.

Neurological tests

Neurological examination includes neurological integrity testing, neurodynamic tests and some other nerve tests.

Integrity of the nervous system

Generally, if symptoms are localized to the upper cervical spine and head, neurological examination can be limited to cranial nerves and C1–C4 nerve roots.

Dermatomes/peripheral nerves.   Light touch and pain sensation of the face, head and neck are tested using cotton wool and pinprick respectively, as described in Chapter 3. Knowledge of the cutaneous distribution of nerve roots (dermatomes) and peripheral nerves enables the clinician to distinguish the sensory loss due to a root lesion from that due to a peripheral nerve lesion. The cutaneous nerve distribution and dermatome areas are shown in Figure 3.18.

Myotomes/peripheral nerves.   The following myotomes are tested and are shown in Figure 3.26.

- V cranial (trigeminal N): clench teeth, note temporalis and masseter muscles
- VII cranial (facial N): wrinkle forehead, close eyes, purse lips, show teeth
- XI cranial (accessory N): sternocleidomastoid and shoulder girdle elevation
- C1–C2: upper cervical flexion
- C2: upper cervical extension
- C3: cervical lateral flexion

- C4 and XI cranial nerve: shoulder girdle elevation.

A working knowledge of the muscular distribution of nerve roots (myotomes) and peripheral nerves enables the clinician to distinguish the motor loss due to a root lesion from that due to a peripheral nerve lesion.

Reflex testing. There are no deep tendon reflexes for C1–C4 nerve roots. The jaw jerk (Vth cranial nerve) is elicited by applying a sharp downward tap on the chin with the mouth slightly open. A slight jerk is normal, excessive jerk suggests bilateral upper motor neurone lesion.

Neurodynamic tests

The following neurodynamic tests may be carried out in order to ascertain the degree to which neural tissue is responsible for the production of the patient's symptom(s):

- passive neck flexion (PNF)
- upper limb tension tests (ULTT)
- straight leg raise (SLR)
- slump.

These tests are described in detail in Chapter 3.

Other nerve tests

Plantar response to test for an upper motor neurone lesion (Walton 1989). Pressure applied from the heel along the lateral border of the plantar aspect of the foot produces flexion of the toes in the normal. Extension of the big toe with downward fanning of the other toes occurs with an upper motor neurone lesion.

Miscellaneous tests. In the case of the upper cervical spine, these are *vascular tests*.

Vertebral artery test. Vertebrobasilar insufficiency test. Minimum testing is sustained cervical rotation to the end of range to both left and right sides, and the position or movement that provokes the symptoms, as described by the patient (Magarey et al 2000). The movements are active and each position is maintained by the clinician giving gentle overpressure for a minimum of 10 seconds. The patient keeps his/her eyes open and the clinician observes for nystagmus. The move-

ment is then released for 10 seconds before the next movement is carried out. If dizziness, nausea or any other symptom associated with vertebrobasilar insufficiency (disturbance in vision, diplopia, nausea, ataxia, 'drop attacks', impairment of trigeminal sensation, sympathoplegia, dysarthria, hemianaesthesia and hemiplegia) (Bogduk 1994) is provoked during any part of the test, it is considered positive and testing is stopped. If the test is positive, this contraindicates manipulation of the cervical spine. Further testing can be performed for patients who present with dizziness and include other cervical movements, namely extension, combined movement of extension with rotation and quick movements.

Differentiation between dizziness produced from the vestibular apparatus of the inner ear and that from the neck movement (due to cervical vertigo or compromised vertebral artery) may be required. In standing, the clinician maintains head position while the patient moves the trunk to produce cervical rotation. Rotation to left and right is each held for at least 10 seconds, with at least a 10-second rest period between directions. The test is completed with repetitive trunk rotation movements to left and right (Magarey 2000). The test is considered positive and stopped immediately if dizziness, nausea or any other symptom associated with vertebrobasilar insufficiency is provoked, which suggests that the patient's symptoms are not caused by a disturbance of the vestibular system. A positive vertebral artery test contraindicates certain treatment techniques to the cervical spine (see Table 2.4).

Further information on vertebrobasilar insufficiency can be found in Refshauge & Gass (2004).

Palpation of pulses. If the compromised circulation is suspected, the clinician palpates the pulses of the carotid, facial and temporal arteries.

Palpation

The cervical spine is palpated, as well as the head, face, thoracic spine and upper limbs, as appropriate. It is useful to record palpation findings on a body chart (see Fig. 2.3) and/or palpation chart (see Fig. 3.38).

The clinician notes the:

- temperature of the area
- localized increased skin moisture
- presence of oedema or effusion
- mobility and feel of superficial tissues, e.g. ganglions, nodules, thickening of deep suboccipital tissues
- presence or elicitation of any muscle spasm
- tenderness of bone, ligaments, muscle, tendon, tendon sheath and nerve. Check for tenderness in suboccipital region. Test for the relevant trigger points shown in Figure 3.39
- increased or decreased prominence of bones
- symptoms (often pain) provoked or reduced on palpation.

Passive accessory intervertebral movements (PAIVMs)

It is useful to use the palpation chart and movement diagrams (or joint pictures) to record findings. These are explained in detail in Chapter 3.

The clinician notes the:

- quality of movement
- range of movement
- resistance through the range and at the end of the range of movement
- behaviour of pain through the range
- provocation of any muscle spasm.

Upper cervical spine (C1–C4) accessory movements are listed in Table 5.3 and for C1 level shown in Figure 5.11 (other levels are shown in the cervicothoracic chapter). A number of

ways of combining movements have been documented (Edwards 1994, 1999) and are described below.

Atlanto-occipital joint. Apply anteroposterior (AP) and/or posteroanterior (PA) unilateral pressures on C1 with the spine positioned in flexion and rotation or extension and rotation, so as to increase and/or decrease the compressive or stretch effect at the atlanto-occipital joint:

- A PA on the right of C1 with the spine in flexion and right rotation will increase the stretch at the right C0–C1 joint (Fig. 5.12); an AP on the right of C1 will decrease the stretch.
- An AP on the left of C1 with the spine in extension and right rotation will increase the stretch on the left C0–C1 joint; a PA on the left of C1 will decrease the stretch.

Atlanto-axial joint. Apply AP and/or PA unilateral vertebral pressures on C1 and/or C2 with the spine positioned in rotation and flexion or rotation and extension so as to increase and/or decrease the compressive or stretch effect at the atlanto-axial joint:

- A PA on the left of C1 with the head in right rotation and flexion will increase the stretch at the left C1–C2 joint; a PA on C2 will decrease this stretch.
- A PA on the left of C2 with the head in left rotation and extension will increase the rotation at the C1–C2 joint; a PA on C1 will decrease the rotation.

Table 5.3 Accessory movements, choice of application and reassessment of the patient's asterisks

Accessory movements	Choice of application	Identify any effect of accessory movements on patient's signs and symptoms
Upper cervical spine: ↕ Central posteroanterior ⌐°⌐ Unilateral posteroanterior →• Med transverse for C1 →• Med/lat transverse for C2-C4 ↖↗ Unilateral anteroposterior	Start position, e.g. in flexion, extension, etc. – speed of force application – direction of the applied force – point of application of applied force	Reassess all asterisks
?Temporomandibular joint	As above	Reassess all asterisks
?Lower cervical spine	As above	Reassess all asterisks
?Thoracic spine	As above	Reassess all asterisks

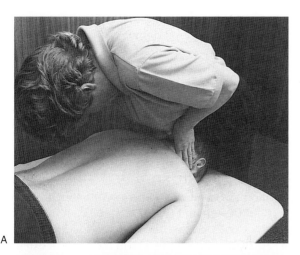

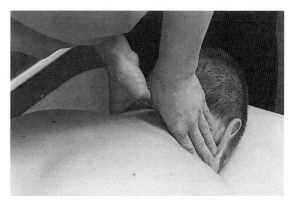

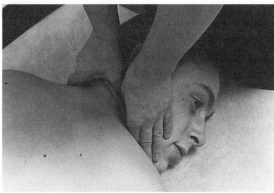

Figure 5.11 Accessory movements to C1. **A** Central posteroanterior. Thumb pressure is applied over the posterior arch of C1 and directed upwards and forwards towards the patient's eyes. **B** Unilateral posteroanterior. Thumb pressure is applied laterally over the posterior arch of C1. **C** Transverse pressure on the right. The head is rotated to the right and thumb pressure is applied to the transverse process of C1.

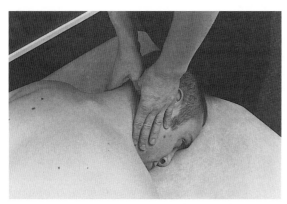

Figure 5.12 Palpation for the C0–C1 joint using combined movements. Thumb pressure over the right of the posterior arch of the atlas is applied with the patient's head in flexion and right rotation.

- An AP on left of C2 with the head in right rotation and flexion will increase the rotation at the C1–C2 joint; an AP on C1 will decrease the rotation.
- An AP on the left of C1 with the head in left rotation and extension will increase the rotation at the C1–C2 joint (Fig. 5.13); an AP on C2 will decrease the rotation.

Following accessory movements to the upper cervical spine the clinician reassesses all the physical asterisks (movements or tests that have been found to reproduce the patient's symptoms) in order to establish the effect of the accessory movements on the patient's signs and symptoms. Accessory movements can then be tested for other regions suspected to be a source of, or contributing to, the symptoms. Again, following accessory movements the clinician reassesses all the physi-

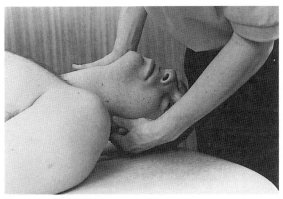

Figure 5.13 Palpation for the C0–C1 joint using combined movements. Thumb pressure over the anterior aspect of the atlas on the left is applied with the head in left rotation and extension.

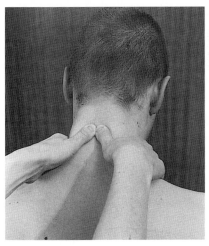

Figure 5.14 A SNAG. A posteroanterior pressure is applied to C4 as the subject moves into cervical flexion.

cal asterisks. Regions likely to be examined are the temporomandibular joint, lower cervical spine and upper thoracic spine (Table 5.2).

Sustained natural apophyseal glides (SNAGs)

The painful cervical spine movements are examined in sitting. Pressure is applied by the clinician to each spinous process and/or transverse process of the cervical vertebrae as the patient moves slowly towards the pain (Mulligan 1999). Figure 5.14 demonstrates a SNAG to the spinous process of C4 as the subject moves into cervical flexion.

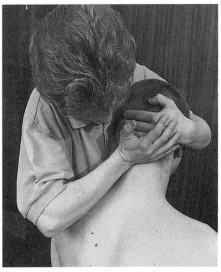

Figure 5.15 Headache SNAG. A posteroanterior pressure is applied to C2 using the heel of the right hand. The left hand supports the head.

The symptomatic level will be one in which the pressure reduces the pain. For further information, refer to Chapter 3.

For patients complaining of headaches, Mulligan (1999) describes four examination techniques.

Headache SNAGs. The clinician applies a posteroanterior pressure to C2 on a stabilized occiput with the patient in sitting (Fig. 5.15). The pressure is sustained for at least 10 seconds while the patient remains still; there is no active movement. The test is considered positive if the headache is relieved, which would indicate a mechanical joint problem.

Reverse headache SNAGs. The clinician moves the occiput anteriorly on the stabilized C2 with the patient in sitting (Fig. 5.16). The movement is sustained for at least 10 seconds while the patient remains still; there is no active movement. Again the test is considered positive if the headache is relieved, which would indicate a mechanical joint problem.

Upper cervical traction. The clinician maintains the patient's cervical lordosis by placing a forearm under the cervical spine with the patient supine (Fig. 5.17). Pronation of the forearm and a gentle pull on the chin produces cervical traction. The

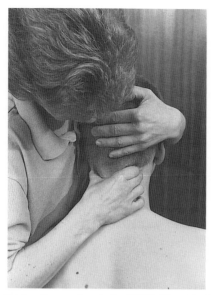

Figure 5.16 Reverse headache SNAG. The right hand palpates the transverse processes of C2. The left hand supports and moves the head anteriorly on the stabilized C2.

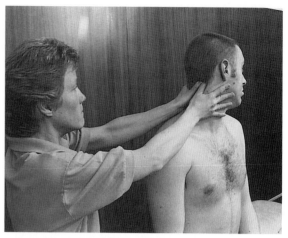

Figure 5.18 SNAGs for restricted cervical rotation at C1–C2. A posteroanterior pressure is applied to the right articular pillar of C1 as the patient moves slowly into left rotation.

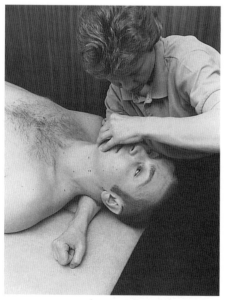

Figure 5.17 Cervical traction. The patient lies supine and the clinician's forearm is placed under the patient's cervical spine. The left hand grips the mandible and applies a gentle traction force.

position is held for at least 10 seconds; relief of symptoms indicates a positive test, which would indicate a mechanical joint problem.

SNAGs for restricted cervical rotation at C1–C2. The painful cervical spine movements are examined in sitting. Pressure to the left or right side of the posterior arch of C1 is applied by the clinician as the patient slowly rotates to the right or left side towards the pain (Fig. 5.18). Pain-free movement indicates a positive test and would indicate a mechanical joint problem.

COMPLETION OF THE EXAMINATION

Having carried out the above tests, the examination of the upper cervical spine is now complete. The subjective and physical examinations produce a large amount of information, which needs to be recorded accurately and quickly. An outline examination chart may be useful for some clinicians and one is suggested in Figure 5.19. It is important, however, that the clinician does not examine in a rigid manner, simply following the suggested sequence outlined in the chart. Each patient presents differently and this should be reflected in the examination process. It is vital at this stage to highlight with an asterisk (*) important findings from the examination. These findings must be

Body chart	Name
	Age
	Date
	24-hour behaviour
	Improving static worsening
	Special questions
	General health
	Weight loss
	RA
	Drugs
	Steroids
	Anticoagulants
Relationship of symptoms	X-ray
	Cord symptoms
	Cauda equina symptoms
	VBI symptoms
Aggravating factors and function	HPC
	PMH
Severe Irritable	
Easing factors	
	SH & FH
	(Patient's perspective, experience,
	expectations. Yellow, blue, black flags)

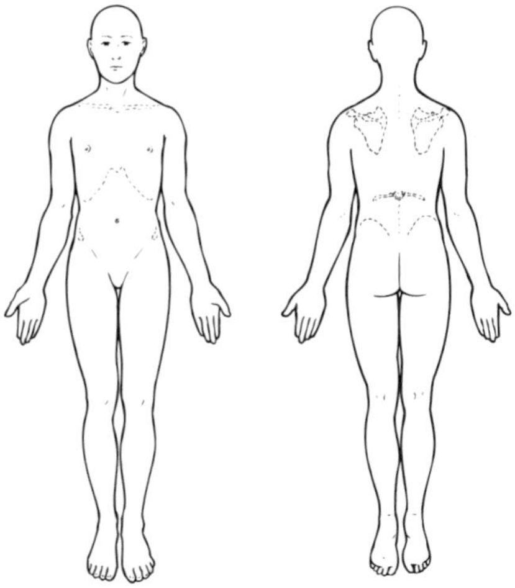

Figure 5.19   Upper cervical spine examination chart.

Physical examination Observation	Isometric muscle testing
	Neurological integrity tests
Joint integrity tests (distraction, anterior/posterior stability C0/C1, Sharp-Perser for C1/C2, lateral stability C1/C2, alar stress tests)	
	Neurodynamic tests
Active and passive physiological movements of upper cervical spine and other relevant regions	
	Other nerve tests (plantar response)
	Miscellaneous tests (VBI testing, pulses)
Muscle strength	Palpation
Muscle control (head flexion)	
	Accessory movements and reassessment of each relevant region
Muscle length	

Figure 5.19 *Continued*

reassessed at, and within, subsequent treatment sessions to evaluate the effects of treatment on the patient's condition.

The physical testing procedures which specifically indicate joint, nerve or muscle tissues, as a source of the patient's symptoms, are summarized in Table 3.10. The strongest evidence that a joint is the source of the patient's symptoms is that active and passive physiological movements, passive accessory movements and joint palpation all reproduce the patient's symptoms, and that following a treatment dose, reassessment identifies an improvement in the patient's signs and symptoms. Weaker evidence includes an alteration in range, resistance or quality of physiological and/or accessory movements and tenderness over the joint, with no alteration in signs and symptoms after treatment. One or more of these findings may indicate a dysfunction of a joint which may or may not be contributing to the patient's condition.

The strongest evidence that a muscle is the source of a patient's symptoms is if active movements, an isometric contraction, passive lengthening and palpation of a muscle all reproduce the symptoms, and that following a treatment dose, reassessment identifies an improvement in the patient's signs and symptoms. Further evidence of muscle dysfunction may be suggested by reduced strength or poor quality during the active physiological movement and the isometric contraction, reduced range, and/or increased/decreased resistance, during the passive lengthening of the muscle, and tenderness on palpation, with no alteration in signs and symptoms after treatment. One or more of these findings may indicate a dysfunction of a muscle which may, or may not, be contributing to the patient's condition.

The strongest evidence that a nerve is the source of the patient's symptoms is when active and/or passive physiological movements reproduce the patient's symptoms, which are then increased or decreased with an additional sensitizing movement, at a distance from the patient's symptoms. In addition, there is reproduction of the patient's symptoms on palpation of the nerve and following neurodynamic testing, sufficient to be considered a treatment dose, results in an improvement in the above signs and symptoms. Further evidence of nerve dysfunction may be

suggested by reduced range (compared to the asymptomatic side) and/or increased resistance to the various arm movements, and tenderness on nerve palpation.

On completion of the physical examination, the clinician:

- Warns the patient of possible exacerbation up to 24–48 hours following the examination.
- Requests the patient to report details on the behaviour of the symptoms following examination at the next attendance.
- Explains the findings of the physical examination and how these findings relate to the subjective assessment. An attempt should be made to clear up any misconceptions patients may have regarding their illness or injury.
- Evaluates the findings, formulates a clinical diagnosis and writes up a problem list. Clinicians may find the management planning forms shown in Figures 3.53 and 3.54 helpful in guiding them through what is often a complex clinical reasoning process.
- Determines the objectives of treatment.
- Devises an initial treatment plan.

In this way, the clinician develops the following hypotheses categories (adapted from Jones & Rivett 2004):

- Function: abilities and restrictions.
- Patients' perspectives on their experience.
- Source of symptoms. This includes the structure or tissue that is thought to be producing the patients' symptoms, the nature of the structure or tissues in relation to the healing process, and the pain mechanisms.
- Contributing factors to the development and maintenance of the problem. There may be environmental, psychosocial, behavioural, physical or heredity factors.
- Precautions/contraindications to treatment and management. This includes the severity and irritability of the patient's symptoms and the nature of the patient's condition.
- Management strategy and treatment plan.
- Prognosis – this can be affected by factors such as the stage and extent of the injury as well as the patient's expectation, personality and lifestyle.

References

Barker S, Kesson M, Ashmore J, Turner G, Conway J, Stevens D 2000 Guidance for pre-manipulative testing of the cervical spine. Manual Therapy 5(1): 37–40

Bogduk N 1994 Cervical causes of headache and dizziness. In: Boyling J D, Palastanga N (eds) Grieve's modern manual therapy, 2nd edn. Churchill Livingstone, Edinburgh, ch 22, p 317

Clinical Standards Advisory Report 1994 Report of a CSAG committee on back pain. HMSO, London

Cole J H, Furness A L, Twomey L T 1988 Muscles in action, an approach to manual muscle testing. Churchill Livingstone, Edinburgh

Dahlberg C, Lanig I S, Kenna M, Long S 1997 Diagnosis and treatment of esophageal perforations in cervical spinal cord injury. Topics in Spinal Cord Injury Rehabilitation 2(3): 41–48

Edeling J 1994 Manual therapy for chronic headache, 2nd edn. Butterworth-Heinemann, Oxford

Edwards B C 1994 Examination of the high cervical spine (occiput-C2) using combined movements. In: Boyling J D, Palastanga N (eds) Grieve's modern manual therapy, 2nd edn. Churchill Livingstone, Edinburgh, ch 41, p 555

Edwards B C 1999 Manual of combined movements: their use in the examination and treatment of mechanical vertebral column disorders, 2nd edn. Butterworth-Heinemann, Oxford

Grieve G P 1994 Counterfeit clinical presentations. Manipulative Physiotherapist 26: 17–19

Headache Classification Committee of the International Headache Society 1988 Classification and diagnostic criteria for headache disorders, cranial neuralgias and facial pain. Cephalalgia 8(7): 9–96

Hislop H, Montgomery J 1995 Daniels and Worthingham's muscle testing, techniques of manual examination, 7th edn. W B Saunders, Philadelphia

Jackson R 1966 The cervical syndrome, 3rd edn. Charles C Thomas, Springfield, IL

Janda V 1994 Muscles and motor control in cervicogenic disorders: assessment and management. In: Grant R (ed) Physical therapy of the cervical and thoracic spine, 2nd edn. Churchill Livingstone, New York, ch 10, p 195

Janda V 2002 Muscles and motor control in cervicogenic disorders. In: Grant R (ed) Physical therapy of the cervical and thoracic spine, 3rd edn. Churchill Livingstone, New York, ch 10, p 182

Jones M A, Rivett D A 2004 Clinical reasoning for manual therapists. Butterworth-Heinemann, Edinburgh

Jull G A 1994 Headaches of cervical origin. In: Grant R (ed) Physical therapy of the cervical and thoracic spine, 2nd edn. Churchill Livingstone, New York, ch 13, p 261

Kendall F P, McCreary E K, Provance P G 1993 Muscles testing and function, 4th edn. Williams & Wilkins, Baltimore, MD

Magarey M, Coughlan B, Rebbeck T 2000 APA pre-manipulative testing protocol for the cervical spine: researched and renewed, part 2 – revised clinical guidelines. International Federation of Orthopaedic Manipulative Therapists, Perth

Maitland G D, Hengeveld E, Banks K, English K 2001 Maitland's vertebral manipulation, 6th edn. Butterworth-Heinemann, Oxford

Mulligan B R 1999 Manual therapy 'NAGs', 'SNAGs', 'MWMs' etc., 4th edn. Plane View Services, New Zealand

Pettman E 1994 Stress tests of the craniovertebral joints. In: Boyling J D, Palastanga N (eds) Grieve's modern manual therapy, 2nd edn. Churchill Livingstone, Edinburgh, ch 38, p 529

Refshauge K, Gass E (eds) 2004 Musculoskeletal physiotherapy clinical science and evidence-based practice. Butterworth-Heinemann, Oxford

Sahrmann S A 2002 Diagnosis and treatment of movement impairment syndromes. Mosby, St Louis

Waddell G 2004 The back pain revolution, 2nd edn. Churchill Livingstone, Edinburgh

Walton J H 1989 Essentials of neurology, 6th edn. Churchill Livingstone, Edinburgh

Watson D H 1994 Cervical headache: an investigation of natural head posture and upper cervical flexor muscle performance. In: Boyling J D, Palastanga N (eds) Grieve's modern manual therapy, 2nd edn. Churchill Livingstone, Edinburgh, ch 24, p 349

Chapter **6**

Examination of the cervicothoracic spine

POSSIBLE CAUSES OF PAIN AND/OR LIMITATION OF MOVEMENT

The cervicothoracic region is defined here as the region between C3 and T4, and includes the joints and their surrounding soft tissues.

- Trauma
  - Whiplash
  - Fracture of vertebral body, spinous or transverse process
  - Ligamentous sprain
  - Muscular strain
- Degenerative conditions
  - Spondylosis: degeneration of intervertebral disc
  - Arthrosis: degeneration of zygapophyseal joints
- Inflammatory conditions
  - Rheumatoid arthritis
  - Ankylosing spondylitis
- Neoplasm
- Infection
- Cervical rib
- Torticollis
- Hypermobility syndrome
- Referral from the upper cervical spine.

Further details of the questions asked during the subjective examination and the tests carried out in the physical examination can be found in Chapters 2 and 3 respectively.

The order of the subjective questioning and the physical tests described below can be altered as appropriate for the patient being examined.

SUBJECTIVE EXAMINATION

Body chart

The following information concerning the area and type of current symptoms can be recorded on a body chart (see Fig. 2.3).

Area of current symptoms

Be exact when mapping out the area of the symptoms. Patients may have symptoms over a large area. As well as symptoms over the cervical spine, they may have symptoms over the head and face, thoracic spine and upper limbs. Ascertain which is the worst symptom and record where the patient feels the symptoms are coming from.

Areas relevant to the region being examined

All other relevant areas are checked for symptoms; it is important to ask about pain or even stiffness, as this may be relevant to the patient's main symptom. Mark unaffected areas with ticks (✓) on the body chart. Check for symptoms in the head, temporomandibular joint, thoracic spine, shoulder, elbow, wrist and hand, and ascertain if the patient has ever experienced any dizziness. This is relevant for symptoms emanating from the cervical spine, where vertebrobasilar insufficiency (VBI) may be provoked. If dizziness is a feature described by the patient, the clinician determines what factors aggravate and what factors ease the symptoms, the duration and severity of the dizziness and its relationship with other symptoms such as disturbance in vision, diplopia, nausea, ataxia, 'drop attacks', impairment of trigeminal sensation, sympathoplegia, dysarthria, hemianaesthesia and hemiplegia (Bogduk 1994). In addition, the vertebral artery tests must be carried out in the physical examination (see below).

Quality of pain

Establish the quality of the pain. If the patient suffers from associated headaches, consider carrying out a full upper cervical spine examination (see Ch. 5). Patients who have suffered a hyperextension injury to the cervical spine may complain of a sore throat, difficulty in swallowing and a feeling of something stuck in their throat resulting from an associated injury to the oesophagus (Dahlberg et al 1997).

Intensity of pain

The intensity of pain can be measured using, for example, a visual analogue scale (VAS), as shown in Figure 2.8. A pain diary may be useful for patients with chronic neck pain with or without headaches to determine the pain patterns and triggering factors.

Depth of pain

Establish the depth of the pain. Does the patient feel it is on the surface or deep inside?

Abnormal sensation

Check for any altered sensation locally in the cervical spine and in other relevant areas such as the upper limbs or face.

Constant or intermittent symptoms

Ascertain the frequency of the symptoms, whether they are constant or intermittent. If symptoms are constant, check whether there is variation in the intensity of the symptoms, as constant unremitting pain may be indicative of neoplastic disease.

Relationship of symptoms

Determine the relationship between the symptomatic areas – do they come together or separately? For example, the patient could have shoulder pain without cervical pain, or they may always be present together.

Behaviour of symptoms

Aggravating factors

For each symptomatic area, discover what movements and/or positions aggravate the patient's symptoms, i.e. what brings them on (or makes them worse), are they able to maintain this position or movement (severity), what happens to other symptom(s) when this symptom is produced (or is made worse), and how long does it take for symptoms to ease once the position or movement is stopped (irritability). These questions help to confirm the relationship between the symptoms.

The clinician also asks the patient about theoretically known aggravating factors for structures that could be a source of the symptoms. Common aggravating factors for the cervical spine are cervical extension, cervical rotation and sustained flexion. Aggravating factors for other regions, which may need to be queried if they are suspected to be a source of the symptoms, are shown in Table 2.3.

The clinician ascertains how the symptoms affect function, such as: static and active postures, e.g. sitting, standing, lying, washing, ironing, dusting, driving, reading, writing, work, sport and social activities. Note details of training regimen for any sports activities. The clinician finds out if the patient is left- or right-handed as there may be increased stress on the dominant side.

Detailed information on each of the above activities is useful in order to help determine the structure(s) at fault and identify functional restrictions. This information can be used to determine the aims of treatment and any advice that may be required. The most notable functional restrictions are highlighted with asterisks (*), explored in the physical examination, and reassessed at subsequent treatment sessions to evaluate treatment intervention.

Easing factors

For each symptomatic area, the clinician asks what movements and/or positions ease the patient's symptoms, how long it takes to ease them and what happens to other symptom(s) when this symptom is relieved. These questions help to confirm the relationship between the symptoms.

The clinician asks the patient about theoretically known easing factors for structures that could be a source of the symptoms. For example, symptoms from the cervical spine may be eased by supporting the head or neck, whereas symptoms arising from a cervical rib may be eased by shoulder girdle elevation and/or depression. The clinician can then analyse the position or movement that eases the symptoms, to help determine the structure at fault.

Twenty-four-hour behaviour of symptoms

The clinician determines the 24-hour behaviour of symptoms by asking questions about night, morning and evening symptoms.

Night symptoms.   The following questions may be asked:

- Do you have any difficulty getting to sleep?
- What position is most comfortable/uncomfortable?
- What is your normal sleeping position?
- What is your present sleeping position?
- Do your symptom(s) wake you at night? If so,
  - Which symptom(s)?
  - How many times in the past week?
  - How many times in a night?
  - How long does it take to get back to sleep?
- How many and what type of pillows are used?
- Is your mattress firm or soft?
- Has the mattress been changed recently?

Morning and evening symptoms.   The clinician determines the pattern of the symptoms first thing in the morning, through the day and at the end of the day. Stiffness in the morning for the first few minutes might suggest cervical spondylosis; stiffness and pain for a few hours is suggestive of an inflammatory process such as rheumatoid arthritis.

Stage of the condition

In order to determine the stage of the condition, the clinician asks whether the symptoms are getting better, getting worse or remaining unchanged.

Special questions

Special questions must always be asked, as they may identify certain precautions or contraindications to the physical examination and/or treatment (Table 2.4). As mentioned in Chapter 2, the clinician must differentiate between conditions that are suitable for conservative management and systemic, neoplastic and other non-neuromuscu-loskeletal conditions, which require referral to a medical practitioner. The reader is referred to Appendix 2.3 for details of various serious patho-logical processes that can mimic neuromuscu-loskeletal conditions (Grieve 1994).

The following information is routinely obtained from patients.

General health. The clinician ascertains the state of the patient's general health – find out if the patient suffers any malaise, fatigue, fever, nausea or vomiting, stress, anxiety or depression.

Weight loss. Has the patient noticed any recent unexplained weight loss?

Rheumatoid arthritis. Has the patient (or a member of his/her family) been diagnosed as having rheumatoid arthritis?

Drug therapy. What drugs are being taken by the patient? Has the patient ever been prescribed long-term (6 months or more) medication or steroid therapy? Has the patient been taking anti-coagulants recently?

X-rays and medical imaging. Has the patient been X-rayed or had any other medical tests recently? Routine spinal X-rays are no longer con-sidered necessary prior to conservative treatment as they only identify the normal age-related degenerative changes, which do not necessarily correlate with the patient's symptoms (Clinical Standards Advisory Report 1994). The medical tests may include blood tests, magnetic resonance imaging, myelography, discography or a bone scan. For further information on these tests, readers are referred to Refshauge & Gass (2004).

Neurological symptoms. Has the patient experi-enced symptoms of spinal cord compression, which are bilateral tingling in hands or feet and/or disturbance of gait?

Vertebrobasilar insufficiency (VBI) symptoms. For symptoms emanating from the cervical spine, the clinician needs to ask about symptoms that may be caused by VBI. Symptoms include: dizzi-ness (most commonly), altered vision (including diplopia), nausea, ataxia, 'drop attacks', altered

---

> **Box 6.1   Risk factors for symptoms related to vertebrobasilar insufficiency (Barker et al 2000)**
>
> - Drop attacks, blackouts, loss of consciousness
> - Nausea, vomiting and general unwell feelings
> - Dizziness or vertigo, particularly if associated with head positioning
> - Disturbances of vision (e.g. decreased, blurred, diplopia)
> - Unsteadiness of gait (ataxia) and general feeling of weakness
> - Tingling or numbness (especially dysaesthesia, i.e. tingling around the lips, hemianaesthesia or any alteration in facial sensation)
> - Difficulty in speaking (dysarthria) or swallowing
> - Hearing disturbance (e.g. tinnitus, deafness)
> - Headache
> - Past history of trauma
> - Cardiac disease, vascular disease, altered blood pressure, previous cerebrovascular accident or transient ischaemic attacks
> - Blood clotting disorders
> - Anticoagulant therapy
> - Oral contraceptives
> - Long-term use of steroids
> - A history of smoking
> - Immediately post partum

facial sensation, difficulty speaking, difficulty swallowing, sympathoplegia, hemianaesthesia and hemiplegia (Bogduk 1994). If present, the clinician determines the aggravating and easing factors in the usual way. These symptoms can also be due to upper cervical instability and diseases of the inner ear. Risk factors associated with VBI are given in Box 6.1 (Barker et al 2000) and include some further screening questions that the clinician may need to ask some patients, particularly prior to treatment with a cervical manipulation.

History of the present condition (HPC)

For each symptomatic area, the clinician needs to know how long the symptom has been present, whether there was a sudden or slow onset and whether there was a known cause that provoked the onset of the symptom. If the onset was slow, the clinician should find out if there has been any change in the patient's lifestyle, e.g. a new job or hobby or a change in sporting activity, which may have affected the stresses on the cervical spine and related areas. To confirm the relationship between the symptoms, the clinician asks what happened to other symptoms when each symptom began.

Past medical history (PMH)

The following information is obtained from the patient and/or the medical notes:

- The details of any relevant medical history, particularly related to the cervical spine, cranium and face.
- The history of any previous attacks: how many episodes, when were they, what was the cause, what was the duration of each episode and did the patient fully recover between episodes? If there have been no previous attacks, has the patient had any episodes of stiffness in the cervical or thoracic spine? Check for a history of trauma or recurrent minor trauma.
- Ascertain the results of any past treatment for the same or similar problem. Past treatment records may be obtained for further information.

Social and family history (SH, FH)

Social and family history that is relevant to the onset and progression of the patient's problem is recorded. This includes the patient's perspectives, experience and expectations, age, employment, home situation, and details of any leisure activities. Factors from this information may indicate direct and/or indirect mechanical influences on the cervical spine. In order to treat the patient appropriately, it is important that the condition is managed within the context of the patient's social and work environment.

The clinician may ask the following types of questions to elucidate psychosocial factors:

- Have you had time off work in the past with your pain?
- What do you understand to be the cause of your pain?
- What are you expecting will help you?

- How is your employer/co-workers/family responding to your pain?
- What are you doing to cope with your pain?
- Do you think you will return to work? When?

While these questions are described in relation to psychosocial risk factors for poor outcomes for patients with low back pain (Waddell 2004), they may be relevant to other patients.

Plan of the physical examination

When all this information has been collected, the subjective examination is complete. It is useful at this stage to highlight with asterisks (*), for ease of reference, important findings and particularly one or more functional restrictions. These can then be re-examined at subsequent treatment sessions to evaluate treatment intervention.

In order to plan the physical examination, the following hypotheses need to be developed from the subjective examination:

- The regions and structures that that need to be examined as a possible cause of the symptoms, e.g. temporomandibular region, upper cervical spine, cervical spine, thoracic spine, acromioclavicular joint, sternoclavicular joint, glenohumeral joint, elbow, wrist and hand, muscles and nerves. Often, it is not possible to examine fully at the first attendance and so examination of the structures must be prioritized over the subsequent treatment sessions.
- Other factors that need to be examined, e.g. working and everyday postures, vertebral artery, muscle weakness.
- In what way should the physical tests be carried out? Will it be easy or hard to reproduce each symptom? Will it be necessary to use combined movements, repetitive movements, etc. to reproduce the patient's symptoms? Are symptom(s) severe and/or irritable? If symptoms are severe, physical tests may be carried out to just before the onset of symptom production or just to the onset of symptom production; no overpressures should be carried out, as the patient would be unable to tolerate this. If symptoms are irritable, physical tests may be examined to just before symptom production or just to the onset of provocation with less physical tests being examined to allow for rest period between tests.

Are there any precautions and/or contraindications to elements of the physical examination that need to be explored further, such as vertebrobasilar insufficiency, neurological involvement, recent fracture, trauma, steroid therapy or rheumatoid arthritis? There may also be certain contraindications to further examination and treatment, e.g. symptoms of cord compression.

A physical planning form can be useful for clinicians to help guide them through the clinical reasoning process (see Fig. 2.10 and Appendix 2.1).

PHYSICAL EXAMINATION

The information from the subjective examination helps the clinician to plan an appropriate physical examination. The severity, irritability and nature of the condition are the major factors that will influence the choice and priority of physical testing procedures. The first and over-arching question the clinician might ask is: 'is this patient's condition suitable for me to manage as a therapist?' For example, a patient presenting with cauda equina compression symptoms may only need neurological integrity testing, prior to an urgent medical referral. The nature of the patient's condition has had a major impact on the physical examination. The second question the clinician might ask is: 'does this patient have a neuromusculoskeletal dysfunction that I may be able to help?' To answer that, the clinician needs to carry out a full physical examination; however, this may not be possible if the symptoms are severe and/or irritable. If the patient's symptoms are severe and/or irritable, the clinician aims to explore movements as much as possible, within a symptom-free range. If the patient has constant and severe and/or irritable symptoms, then the clinician aims to find physical tests that ease the symptoms. If the patient's symptoms are non-severe and non-irritable, then the clinician aims to find physical tests that reproduce each of the patient's symptoms.

Each significant physical test that either provokes or eases the patient's symptoms is highlighted in the patient's notes by an asterisk (*) for easy reference. The highlighted tests are often referred to as 'asterisks' or 'markers'.

The order and detail of the physical tests described below need to be appropriate to the patient being examined; some tests will be irrelevant, some tests will be carried out briefly, while it will be necessary to investigate others fully. It is important that readers understand that the techniques shown in this chapter are some of many; the choice depends mainly on the relative size of the clinician and patient, as well as the clinician's preference. For this reason, novice clinicians may initially want to copy what is shown, but then quickly adapt to what is best for them.

Observation

Informal observation

The clinician needs to observe the patient in dynamic and static situations; the quality of movement is noted, as are the postural characteristics and facial expression. Informal observation will have begun from the moment the clinician begins the subjective examination and will continue to the end of the physical examination.

Formal observation

Observation of posture. The clinician examines the patient's spinal posture in sitting and standing, noting the posture of the head and neck, thoracic spine and upper limbs. The clinician passively corrects any asymmetry to determine its relevance to the patient's problem. A specific posture relevant to the cervicothoracic spine is the shoulder crossed syndrome (Janda 1994, 2002), which has been described in Chapter 3.

It should be noted that pure postural dysfunction rarely influences one region of the body in isolation and it may be necessary to observe the patient more fully for a full postural examination.

Observation of muscle form. The clinician observes the muscle bulk and muscle tone of the patient, comparing left and right sides. It must be remembered that handedness and level and frequency of physical activity may well produce differences in muscle bulk between sides. Some muscles are thought to shorten under stress, while other muscles weaken, producing muscle imbalance (see Table 3.2). Patterns of muscle imbalance are thought to be the cause of the shoulder crossed syndrome mentioned above, as well as other abnormal postures outlined in Table 6.1.

Observation of soft tissues. The clinician observes the quality and colour of the patient's skin and any area of swelling or presence of scarring, and takes cues for further examination.

Table 6.1 Possible muscle imbalance causing altered posture (Janda 1994)

Posture	Muscle tightness
Straight neck–shoulder line (gothic-shaped shoulders) and elevation of the shoulder girdle	Levator scapula and upper trapezius
Prominence of pectoralis major, protraction of the shoulder girdles and slight medial rotation of the arms	Pectoral muscles
Prominence of the insertion of sternocleidomastoid and forward head posture	Sternocleidomastoid

Posture	Muscle weakness
Winging of the scapula	Serratus anterior
Flat or hollowed interscapular space	Rhomboids and middle trapezius
Forward head position	Deep neck flexors

Observation of the patient's attitudes and feelings. The age, gender and ethnicity of patients and their cultural, occupational and social backgrounds will all affect their attitudes and feelings towards themselves, their condition and the clinician. The clinician needs to be aware of and sensitive to these attitudes, and to empathize and communicate appropriately so as to develop a rapport with the patient and thereby enhance the patient's compliance with the treatment.

Active physiological movements

For active physiological movements, the clinician notes the:

- Quality of movement
- Range of movement
- Behaviour of pain through the range of movement
- Resistance through the range of movement and at the end of the range of movement
- Provocation of any muscle spasm.

A movement diagram can be used to depict this information. The active movements with overpressure listed below and shown in Figure 6.1 are tested with the patient in sitting. The clinician establishes the patient's symptoms at rest and prior to each movement, and corrects any move-

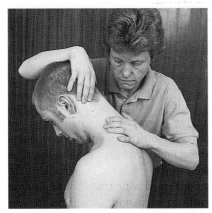

A Flexion. The left hand stabilizes the trunk while the right hand moves the head down so that the chin moves towards the chest.

Figure 6.1 (A–G) Overpressures to the cervical spine.

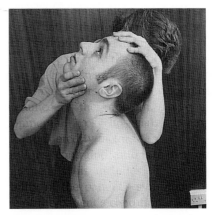

B Extension. The left hand rests over the head to the forehead while the right hand holds over the mandible. Both hands then apply a force to cause the head and neck to extend backwards.

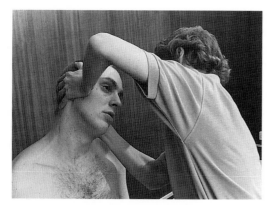

C Lateral flexion. Both hands rest over the patient's head around the ears and apply a force to cause the head and neck to tilt laterally.

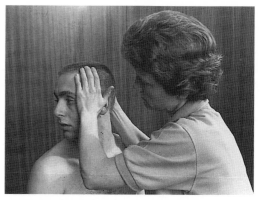

D Rotation. The left hand lies over the zygomatic arch while the right hand rests over the occiput. Both hands then apply pressure to cause the head and neck to rotate.

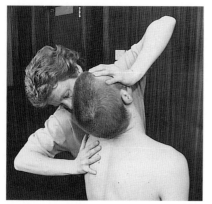

E Left extension quadrant. This is a combination of extension, left rotation and left lateral flexion. The patient actively extends and, as soon as the movement is complete, the clinician passively moves the head into left rotation by applying gentle pressure over the right zygomatic arch. Lateral flexion overpressure is then added by applying a downward force through the zygomatic arch. The trunk is stabilized by the right hand over the left scapula region.

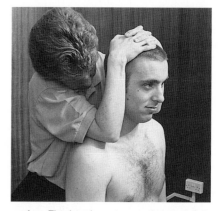

F Compression. The hands rest over the top of the patient's head and apply a downward force.

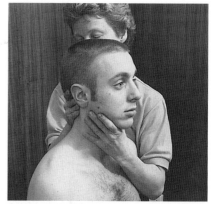

G Distraction. The left hand holds underneath the mandible while the right hand grasps underneath the occiput. Both hands then apply a force to lift the head upwards.

Figure 6.1 *Continued*

Table 6.2 Active physiological movements with possible modifications

Active movements	Modifications
Cervical spine	Repeated movements
Flexion	Speed altered
Extension	Movements combined (Edwards 1980, 1985, 1999), e.g.
L lateral flexion	– extension quadrant: extension, ipsilateral rotation and lateral flexion
R lateral flexion	– flexion then rotation
L rotation	– extension then rotation
R rotation	– flexion then lateral flexion then rotation (Fig. 6.2)
Compression	– extension then lateral flexion
Distraction	Compression or distraction sustained
Upper cervical extension/protraction (pro)	Injuring movement
Repetitive protraction (rep pro)	Differentiation tests
Repetitive flexion (rep flex)	Function
Upper cervical flexion/retraction (ret)	
Repetitive retraction (rep ret)	
Repetitive retraction and extension (rep ext)	
L repetitive lateral flexion (rep lat flex)	
R repetitive lateral flexion (rep lat flex)	
L repetitive rotation (rep rot)	
R repetitive rotation (rep rot)	
Retraction and extension lying supine	
Repetitive retraction and extension lying supine	
Static (maximum of 3 min) retraction and extension lying supine or prone	
?Temporomandibular	
?Shoulder	
?Elbow	
?Wrist and hand	

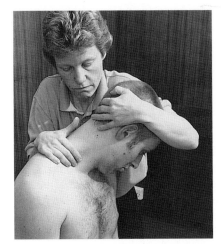

Figure 6.2 Combined movement to the cervical spine. The right hand supports the trunk while the left hand moves the head into flexion then lateral flexion then rotation.

ment deviation to determine its relevance to the patient's symptoms.

For the cervical spine the active movements and possible modifications are shown in Table 6.2. It is mentioning here the work of Robin McKenzie. If all movements are full and symptom-free on overpressure and symptoms are aggravated by certain postures, the condition is categorized as a postural syndrome. McKenzie (1990) suggests that maintaining certain postures that place some structures under prolonged stress will eventually produce symptoms. If on repeated movements there is no change in area of symptoms then the condition is categorized as a dysfunction syndrome (McKenzie 1990). If on repeated movements, peripheralization and centralization syndrome is manifested then this is characterized as a derangement syn-

Table 6.3   Derangement syndromes of the cervical spine (McKenzie 1990)

Derangement	Clinical presentation
1	Central or symmetrical pain around C5–C7 Rarely scapula or shoulder pain No deformity Extension limited Rapidly reversible
2	Central or symmetrical pain around C5–C7 With or without scapula, shoulder or upper arm pain Kyphotic deformity Extension limited Rarely rapidly reversible
3	Unilateral or asymmetrical pain around C3–C7 With or without scapula, shoulder or upper arm pain No deformity Extension, rotation and lateral flexion may be individually or collectively limited Rapidly reversible
4	Unilateral or asymmetrical pain around C5–C7 With or without scapula, shoulder or upper arm pain With deformity of torticollis Extension, rotation and lateral flexion limited Rapidly reversible
5	Unilateral or asymmetrical pain around C5–C7 With or without scapula or shoulder pain and with arm symptoms distal to the elbow No deformity Extension and ipsilateral lateral flexion limited Rapidly reversible
6	Unilateral or asymmetrical pain around C5–C7 With arm symptoms distal to the elbow with deformity – cervical kyphosis or torticollis Extension and ipsilateral lateral flexion limited With neurological motor deficit Not rapidly reversible
7	Symmetrical or asymmetrical pain around C4–C6 With or without anterior/anterolateral neck pain Dysphagia common No deformity Flexion limited Rapidly reversible

drome; there are seven types of derangement syndromes described (Table 6.3).

Numerous differentiation tests (Maitland et al 2001) can be performed; the choice depends on the patient's signs and symptoms. For example, when turning the head around to the left reproduces the patient's left-sided infrascapular pain, differentiation between the cervical and thoracic spine may be required. The clinician can increase and decrease the rotation at the cervical and thoracic regions to find out what effect this has on the infrascapular pain. The patient turns the head and trunk around to the left; the clinician maintains the position of the cervical spine and derotates the thoracic spine, noting the pain response. If symptoms remain the same or increase, this might suggest the cervical spine is the source of the symptoms. The position of cervical and thoracic

Table 6.4   Joint clearing tests

Joint	Physiological movement	Accessory movement
Thoracic spine	Rotation and quadrants	All movements
Temporomandibular joint	Open/close jaw, side to side movement, protraction/retraction	All movements
Shoulder girdle	Elevation, depression, protraction and retraction	
Shoulder joint	Flexion and hand behind back	
Acromioclavicular joint	All movements (particularly horizontal flexion)	
Sternoclavicular joint	All movements	
Elbow joint	All movements	
Wrist joint	Flexion/extension and radial/ulnar deviation	
Thumb	Extension carpometacarpal and thumb opposition	
Fingers	Flexion at interphalangeal joints and grip	

rotation is then resumed and this time the clinician maintains the position of the thoracic spine and derotates the cervical spine, noting the pain response. If the symptoms remain the same or increase, this implicates the thoracic spine, and this may be further tested by increasing the overpressure to the thoracic spine, which would be expected to increase the symptoms.

It may be necessary to examine other regions to determine their relevance to the patient's symptoms; they may be the source of the symptoms, or they may be contributing to the symptoms. The most likely regions are the temporomandibular, shoulder, elbow, wrist and hand. The joints within these regions can be tested fully (see relevant chapter) or partially with the use of clearing tests (Table 6.4).

Some functional ability has already been tested by the general observation of the patient during the subjective and physical examinations, e.g. the postures adopted during the subjective examination and the ease or difficulty of undressing prior to the examination. Any further functional testing can be carried out at this point in the examination and may include sitting postures, aggravating movements of the upper limb, etc. Clues for appropriate tests can be obtained from the subjective examination findings, particularly aggravating factors.

Capsular pattern.   The capsular pattern (Cyriax 1982) for the cervical spine is as follows: lateral flexion and rotation are equally limited, flexion is full but painful and extension is limited.

Passive physiological movements

This can take the form of passive physiological intervertebral movements (PPIVMs), which examine the movement at each segmental level. PPIVMs can be a useful adjunct to passive accessory intervertebral movements (PAIVMs) to identify segmental hypomobility and hypermobility. With the patient supine, the clinician palpates the gap between adjacent spinous processes and articular pillars to feel the range of intervertebral movement during flexion, extension, lateral flexion and rotation. Figure 6.3 demonstrates a rotation PPIVM at the C4/5 segmental level.

It may be necessary to examine other regions to determine their relevance to the patient's symptoms; they may be the source of the symptoms, or they may be contributing to the symptoms. The most likely regions are the temporomandibular, shoulder, elbow, wrist and hand.

Muscle tests

Muscle tests include those examining muscle strength, control, length and isometric muscle contraction.

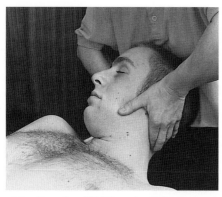

Figure 6.3   Rotation PPIVM at the C4/5 segmental level. The clinician places the index finger, reinforced by the middle finger, over the left C4/5 zygapophyseal joint and feels the opening up at this level as the head is passively rotated to the right.

Muscle strength

The clinician tests the cervical flexors, extensors, lateral flexors and rotators and any other relevant muscle groups. For details of these general tests readers are directed to Cole et al (1988), Hislop & Montgomery (1995) or Kendall et al (1993).

Greater detail may be required to test the strength of muscles, in particular those thought prone to become weak (Janda 1994, Sahrmann 2002); these include serratus anterior, subscapularis, middle and lower fibres of trapezius and the deep neck flexors. Testing the strength of these muscles is described in Chapter 3.

Muscle control

The relative strength of muscles is considered more important than the overall strength of a muscle group (Janda 1994, 2002, Sahrmann 2002). Relative strength is assessed indirectly by observing posture, as already mentioned, by the quality of active movement, noting any changes in muscle recruitment patterns, and by palpating muscle activity in various positions.

Weak deep neck flexors have been found to be associated with cervicogenic headaches (Watson 1994). These muscles are tested by the clinician observing the pattern of movement that occurs when the patient flexes his/her head from a supine position. When the deep neck flexors are

weak, the sternocleidomastoid initiates the movement, causing the jaw to lead the movement, and the upper cervical spine hyperextends. After about 10° of head elevation, the cervical spine then curls up into flexion. A pressure biofeedback unit (PBU, Chattanooga, Australia) can be used to measure the function of the deep neck flexors more objectively (Jull 1994). The patient lies supine with a towel under the head to position the cervical spine in neutral. The PBU is placed under the cervical spine and inflated to around 20 mmHg (see Fig. 5.10). The patient then is asked to tuck in the chin, which will normally increase the pressure by 6–10 mmHg. Normal function of the deep neck flexors is the ability to hold this contraction for 10 seconds and repeat the contraction 10 times (Jull, personal communication, 1999).

Muscle imbalance around the scapula has been described by a number of workers (Janda 1994, 2002, Jull & Janda 1987) and can be assessed by observation of upper limb movements. For example, the clinician can observe the patient performing a slow push-up from the prone position. Any excessive or abnormal movement of the scapula is noted; muscle weakness may cause the scapula to rotate and glide laterally and/or move superiorly. Serratus anterior weakness, for example, will cause the scapula to wing (the medial border moves away from the thorax). Another movement that can be useful to analyse is shoulder abduction performed slowly, with the patient in sitting and the elbow flexed. Once again, the clinician observes the quality of movement of the shoulder joint and scapula and notes any abnormal or excessive movement.

Muscle length

The clinician tests the length of muscles, in particular those thought prone to shorten (Janda 1994); that is: levator scapula, upper trapezius, sternocleidomastoid, pectoralis major and minor, scalenes and the deep occipital muscles. Testing the length of these muscles is described in Chapter 3.

Isometric muscle testing

Test neck flexors, extensors, lateral flexors and rotators in resting position and, if indicated, in different parts of the physiological range. In addition the clinician observes the quality of the muscle contraction to hold this position (this can be done with the patient's eyes shut). The patient may, for example, be unable to prevent the joint from moving or may hold with excessive muscle activity; either of these circumstances would suggest a neuromuscular dysfunction.

Neurological tests

Neurological examination includes neurological integrity testing, neurodynamic tests and some other nerve tests.

Integrity of nervous system

As a general guide, a neurological examination is indicated if symptoms are felt below the acromion.

Dermatomes/peripheral nerves.   Light touch and pain sensation of the upper limb are tested using cotton wool and pinprick respectively, as described in Chapter 3. Knowledge of the cutaneous distribution of nerve roots (dermatomes) and peripheral nerves enables the clinician to distinguish the sensory loss due to a root lesion from that due to a peripheral nerve lesion. The cutaneous nerve distribution and dermatome areas are shown in Figures 3.18–3.20.

Myotomes/peripheral nerves. The following myotomes are tested and are shown in Figure 3.26:

- C4: shoulder girdle elevation
- C5: shoulder abduction
- C6: elbow flexion
- C7: elbow extension
- C8: thumb extension
- T1: finger adduction.

A working knowledge of the muscular distribution of nerve roots (myotomes) and peripheral nerves enables the clinician to distinguish the motor loss due to a root lesion from that due to a peripheral nerve lesion. The peripheral nerve distributions are shown in Figures 3.23 and 3.24.

Reflex testing.   The following deep tendon reflexes are tested (see also Fig. 3.28):

- C5–C6: biceps
- C7: triceps and brachioradialis.

Neurodynamic tests

The following neurodynamic tests may be carried out in order to ascertain the degree to which neural tissue is responsible for the production of the patient's symptom(s):

- Passive neck flexion (PNF)
- Upper limb tension tests (ULTT)
- Straight leg raise (SLR)
- Slump.

These tests are described in detail in Chapter 3.

Other nerve tests

Plantar response to test for an upper motor neurone lesion (Walton 1989).   Pressure applied from the heel along the lateral border of the plantar aspect of the foot produces flexion of the toes in the normal. Extension of the big toe with downward fanning of the other toes occurs with an upper motor neurone lesion.

Tinel's sign.   The clinician taps the skin overlying the brachial plexus. Reproduction of distal pain/paraesthesia denotes a positive test indicating regeneration of an injured sensory nerve (Walton 1989).

Miscellaneous tests

In the case of the cervicothoracic spine, these are *vascular tests*.

Vertebrobasilar insufficiency test

Minimum testing is sustained cervical rotation to the end of range to both left and right sides, and the position or movement that provokes the symptoms, as described by the patient (Magarey et al 2000). The movements are active and each position is maintained by the clinician giving gentle overpressure for a minimum of 10 seconds. The patient keeps their eyes open and the clinician observes for nystagmus. The movement is then released for 10 seconds before the next movement is carried out. If dizziness, nausea or any other symptom associated with vertebrobasilar insufficiency (disturbance in vision, diplopia, nausea, ataxia, 'drop attacks', impairment of trigeminal sensation, sympathoplegia, dysarthria, hemianaesthesia and hemiplegia) (Bogduk 1994) is provoked during any part of the test, it is considered positive and testing is stopped. If the test is positive, manipulation of the cervical spine is contraindicated. Further testing can be performed for patients who present with dizziness and include other cervical movements, namely extension, combined movement of extension with rotation and quick movements.

Differentiation between dizziness produced from the vestibular apparatus of the inner ear and that from the neck movement (due to cervical vertigo or compromised vertebral artery) may be required. In standing, the clinician maintains head position while the patient moves the trunk to produce cervical rotation. Rotation to left and right is each held for at least 10 seconds, with at least a 10-second rest period between directions. The test is completed with repetitive trunk rotation movements to left and right (Magarey et al 2000). The test is considered positive and stopped immediately if dizziness, nausea or any other symptom associated with VBI is provoked, which suggests that the patient's symptoms are not caused by a disturbance of the vestibular system. A positive vertebral artery test contraindicates certain treatment techniques to the cervical spine (Table 2.4).

Further information on vertebrobasilar insufficiency can be found in Refshauge & Gass (2004).

Palpation of pulses. If the circulation is suspected of being compromised, the clinician palpates the pulses of the carotid, facial and temporal arteries.

Test for thoracic outlet syndrome. There are several tests for this syndrome, which are described in Chapter 8.

Palpation

The clinician palpates the cervicothoracic spine and, if appropriate, the patient's upper cervical spine, lower thoracic spine and any other relevant areas. It is useful to record palpation findings on a body chart (see Fig. 2.3) and/or palpation chart (see Fig. 3.38).

The clinician should note the following:

- The temperature of the area
- Increased skin moisture
- The presence of oedema or effusion
- Mobility and feel of superficial tissues, e.g. ganglions, nodules
- The presence or elicitation of any muscle spasm
- Tenderness of bone, ligaments, muscle, tendon, tendon sheath, trigger points (shown in Fig. 3.39) and nerve; palpable nerves in the upper limb are as follows:
  - The suprascapular nerve can be palpated along the superior border of the scapula in the suprascapular notch
  - The brachial plexus can be palpated in the posterior triangle of the neck; it emerges at the lower third of sternocleidomastoid
  - The suprascapular nerve can be palpated along the superior border of the scapula in the suprascapular notch
  - The dorsal scapular nerve can be palpated medial to the medial border of the scapula
  - The median nerve can be palpated over the anterior elbow joint crease, medial to the biceps tendon, also at the wrist between palmaris longus and flexor carpi radialis
  - The radial nerve can be palpated around the spiral groove of the humerus, between brachioradialis and flexor carpi radialis, in the forearm and also at the wrist in the snuffbox
- Increased or decreased prominence of bones
- Symptoms (often pain) provoked or reduced on palpation.

Passive accessory intervertebral movements (PAIVMs)

It is useful to use the palpation chart and movement diagrams (or joint pictures) to record findings. These are explained in detail in Chapter 3.

The clinician should note the following:

- Quality of movement
- Range of movement

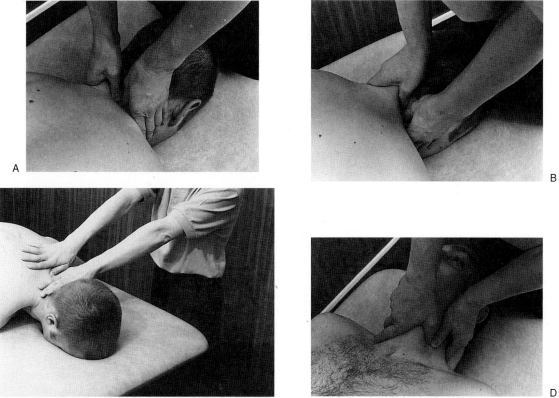

Figure 6.4   Cervical accessory movements. A Central posteroanterior. Thumb pressure is applied to the spinous process. B Unilateral posteroanterior. Thumb pressure is applied to the articular pillar. C Transverse. Thumb pressure is applied to the lateral aspect of spinous process. D Unilateral anteroposterior. In the supine position, thumb pressure is applied to the anterior aspect of the transverse process.

- Resistance through the range and at the end of the range of movement
- Behaviour of pain through the range
- Provocation of any muscle spasm.

The cervical and upper thoracic spine (C2–T4) accessory movements are shown in Figure 6.4 and are listed in Table 6.5.

Following accessory movements to the cervicothoracic region, the clinician reassesses all the physical asterisks (movements or tests that have been found to reproduce the patient's symptoms), in order to establish the effect of the accessory movements on the patient's signs and symptoms. Accessory movements can then be tested for other regions suspected to be a source of, or contributing to, the patient's symptoms. Again, following accessory movements to any one region, the clin-

ician reassesses all the asterisks. Regions likely to be examined are the upper cervical spine, lower thoracic spine, shoulder, elbow, wrist and hand (Table 6.4).

Natural apophyseal glides (NAGs)

These can be applied to the apophyseal joints between C2 and T3. The patient sits and the clinician supports the patient's head and neck and applies a static or oscillatory force to the spinous process or articular pillar in the direction of the facet joint plane of each vertebra (Mulligan 1999). Figure 6.6 demonstrates a unilateral NAG on C6. This is repeated six to ten times. The patient should feel no pain, but may feel slight discomfort. The technique aims to facilitate the glide of

Table 6.5   Accessory movements, choice of application and reassessment of the patient's asterisks

Accessory movements		Choice of application	Identify any effect of accessory movements on patient's signs and symptoms
C2–T4		Alter speed of force application start position, e.g.	Reassess all asterisks
↕	central posteroanterior		
⌐° °⌐ ↓	unilateral posteroanterior	– in flexion	
◄•►	transverse	– in extension	
↳° °↲	unilateral anteroposterior (C2–T1 only)	– in lateral flexion (Fig. 6.5)	
Ribs 1–4 (see Fig. 7.8)		– in flexion and rotation	
◄••► Caud	longitudinal caudad 1st rib	– in flexion and lateral flexion	
↕	anteroposterior	– in extension and rotation	
↓	posteroanterior	– in extension and lateral flexion	
--•► Med	medial glide	Direction of the applied force	
		Point of application of applied force	
Upper cervical spine		As above	Reassess all asterisks
Lower thoracic spine		As above	Reassess all asterisks
Shoulder region		As above	Reassess all asterisks
Elbow region As above		Reassess all asterisks	
Wrist and hand		As above	Reassess all asterisks

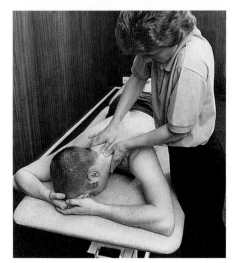

Figure 6.5   Palpation of accessory movements using a combined movement. Thumb pressure over the left articular pillar of C5 is carried out with the cervical spine positioned in right lateral flexion.

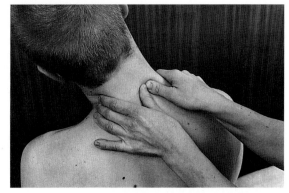

Figure 6.6   Unilateral NAG on C6. Thumb pressure is applied to the right articular pillar of C6 (in the line of the facet joint plane) as the patient laterally flexes to the left.

Reversed natural apophyseal glides (reversed NAGs)

The patient sits and the clinician supports the head and neck and applies a force to the articular pillars of a vertebra using the index and thumb of a fisted hand (Fig. 6.7). A force is then applied to the pillars in the direction of the facet plane in order to facilitate the glide of the superior facet upwards and

the inferior facet of the vertebra upwards and forwards on the vertebra below. In the example given, if the C6 NAG on the right reduces pain on left lateral flexion it suggests the symptomatic joint is the right C6–C7 apophyseal joint.

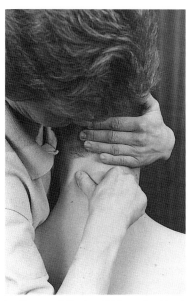

Figure 6.7 Reversed flexion NAG to C4. The left hand supports the head and neck. The index and thumb of the fisted right hand apply an anterior force to the articular pillars of C4 in the direction of the facet plane.

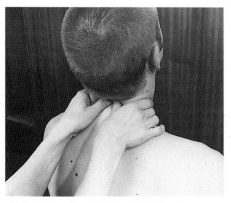

Figure 6.8 Extension SNAG to C5. Thumb pressure is applied to the spinous process of C5, in the direction of the facet plane, as the patient slowly extends.

forwards on the inferior facet of the vertebra above. If a reversed NAG to C4 reduces the patient's pain on extension, for example, this would suggest that the symptomatic level is C3–C4.

Sustained natural apophyseal glides (SNAGs)

The painful cervical spine movements are examined in sitting. The clinician applies a force to the spinous process and/or transverse process in the direction of the facet joint plane of each cervical vertebra as the patient moves slowly towards the pain. All cervical movements can be tested in this way. Figure 6.8 demonstrates a C5 extension SNAG. The technique aims to facilitate the glide of the inferior facet of the vertebra upwards and forwards on the vertebra below. In the above example, if the C5 SNAG reduces the pain it suggests that the symptomatic level is C5–C6. For further details on these techniques, see Chapter 3 and Mulligan (1999).

COMPLETION OF THE EXAMINATION

Having carried out the above tests, the examination of the cervical spine is now complete. The subjective and physical examinations produce a large amount of information, which needs to be recorded accurately and quickly. An outline examination chart may be useful for some clinicians and one is suggested in Figure 6.9. It is important, however, that the clinician does not examine in a rigid manner, simply following the suggested sequence outlined in the chart. Each patient presents differently and this needs to be reflected in the examination process. It is vital at this stage to highlight with an asterisk (*) important findings from the examination. These findings must be reassessed at, and within, subsequent treatment sessions to evaluate the effects of treatment on the patient's condition.

The physical testing procedures which specifically indicate joint, nerve or muscle tissues, as a source of the patient's symptoms, are summarized in Table 3.10. The strongest evidence that a joint is the source of the patient's symptoms is that active and passive physiological movements, passive accessory movements and joint palpation all reproduce the patient's symptoms, and that following a treatment dose, reassessment identifies an improvement in the patient's signs and symptoms. Weaker evidence includes an alteration in range, resistance or quality of physiological and/or accessory movements and tenderness over the joint, with no alteration in signs and symptoms after treatment. One or more of these findings may indicate a dysfunction of a joint which may or may not be contributing to the patient's condition.

Body chart	Name
	Age
	Date
	24-hour behaviour
	Improving static worsening
	Special questions General health Weight loss RA Drugs Steroids Anticoagulants X-ray Cord symptoms Cauda equina symptoms VBI symptoms
Relationship of symptoms	
Aggravating factors and function	HPC
	PMH
Severe Irritable	
Easing factors	SH & FH (Patient's perspective, experience, expectations. Yellow, blue, black flags)

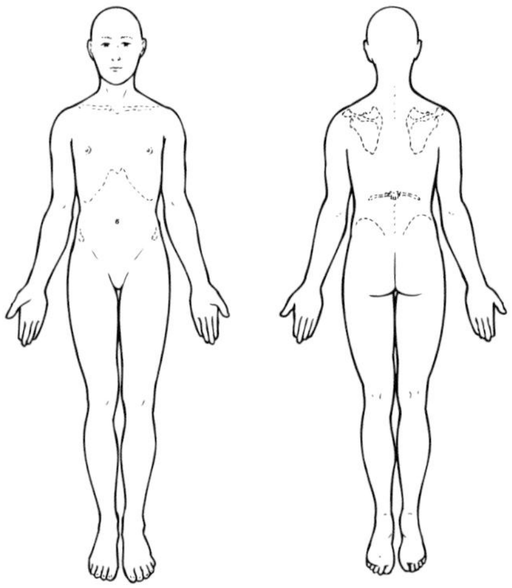

Figure 6.9   Cervicothoracic spine examination chart.

Physical examination	Isometric muscle testing
Observation	
	Neurological integrity tests
Active and passive physiological movements for cervicothoracic spine and other relevant regions	
	Neurodynamic tests
	Other nerve tests (plantar response, Tinel's sign)
	Miscellaneous tests (VBI testing, pulses, thoracic outlet tests)
Capsular pattern yes/no	Palpation
Muscle strength	
Muscle control	Accessory movements and reassessment of each relevant region
Muscle length	

Figure 6.9 *Continued*

The strongest evidence that a muscle is the source of a patient's symptoms is if active movements, an isometric contraction, passive lengthening and palpation of a muscle all reproduce the patient's symptoms, and that following a treatment dose, reassessment identifies an improvement in the patient's signs and symptoms. Further evidence of muscle dysfunction may be suggested by reduced strength or poor quality during the active physiological movement and the isometric contraction, reduced range, and/or increased/decreased resistance, during the passive lengthening of the muscle, and tenderness on palpation, with no alteration in signs and symptoms after treatment. One or more of these findings may indicate a dysfunction of a muscle which may or may not be contributing to the patient's condition.

The strongest evidence that a nerve is the source of the patient's symptoms is when active and/or passive physiological movements reproduce the patient's symptoms, which are then increased or decreased with an additional sensitizing movement, at a distance from the patient's symptoms. In addition, there is reproduction of the patient's symptoms on palpation of the nerve and neurodynamic testing, sufficient to be considered a treatment dose, results in an improvement in the above signs and symptoms. Further evidence of nerve dysfunction may be suggested by reduced range (compared to the asymptomatic side) and/or increased resistance to the various arm movements, and tenderness on nerve palpation.

On completion of the physical examination the clinician:

- Warns the patient of possible exacerbation up to 24–48 hours following the examination.
- Requests the patient to report details on the behaviour of the symptoms following examination at the next attendance.

- Explains the findings of the physical examination and how these findings relate to the subjective assessment. An attempt should be made to clear up any misconceptions patients may have regarding their illness or injury.
- Evaluates the findings, formulates a clinical diagnosis and writes up a problem list. Clinicians may find the management planning forms shown in Figures 3.53 and 3.54 helpful in guiding them through what is often a complex clinical reasoning process.
- Determines the objectives of treatment.
- Devises an initial treatment plan.

In this way, the clinician develops the following hypotheses categories (adapted from Jones & Rivett 2004):

- Function: abilities and restrictions.
- Patients' perspectives on their experience.
- Source of symptoms. This includes the structure or tissue that is thought to be producing the patients' symptoms, the nature of the structure or tissues in relation to the healing process, and the pain mechanisms involved.
- Contributing factors to the development and maintenance of the problem. There may be environmental, psychosocial, behavioural, physical or heredity factors.
- Precautions/contraindications to treatment and management. This includes the severity and irritability of the patient's symptoms and the nature of the patient's condition.
- Management strategy and treatment plan.
- Prognosis – this can be affected by factors such as the stage and extent of the injury as well as the patient's expectation, personality and lifestyle.

References

Barker S, Kesson M, Ashmore J, Turner G, Conway J, Stevens D 2000 Guidance for pre-manipulative testing of the cervical spine. Manual Therapy 5(1): 37–40

Bogduk N 1994 Cervical causes of headache and dizziness. In: Boyling J D, Palastanga N (eds) Grieve's modern manual therapy, 2nd edn. Churchill Livingstone, Edinburgh, ch 22, p 317

Clinical Standards Advisory Report 1994 Report of a CSAG committee on back pain. HMSO, London

Cole J H, Furness A L, Twomey L T 1988 Muscles in action, an approach to manual muscle testing. Churchill Livingstone, Edinburgh

Cyriax J 1982 Textbook of orthopaedic medicine – diagnosis of soft tissue lesions, 8th edn. Baillière Tindall, London

Dahlberg C, Lanig I S, Kenna M, Long S 1997 Diagnosis and treatment of esophageal perforations in cervical spinal cord injury. Topics in Spinal Cord Injury Rehabilitation 2(3): 41–48

Edwards B C 1980 Combined movements in the cervical spine (C2–7): their value in examination and technique choice. Australian Journal of Physiotherapy 26(5): 165–169

Edwards B C 1985 Combined movements in the cervical spine (their use in establishing movement patterns). In: Glasgow E F, Twomey L T, Scull E R, Kleynhans A M, Idczak R M (eds) Aspects of manipulative therapy. Churchill Livingstone, Melbourne, ch 19, p 128

Edwards B C 1999 Manual of combined movements: their use in the examination and treatment of mechanical vertebral column disorders, 2nd edn. Butterworth-Heinemann, Oxford

Grieve G P 1994 Counterfeit clinical presentations. Manipulative Physiotherapist 26: 17–19

Hislop H, Montgomery J 1995 Daniels and Worthingham's muscle testing, techniques of manual examination, 7th edn. W B Saunders, Philadelphia

Janda V 1994 Muscles and motor control in cervicogenic disorders: assessment and management. In: Grant R (ed) Physical therapy of the cervical and thoracic spine, 2nd edn. Churchill Livingstone, New York, ch 10, p 195

Janda V 2002 Muscles and motor control in cervicogenic disorders. In: Grant R (ed) Physical therapy of the cervical and thoracic spine, 3rd edn. Churchill Livingstone, New York, ch 10, p 182

Jones M A, Rivett D A 2004 Clinical reasoning for manual therapists. Butterworth-Heinemann, Edinburgh

Jull G A 1994 Headaches of cervical origin. In: Grant R (ed) Physical therapy of the cervical and thoracic spine, 2nd edn. Churchill Livingstone, New York, ch 13, p 261

Jull G A, Janda V 1987 Muscles and motor control in low back pain: assessment and management. In: Twomey L T, Taylor J R (eds) Physical therapy of the low back. Churchill Livingstone, New York, ch 10, p 253

Kendall F P, McCreary E K, Provance P G 1993 Muscles testing and function, 4th edn. Williams & Wilkins, Baltimore, MD

McKenzie R A 1990 The cervical and thoracic spine: mechanical diagnosis and therapy. Spinal Publications, New Zealand

Magarey M, Coughlan B, Rebbeck T 2000 APA pre-manipulative testing protocol for the cervical spine: researched and renewed, part 2 – revised clinical guidelines. International Federation of Orthopaedic Manipulative Therapists, Perth

Maitland G D, Hengeveld E, Banks K, English K 2001 Maitland's vertebral manipulation, 6th edn. Butterworth-Heinemann, Oxford

Mulligan B R 1999 Manual therapy 'NAGs', 'SNAGs', 'MWMs' etc., 4th edn. Plane View Services, New Zealand

Refshauge K, Gass E (eds) 2004 Musculoskeletal physiotherapy clinical science and evidence-based practice. Butterworth-Heinemann, Oxford

Sahrmann S A 2002 Diagnosis and treatment of movement impairment syndromes. Mosby, St Louis

Waddell G 2004 The back pain revolution, 2nd edn. Churchill Livingstone, Edinburgh

Walton J H 1989 Essentials of neurology, 6th edn. Churchill Livingstone, Edinburgh

Watson D H 1994 Cervical headache: an investigation of natural head posture and upper cervical flexor muscle performance. In: Boyling J D, Palastanga N (eds) Grieve's modern manual therapy, 2nd edn. Churchill Livingstone, Edinburgh, ch 24, p 349

Chapter **7**

Examination of the thoracic spine

POSSIBLE CAUSES OF PAIN AND/OR LIMITATION OF MOVEMENT

- Trauma
  - Fracture of spinous process, transverse process, vertebral arch or vertebral body; fracture dislocation
  - Ligamentous sprain
  - Muscular strain
- Degenerative conditions
  - Spondylosis: degeneration of the intervertebral disc
  - Arthrosis: degeneration of the zygapophyseal joints
  - Scheuermann's disease
- Inflammatory: ankylosing spondylitis
- Metabolic
  - Osteoporosis
  - Paget's disease
  - Osteomalacia
- Infections
  - Tuberculosis of the spine
- Tumours, benign and malignant
- Syndromes
  - T4 syndrome
  - Thoracic outlet syndrome
- Postural thoracic pain
- Referral of symptoms from the cervical or lumbar spine or from the viscera (such as the gall bladder, heart, spleen, lung and pleura).

The thoracic spine examination is appropriate for patients with symptoms in the spine or thorax between T3 and T10. This region includes the intervertebral joints between T3 and T10 as well as the costovertebral, costotransverse, sternocostal, costochondral and interchondral joints with their surrounding soft tissues.

To test the upper thoracic spine above T4, it is more appropriate to carry out an adapted cervical spine examination. Similarly, to test the lower thoracic spine below T9, it is more appropriate to carry out an adapted lumbar spine examination.

Further details of the questions asked during the subjective examination and the tests carried out in the physical examination can be found in Chapters 2 and 3 respectively.

The order of the subjective questioning and the physical tests described below can be altered as appropriate for the patient being examined.

SUBJECTIVE EXAMINATION

Body chart

The following information concerning the type and area of current symptoms can be recorded on a body chart (see Fig. 2.3).

Area of current symptoms

Be exact when mapping out the area of the symptoms. The area of symptoms may follow the course of a rib or it may run horizontally across the chest; symptoms may be felt posteriorly over the thoracic spine and anteriorly over the sternum. The clinician needs to be aware that the cervical spine (between C3 and C7), intervertebral discs and their surrounding ligaments can refer pain to the scapula and upper arm (Cloward 1959). The upper thoracic spine can refer symptoms to the upper limbs, and the lower thoracic spine to the lower limbs. Ascertain which is the worst symptom and record where the patient feels the symptoms are coming from.

Areas relevant to the region being examined

All other relevant areas are checked for symptoms; it is important to ask about pain or even stiffness, as this may be relevant to the patient's main symptom. Mark unaffected areas with ticks (✓) on the body chart. Check for symptoms in the cervical spine and upper limbs if it is an upper thoracic problem, or in the lumbar spine and lower limbs if it is a lower thoracic problem. If the patient has symptoms that may emanate from the cervical spine, ask whether there is any dizziness. Further questions about dizziness and testing for vertebrobasilar insufficiency are described more fully in Chapter 6.

Quality of pain

Establish the quality of the pain.

Intensity of pain

The intensity of pain can be measured using, for example, a visual analogue scale (VAS) as shown in Figure 2.8. A pain diary may be useful for patients with chronic thoracic pain to determine the pain patterns and triggering factors over a period of time.

Depth of pain

Establish the depth of the pain. Does the patient feel it is on the surface or deep inside?

Abnormal sensation

Check for any altered sensation over the thoracic spine, rib cage and other relevant areas.

Constant or intermittent symptoms

Ascertain the frequency of the symptoms, whether they are constant or intermittent. If symptoms are constant, check whether there is variation in the intensity of the symptoms, as constant unremitting pain may be indicative of neoplastic disease.

Relationship of symptoms

Determine the relationship between the symptomatic areas – do they come together or separately? For example, the patient could have shoulder pain without thoracic spine pain, or they may always be present together.

Behaviour of symptoms

Aggravating factors

For each symptomatic area, discover what movements and/or positions aggravate the patient's symptoms, i.e. what brings them on (or makes them worse), are they able to maintain this position or movement (severity), what happens to other symptom(s) when this symptom is produced (or is made worse), and how long does it take for symptoms to ease once the position or movement is stopped (irritability). These questions help to confirm the relationship between the symptoms.

The clinician also asks the patient about theoretically known aggravating factors for structures that could be a source of the symptoms. Common aggravating factors for the thoracic spine are rotation of the thorax and deep breathing. Aggravating factors for other regions, which may need to be queried if they are suspected to be a source of the symptoms, are shown in Table 2.3.

The clinician ascertains how the symptoms affect function, such as: static and active postures, e.g. sitting, standing, lying, washing, ironing, dusting, driving (and reversing the car, which requires trunk rotation), reading, writing, work, sport and social activities. Note details of training regimen for any sports activities. The clinician finds out if the patient is left- or right-handed as there may be increased stress on the dominant side.

Detailed information on each of the above activities is useful in order to help determine the structure(s) at fault and identify functional restrictions. This information can be used to determine the aims of treatment and any advice that may be required. The most notable functional restrictions are highlighted with asterisks (*), explored in the physical examination, and reassessed at subsequent treatment sessions to evaluate treatment intervention.

Easing factors

For each symptomatic area, the clinician asks what movements and/or positions ease the patient's symptoms, how long it takes to ease them and what happens to other symptom(s) when this symptom is relieved. These questions help to confirm the relationship between the symptoms.

The clinician asks the patient about theoretically known easing factors for structures that could be a source of the symptoms. For example, symptoms from the thoracic spine may be eased by thoracic extension, whereas symptoms arising from the cervical spine may be eased by supporting the head. The clinician can then analyse the position or movement that eases the symptoms to help determine the structure at fault.

Twenty-four-hour behaviour of symptoms

The clinician determines the 24-hour behaviour of symptoms by asking questions about night, morning and evening symptoms.

Night symptoms. The following questions may be asked:

- Do you have any difficulty getting to sleep?
- What position is most comfortable/uncomfortable?
- What is your normal sleeping position?
- What is your present sleeping position?
- Do your symptom(s) wake you at night? If so,
  - Which symptom(s)?
  - How many times in the past week?
  - How many times in a night?
  - How long does it take to get back to sleep?
- How many and what type of pillows are used?
- Is your mattress firm or soft and has it been changed recently?

Morning and evening symptoms. The clinician determines the pattern of the symptoms first thing in the morning, through the day and at the end of the day. Stiffness in the morning for the first few minutes might suggest spondylosis; stiffness and pain for a few hours are suggestive of an inflammatory process such as ankylosing spondylitis.

Stage of the condition

In order to determine the stage of the condition, the clinician asks whether the symptoms are getting better, getting worse or remaining unchanged.

Special questions

Special questions must always be asked, as they may identify certain precautions or contraindications to the physical examination and/or treatment (Table 2.4). As mentioned in Chapter 2, the clinician must differentiate between conditions that are suitable for conservative management and systemic, neoplastic and other non-neuromuscloskeletal conditions, which require referral to a medical practitioner. The reader is referred to Appendix 2.3 for details of various serious pathological processes that can mimic neuromuscloskeletal conditions (Grieve 1994).

The following information is routinely obtained from patients.

General health. The clinician ascertains the state of the patient's general health to find out if the patient suffers from any cough, breathlessness, chest pain, malaise, fatigue, fever, nausea or vomiting, stress, anxiety or depression.

Weight loss. Has the patient noticed any recent unexplained weight loss?

Rheumatoid arthritis. Has the patient (or a member of his/her family) been diagnosed as having rheumatoid arthritis?

Drug therapy. What drugs are being taken by the patient? Has the patient been prescribed long-term (6 months or more) medication/steroids? Has the patient been taking anticoagulants recently?

X-ray and medical imaging. Has the patient been X-rayed or had any other medical tests recently? Routine spinal X-rays are no longer considered necessary prior to conservative treatment as they only identify the normal age-related degenerative changes, which do not necessarily correlate with the patient's symptoms (Clinical Standards Advisory Report 1994). The medical tests may include blood tests, magnetic resonance imaging, myelography, discography or a bone scan.

Neurological symptoms. Has the patient experienced symptoms of spinal cord compression which are bilateral tingling in hands or feet and/or disturbance of gait?

Vertebrobasilar insufficiency (VBI). For symptoms emanating from the cervical spine, the clinician should ask about symptoms that may be caused by vertebrobasilar insufficiency. VBI symptoms include: dizziness (most commonly), altered vision (including diplopia), nausea, ataxia, drop attacks, altered facial sensation, difficulty speaking, difficulty swallowing, sympathoplegia, hemianaesthesia and hemiplegia (Bogduk 1994). If present, the clinician determines the aggravating and easing factors in the usual way. These symptoms can also be due to upper cervical instability and diseases of the inner ear.

History of the present condition (HPC)

For each symptomatic area, the clinician needs to know how long the symptom has been present, whether there was a sudden or slow onset and whether there was a known cause that provoked the onset of the symptom. If the onset was slow, the clinician finds out if there has been any change in the patient's lifestyle, e.g. a new job or hobby or a change in sporting activity, which may have affected the stresses on the thoracic spine and related areas. To confirm the relationship between symptoms, the clinician asks what happened to other symptoms when each symptom began.

Past medical history (PMH)

The following information is obtained from the patient and/or the medical notes:

- The details of any relevant medical history.
- The history of any previous attacks: how many episodes, when were they, what was the cause, what was the duration of each episode and did the patient fully recover between episodes? If there have been no previous attacks, has the patient had any episodes of stiffness in the cervical, thoracic or lumbar spine or any other relevant region? Check for a history of trauma or recurrent minor trauma.
- Ascertain the results of any past treatment for the same or similar problem. Past treatment records may be obtained for further information.

Social and family history (SH, FH)

Social and family history that is relevant to the onset and progression of the patient's problem is recorded. This includes the patient's perspectives, experience and expectations, their age, employment, home situation, and details of any leisure activities. Factors from this information may indicate direct and/or indirect mechanical influences on the thoracic spine. In order to treat the patient appropriately, it is important that the condition is managed within the context of the patient's social and work environment.

The clinician may ask the following types of questions to elucidate psychosocial factors:

- Have you had time off work in the past with your pain?
- What do you understand to be the cause of your pain?
- What are you expecting will help you?
- How is your employer/co-workers/family responding to your pain?
- What are you doing to cope with your pain?
- Do you think you will return to work? When?

While these questions are described in relation to psychosocial risk factors for poor outcomes for patients with low back pain (Waddell 2004), they may be relevant to other patients.

Plan of the physical examination

When all this information has been collected, the subjective examination is complete. It is useful at this stage to highlight with asterisks (*), for ease of reference, important findings and particularly one or more functional restrictions. These can then be re-examined at subsequent treatment sessions to evaluate treatment intervention.

In order to plan the physical examination, the following hypotheses should be developed from the subjective examination:

- The regions and structures that need to be examined as a possible cause of the symptoms, e.g. thoracic spine, cervical spine, lumbar spine, upper limb joints, lower limb joints, muscles and nerves. Often, it is not possible to examine fully at the first attendance and so examination of the structures must be prioritized over subsequent treatment sessions.
- Other factors that need to be examined, e.g. working and everyday postures, vertebral artery, muscle weakness.
- In what way should the physical tests be carried out? Will it be easy or hard to reproduce each symptom? Will it be necessary to use combined movements, repetitive movements, etc. to reproduce the patient's symptoms? Are symptom(s) severe and/or irritable? If symptoms are severe, physical tests may be carried out to just before the onset of symptom production or just to the onset of symptom production; no overpressures will be carried out, as the patient would be unable to tolerate this. If symptoms are irritable, physical tests may be examined to just before symptom production or just to the onset of provocation with less physical tests being examined to allow for rest period between tests.

Are there any precautions and/or contraindications to elements of the physical examination that need to be explored further, such vertebrobasilar insufficiency, neurological involvement, recent fracture, trauma, steroid therapy or rheumatoid arthritis; there may also be certain contraindications to further examination and treatment, e.g. symptoms of cord compression.

A physical planning form can be useful for clinicians to help guide them through the clinical reasoning process (see Fig. 2.10 and Appendix 2.1).

PHYSICAL EXAMINATION

The information from the subjective examination helps the clinician to plan an appropriate physical examination. The severity, irritability and nature of the condition are the major factors that will influence the choice and priority of physical testing procedures. The first and over-arching question the clinician might ask is: 'is this patient's condition suitable for me to manage as a therapist?' For example, a patient presenting with cauda equina compression symptoms may only need neurological integrity testing, prior to an urgent medical referral. The nature of the patient's condition has had a major impact on the physical examination. The second question the clinician might ask is: 'does this patient have a neuromusculoskeletal dysfunction that I may be able to help?' To answer that, the clinician needs to carry out a full physical examination; however, this may not be possible if the symptoms are severe and/or irritable. If the patient's symptoms are severe and/or irritable, the clinician aims to explore movements as much as possible, within a symptom-free range. If the patient has constant and severe and/or irritable symptoms, then the clinician aims to find physical tests that ease the symptoms. If the patient's symptoms are non-severe and non-irritable, then the clinician aims to find physical tests that reproduce each of the patient's symptoms.

Each significant physical test that either provokes or eases the patient's symptoms is highlighted in the patient's notes by an asterisk (*) for easy reference. The highlighted tests are often referred to as 'asterisks' or 'markers'.

The order and detail of the physical tests described below should be appropriate to the patient being examined; some tests will be irrelevant, some tests will be carried out briefly, while it will be necessary to fully investigate others. It is important that readers understand that the techniques shown in this chapter are only some of many; the choice depends mainly on the relative size of the clinician and patient, as well as the clinician's preference. For this reason, novice clinicians may initially want to copy what is shown, but then quickly adapt to what is best for them.

Observation

Informal observation

The clinician should observe the patient in dynamic and static situations; the quality of movement is noted, as are the postural characteristics and facial expression. Informal observation will have begun from the moment the clinician begins the subjective examination and will continue to the end of the physical examination.

Formal observation

Observation of posture. The clinician examines the spinal posture of the patient in sitting and standing, noting the level of the pelvis, scoliosis, kyphosis or lordosis and the posture of the upper and lower limbs. Typical postures include the following and are described in more detail in Chapter 3 and in Figures 3.2–3.8:

- Shoulder crossed syndrome (Janda 1994, 2002)
- Lower (or pelvic) crossed syndrome (Jull & Janda 1987) or the kyphosis-lordosis posture (Kendall et al 1993)
- Layer syndrome (Jull & Janda 1987)
- Flat back (Kendall et al 1993)
- Sway back (Kendall et al 1993)
- Handedness pattern (Kendall et al 1993).

The clinician passively corrects any asymmetry to determine its relevance to the patient's problem. In addition, the clinician observes for any chest deformity, such as pigeon chest, where the sternum lies forward and downwards, funnel chest, where the sternum lies posteriorly (which may be associated with an increased thoracic kyphosis), or barrel chest, where the sternum lies forward and upwards (associated with emphysema) (Magee 1997). The clinician notes the movement of the rib cage during quiet respiration.

Observation of muscle form. The clinician observes the muscle bulk and muscle tone of the patient, comparing left and right sides. It must be remembered that handedness and level and frequency of physical activity may well produce differences in muscle bulk between sides. Some muscles are thought to shorten under stress, while other muscles weaken, producing muscle imbalance (see Table 3.2). Patterns of muscle imbalance are thought to be the cause of the altered postures mentioned above, as well as other abnormal postures outlined in Table 6.2.

Observation of soft tissues. The clinician observes the quality and colour of the patient's skin and any area of swelling or presence of scarring, and takes cues for further examination.

Observation of gait. The typical gait patterns that might be expected in patients with low thoracic pain or lumbar spine pain are the gluteus maximus gait, Trendelenburg's gait and the short-leg gait. These are described more fully in Chapter 3.

Observation of the patient's attitudes and feelings. The age, gender and ethnicity of patients and their cultural, occupational and social backgrounds will all affect their attitudes and feelings towards themselves, their condition and the clinician. The clinician needs to be aware of and sensitive to these attitudes, and to empathize and communicate appropriately so as to develop a rapport with the patient and thereby enhance the patient's compliance with the treatment.

Active physiological movements

For active physiological movements, the clinician notes the:

- quality of the movement
- range of the movement
- behaviour of the pain through the range of movement
- resistance through the range of movement and at the end of the range of movement
- provocation of any muscle spasm.

A movement diagram can be used to depict this information. The active movements with overpressure listed below (Fig. 7.1) are tested with the patient in sitting. The clinician establishes the patient's symptoms at rest prior to each movement and corrects any movement deviation to determine its relevance to the patient's symptoms.

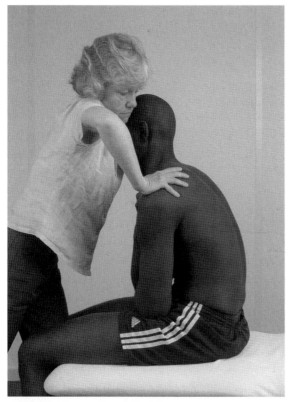

A Flexion. Both hands on top of the shoulders push down to increase thoracic flexion.

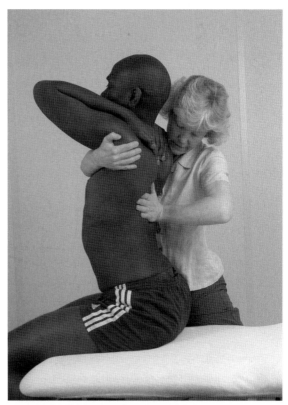

B Extension. One arm wraps around front of thorax and extends the thorax over the hand applying a posteroanterior force in an attempt to produce thoracic flexion down to a particular thoracic level. This is not fully achieved; there is some extension movement occurring in the lumbar spine.

Figure 7.1(A–F)   Overpressures to the thoracic spine. These movements are all carried out with the patient's arms crossed.

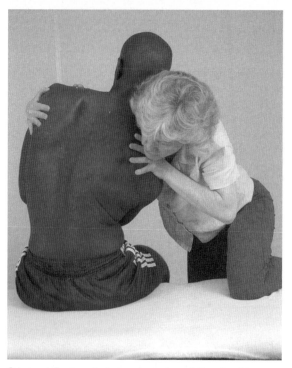

C Lateral flexion. Both hands on top of the shoulders apply a force to increase thoracic lateral flexion.

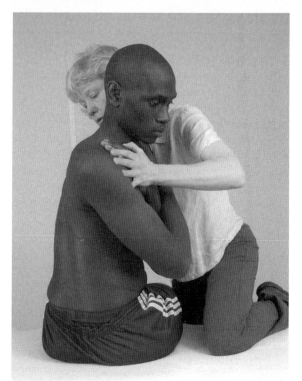

D Rotation. The right hand rests behind the patient's left shoulder and the left hand lies on the front of the right shoulder. Both hands then apply a force to increase right thoracic rotation.

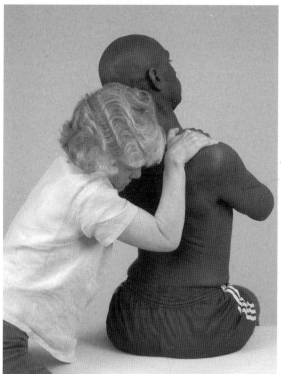

E Right extension quadrant. This movement is a combination of extension, right rotation and right lateral flexion. Both hands are placed on top of the shoulders; the patient then actively extends and the clinician then passively rotates and laterally flexes the thoracic spine to the left.

Figure 7.1 *Continued*

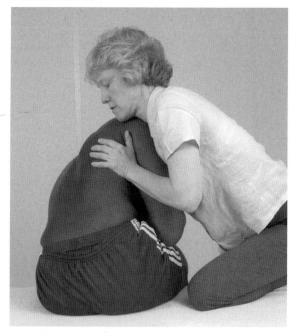

F Combined flexion/right rotation. The right hand grips around the posterior aspect of the patient's left shoulder while the left hand rests over the left side of the thorax. Both hands then apply a force to cause flexion and this position is maintained while right rotation of the thoracic spine is added.

Table 7.1   Active movements and possible modifications

Active physiological movements	Modifications
Thoracic spine	Repeated
Flexion	Speed altered
Extension	Combined (Edwards
L lateral flexion	1999) e.g.
R lateral flexion	– flexion then rotation
L rotation	(Fig. 7.2)
R rotation	– extension then rotation
Repetitive flexion (rep flex)	Compression or distraction
Repetitive extension (rep ext)	Sustained
Repetitive rotation L (rep rot)	Injuring movement Differentiation tests
Repetitive rotation R (rep rot)	Function
?Cervical spine	
?Upper limb	
?Lumbar spine	
?Lower limbs	

Table 7.2   Derangement syndromes of the thoracic spine (McKenzie 1990)

Derangement	Clinical presentation
1	Central or symmetrical pain around T1–T12 No deformity Rapidly reversible
2	Acute kyphosis due to trauma (rare)
3	Unilateral or asymmetrical pain around thoracic region with or without radiation laterally around chest wall Rapidly reversible

Active movements of the thoracic spine and possible modifications are shown in Table 7.1. It is worth mentioning here the work of Robin McKenzie. If all movements are full and symptom-free on overpressure, and symptoms are aggravated by certain postures, the condition is categorized as a postural syndrome (McKenzie 1990). If on repeated movement there is no change in area of symptoms, the condition is categorized as a dysfunction syndrome (McKenzie 1990). If on repeated movement, peripheralization and centralization syndrome is manifested, this is characterized as a derangement syndrome; three types of derangement syndromes are described (Table 7.2).

Numerous differentiation tests (Maitland et al 2001) can be performed; the choice depends on the patient's signs and symptoms. For example, when turning the head around to the left reproduces the patient's left-sided infrascapular pain, differentiation between the cervical and thoracic spine may be required. The clinician can increase and decrease the rotation at the cervical and thoracic regions to find out what effect this has on the infra-

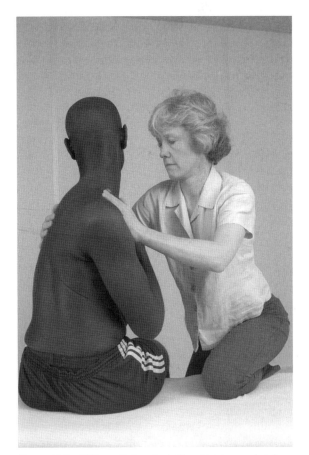

Figure 7.2   Differentiation test. The clinician maintains right rotation of the thoracic spine while the patient turns the head to the left.

scapular pain. The patient turns the head and trunk around to the left; the clinician maintains the position of the cervical spine and derotates the thoracic spine, noting the pain response. If symptoms remain the same or increase, this might suggest the cervical spine is the source of the symptoms. The position of cervical and thoracic rotation is then resumed and this time the clinician maintains the position of the thoracic spine and derotates the cervical spine, noting the pain response. If the symptoms remain the same or increase, this implicates the thoracic spine, and this may be further tested by increasing the overpressure to the thoracic spine, which would be expected to increase the symptoms.

It may be necessary to examine other regions to determine their relevance to the patient's symptoms; they may be the source of the symptoms, or they may be contributing to the symptoms. The regions most likely are the cervical spine and upper limb, or the lumbar spine and lower limbs might be involved. The joints within these regions can be tested fully (see relevant chapter) or partially with the use of clearing tests (see Table 3.5).

Some functional ability has already been tested by the general observation of the patient during the subjective and physical examinations, e.g. the postures adopted during the subjective examination and the ease or difficulty of undressing prior to the examination. Any further functional testing can be carried out at this point in the examination and may include sitting postures, inspiration, expiration, cough, lifting, etc. Clues for appropriate tests can be obtained from the subjective examination findings, particularly aggravating factors.

Capsular pattern. No clear capsular pattern is apparent in the thoracic spine.

Passive physiological movements

These can take the form of passive physiological intervertebral movements (PPIVMs), which examine the movement at each segmental level. PPIVMs can be a useful adjunct to passive accessory intervertebral movements (PAIVMs) to identify segmental hypomobility and hypermobility. They can be performed in the supine position or

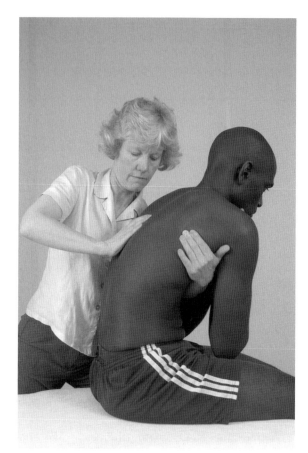

Figure 7.3 PPIVMs for flexion and extension of the thoracic spine. The clinician's right index finger is placed in the gap between adjacent spinous processes and the patient is passively flexed and then extended by grasping around the thorax with the left hand.

sitting. The clinician palpates between adjacent spinous processes or transverse processes to feel the range of intervertebral movement during thoracic flexion, extension, rotation, lateral flexion and lateral glide. Figure 7.3 demonstrates PPIVMs for flexion and extension of the thoracic spine.

It may be necessary to examine other regions to determine their relevance to the patient's symptoms; they may be the source of the symptoms, or they may be contributing to the symptoms. The regions most likely are the cervical spine and upper limb, or the lumbar spine and lower limbs might be involved.

Muscle tests

The muscles that need to be tested will depend on the area of the signs and symptoms and may include muscles of the cervical spine and upper limbs or the lumbar spine and lower limbs. Muscles tests include examining muscle strength, control, length and isometric muscle testing.

Muscle strength

The clinician may test the trunk flexors, extensors, lateral flexors and rotators and other relevant muscle groups as necessary. For details of these general tests readers are directed to Cole et al (1988), Hislop & Montgomery (1995) and Kendall et al (1993).

Greater detail may be required to test the strength of muscles, in particular those thought prone to become weak (Table 3.2). Details of testing the strength of these muscles are given in Chapter 3.

Muscle control

The relative strength of muscles is considered to be more important than the overall strength of a muscle group (Janda 1994, 2002, Sahrmann 2002). Relative strength is assessed indirectly by observing posture, as already mentioned, by the quality of movement, noting any changes in muscle recruitment patterns, and by palpating muscle activity in various positions.

Muscle imbalance around the scapula has been described by a number of workers (Janda 1994, Jull & Janda 1987, Sahrmann 2002) and can be assessed by observation of upper limb movements, e.g. observation of the patient performing a slow push-up from the prone position. The clinician watches for any excessive or abnormal movement of the scapula; muscle weakness may cause the scapula to rotate and glide laterally and/or move superiorly. Serratus anterior weakness, for example, may cause the scapula to wing (the medial border moves away from the thorax). Another movement that can be analysed is shoulder abduction performed slowly, with the patient sitting and the elbow flexed. Once again the clinician observes the quality of movement of the shoulder joint and scapula, and notes any abnormal or excessive movement.

The lateral abdominal muscles may be tested if appropriate. A method of measuring isolated isometric muscle contraction for this muscle group has been described by Jull & Richardson (1994) and is described in Chapter 11.

Muscle length

The clinician tests the length of muscles, in particular those thought prone to shorten (Janda 1994). Details of testing the length of these muscles are given in Chapter 3.

Isometric muscle testing

The clinician tests the trunk flexors, extensors, lateral flexors and rotators (and any other relevant muscle groups) in resting position and, if indicated, in different parts of the physiological range. In addition the clinician observes the quality of the muscle contraction to hold this position (this can be done with the patient's eyes shut). The patient may, for example, be unable to prevent the joint from moving or may hold with excessive muscle activity; either of these circumstances would suggest a neuromuscular dysfunction.

Neurological tests

Neurological examination includes neurological integrity testing, neurodynamic tests and some other nerve tests.

Neurological integrity

The distribution of symptoms will determine the appropriate neurological examination to be carried out. Symptoms confined to the mid-thoracic region require dermatome/cutaneous nerve test only, since there is no myotome or reflex that can be tested. If symptoms spread proximally or distally, a neurological examination of the upper or lower limbs respectively is indicated; testing is described in Chapter 3.

Dermatomes/peripheral nerves. Light touch and pain sensation of the thorax are tested using cotton wool and pinprick respectively, as described in

Chapter 3. Knowledge of the cutaneous distribution of nerve roots (dermatomes) and peripheral nerves enables the clinician to distinguish the sensory loss due to a root lesion from that due to a peripheral nerve lesion. The cutaneous nerve distribution and dermatome areas are shown in Figure 3.19.

Neurodynamic tests

The following neurodynamic tests may be carried out in order to ascertain the degree to which neural tissue is responsible for the production of the patient's symptom(s):

- Passive neck flexion (PNF)
- Upper limb tension tests (ULTT)
- Straight leg raise (SLR)
- Passive knee bend (PKB)
- Slump.

These tests are described in detail in Chapter 3.

Other nerve tests

Plantar response to test for an upper motor neurone lesion (Walton 1989). Pressure applied from the heel along the lateral border of the plantar aspect of the foot produces flexion of the toes in the normal. Extension of the big toe with downward fanning of the other toes occurs with an upper motor neurone lesion.

Miscellaneous tests

Respiratory tests

These tests are appropriate for patients whose spinal dysfunction is such that respiration is affected and may include conditions such as severe scoliosis and ankylosing spondylitis.

Auscultation and examination of the patient's sputum may be required, as well as measurement of the patient's exercise tolerance.

Vital capacity can be measured using a hand-held spirometer. Normal ranges are 2.5–6 L for men and 2–5 L for women (Johnson 1990).

Maximum inspiratory and expiratory pressures ($P_{I\,max}$/MIP, $P_{E\,max}$/MEP) reflect respiratory muscle strength and endurance. A maximum static inspiratory or expiratory effort can be measured by a hand-held mouth pressure monitor (Micromedical

Ltd, Chatham, Kent, UK). Normal values (Wilson et al 1984) are:

$$P_{I\,max} - > 100 \text{ cmH}_2\text{O for males}$$
$$> 70 \text{ cmH}_2\text{O for females}$$
$$P_{E\,max} - > 140 \text{ cmH}_2\text{O for males}$$
$$> 90 \text{ cmH}_2\text{O for females.}$$

Vascular tests

Tests for thoracic outlet syndrome are described in Chapter 8.

Palpation

The clinician palpates the thoracic spine and, if appropriate, the cervical/lumbar spine and upper/lower limbs. It is useful to record palpation findings on a body chart (see Fig. 2.3) and/or palpation chart (See Fig. 3.38).

The clinician should note the following:

- The temperature of the area
- Any increase in skin moisture
- The presence of oedema or effusion
- Mobility and feel of superficial tissues, e.g. ganglions, nodules and scarring
- The presence or elicitation of any muscle spasm
- Tenderness of bone, ligaments, muscle, tendon, tendon sheath, trigger points (shown in Fig. 3.39) and nerve; palpable nerves in the upper limb are as follows:
  - The suprascapular nerve can be palpated along the superior border of the scapula in the suprascapular notch
  - The brachial plexus can be palpated in the posterior triangle of the neck; it emerges at the lower third of sternocleidomastoid
  - The suprascapular nerve can be palpated along the superior border of the scapula in the suprascapular notch
  - The dorsal scapular nerve can be palpated medial to the medial border of the scapula
  - The median nerve can be palpated over the anterior elbow joint crease, medial to the biceps tendon, also at the wrist between palmaris longus and flexor carpi radialis
  - The radial nerve can be palpated around the spiral groove of the humerus, between brachioradialis and flexor carpi radialis, in the forearm and also at the wrist in the snuff box

- Increased or decreased prominence of bones
- Symptoms (usually pain) provoked or reduced on palpation.

Passive accessory intervertebral movements (PAIVMs)

It is useful to use the palpation chart and movement diagrams (or joint pictures) to record findings. These are explained in detail in Chapter 3.

The clinician should note the following:

- The quality of movement
- The range of movement
- The resistance through the range and at the end of the range of movement
- The behaviour of pain through the range
- Any provocation of muscle spasm.

The thoracic spine (T1–T12) accessory movements and rib accessory movements are shown in Figures 7.4–7.7 and listed in Table 7.3. Following accessory movements to the thoracic region, the clinician reassesses all the physical asterisks (movements or tests that have been found to reproduce the patient's symptoms) in order to establish the effect of the accessory movements on the patient's signs and symptoms. Accessory movements can then be tested for other regions suspected to be a source of, or contributing to, the patient's symptoms. Again, following accessory movements to any one region, the clinician reassesses all the asterisks. Regions likely to be examined are the cervical spine and upper limb joints or the lumbar spine and lower limb joints.

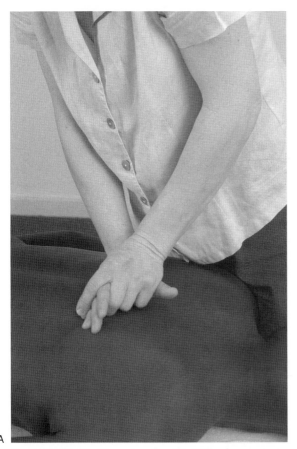
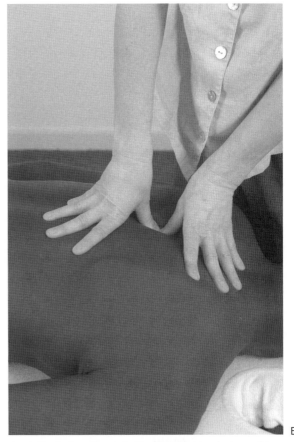

A   B

Figure 7.4(A–C) Thoracic spine (T1–T12) accessory movements. **A** Central posteroanterior. A pisiform grip is used to apply pressure to the spinous process. **B** Unilateral posteroanterior. Thumb pressure is applied to the transverse process.

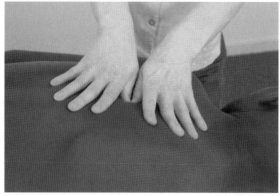

C

Figure 7.4 *Continued* **C** Transverse. Thumb pressure is applied to the lateral aspect of the spinous process.

Sustained natural apophyseal glides (SNAGs)

These examination techniques can be applied to thoracic flexion, extension and rotation. The painful thoracic spine movements are examined in sitting and/or standing. Pressure to the spinous process and/or transverse process of the thoracic vertebrae is applied by the clinician as the patient moves slowly towards the pain. Figure 7.8 demonstrates an extension SNAG on the T6 spinous process. In this example, the technique aims to facilitate the glide of the inferior facets of T6 upwards on T7, so that, if there is a reduction in pain, the T6–T7 segmental level is implicated as a source of the pain. For further details on these techniques, see Chapter 3 and Mulligan (1999).

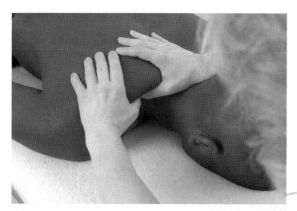

A Longitudinal caudad 1st rib. Thumb pressure is applied to the superior aspect of the 1st rib and pressure is applied downwards towards the feet.

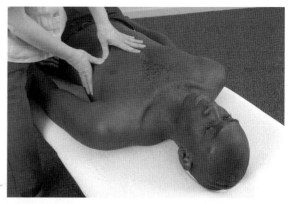

B Anteroposterior. Thumb pressure is applied to the anterior aspect of the rib.

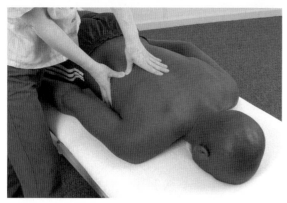

C Posteroanterior. Thumb pressure is applied to the posterior aspect of the rib.

Figure 7.5 Accessory movements to ribs 1–12.

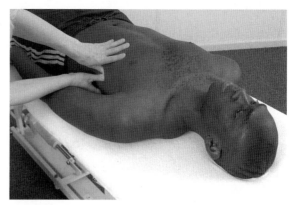

D Medial glide. Thumb pressure is applied to the lateral aspect of the rib.

Table 7.3 Accessory movements, choice of application and reassessment of the patient's asterisks

Accessory movements	Choice of application	Identify any effect of accessory movements on patient's signs and symptoms
Thoracic spine ↕ central posteroanterior ⌐˙˙⌐ unilateral posteroanterior ⇄ transverse **Accessory movements to ribs 1–12** (Fig. 7.5): ↔ Caud longitudinal caudad 1st rib ↕ anteroposterior ↕ posteroanterior → Med medial glide **Costochondral, interchondral and sternocostal joints** (Fig. 7.6) ↕ anteroposterior	Start position e.g. – in flexion (Fig. 7.7) – in extension – in lateral flexion – in flexion and rotation – in extension and rotation Speed of force application Direction of the applied force Point of application of applied force	Reassess all asterisks
?Cervical spine	As above	Reassess all asterisks
?Upper limb joints	As above	Reassess all asterisks
?Lumbar spine	As above	Reassess all asterisks
?Lower limb joints	As above	Reassess all asterisks

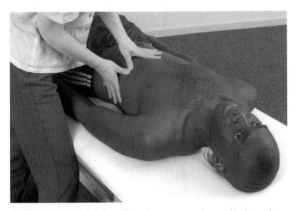 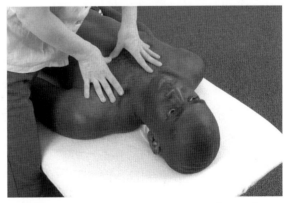

A Costochondral joint. Thumb pressure is applied to the 8th, 9th or 10th costochondral joints.

B Sternocostal joint. Thumb pressure is applied to the sternocostal joint.

Figure 7.6 Anteroposterior accessory movement to the costochondral and sternocostal joints.

COMPLETION OF THE EXAMINATION

Having carried out the above tests, the examination of the thoracic spine is now complete. The subjective and physical examinations produce a large amount of information, which should be recorded accurately and quickly. An outline examination chart may be useful for some clinicians and one is suggested in Figure 7.9. It is important, however, that the clinician does not examine in a rigid manner, simply following the suggested sequence outlined in the chart. Each patient presents differently and this should be reflected in the examination process. It is vital at this stage to highlight with an asterisk (*) important findings from the examination. These findings must be

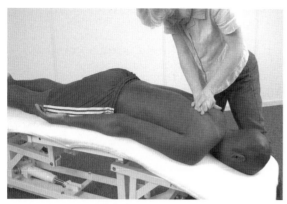

Figure 7.7   Palpation of the thoracic spine using a combined movement. The clinician applies a central PA to T6 with the spine positioned in flexion.

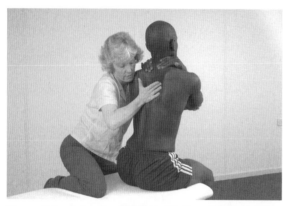

Figure 7.8   Extension SNAG on T6. The clinician applies a posteroanterior pressure to the spinous process of T6 using the heel of the right hand while the patient moves slowly into extension, guided by the clinician's left arm.

reassessed at, and within, subsequent treatment sessions to evaluate the effects of treatment on the patient's condition.

The physical testing procedures which specifically indicate joint, nerve or muscle tissues, as a source of the patient's symptoms, are summarized in Table 3.10. The strongest evidence that a joint is the source of the patient's symptoms is that active and passive physiological movements, passive accessory movements and joint palpation all reproduce the patient's symptoms, and that following a treatment dose, reassessment identifies an improvement in the patient's signs and symptoms. Weaker evidence includes an alteration in range, resistance or quality of physiological

and/or accessory movements and tenderness over the joint, with no alteration in signs and symptoms after treatment. One or more of these findings may indicate a dysfunction of a joint which may, or may not, be contributing to the patient's condition.

The strongest evidence that a muscle is the source of a patient's symptoms is if active movements, an isometric contraction, passive lengthening and palpation of a muscle all reproduce the patient's symptoms, and that following a treatment dose, reassessment identifies an improvement in the patient's signs and symptoms. Further evidence of muscle dysfunction may be suggested by reduced strength or poor quality during the active physiological movement and the isometric contraction, reduced range, and/or increased/decreased resistance, during the passive lengthening of the muscle, and tenderness on palpation, with no alteration in signs and symptoms after treatment. One or more of these findings may indicate a dysfunction of a muscle which may or may not be contributing to the patient's condition.

The strongest evidence that a nerve is the source of the patient's symptoms is when active and/or passive physiological movements reproduce the symptoms, which are then increased or decreased with an additional sensitizing movement, at a distance from the patient's symptoms. In addition, there is reproduction of the patient's symptoms on palpation of the nerve, and following neurodynamic testing, sufficient to be considered a treatment dose, an improvement is seen in the above signs and symptoms. Further evidence of nerve dysfunction may be suggested by reduced range (compared to the asymptomatic side) and/or increased resistance to the various arm movements, and tenderness on nerve palpation.

On completion of the physical examination the clinician should:

- Warn the patient of possible exacerbation up to 24–48 hours following the examination.
- Request the patient to report details on the behaviour of the symptoms following examination at the next attendance.
- Explain the findings of the physical examination and how these findings relate to the sub-

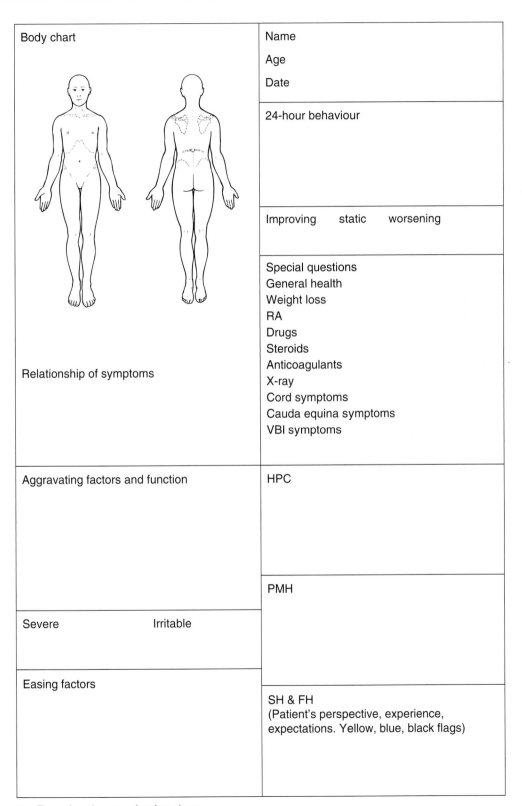

Body chart	Name
	Age
	Date

24-hour behaviour

Improving   static   worsening

Special questions
General health
Weight loss
RA
Drugs
Steroids
Anticoagulants
X-ray
Cord symptoms
Cauda equina symptoms
VBI symptoms

Relationship of symptoms

Aggravating factors and function

HPC

PMH

Severe   Irritable

Easing factors

SH & FH
(Patient's perspective, experience,
expectations. Yellow, blue, black flags)

Figure 7.9   Thoracic spine examination chart.

Physical examination Observation	Isometric muscle testing
	Neurological integrity tests (dermatomes only)
Active and passive physiological movements of thoracic spine and other relevant regions	Neurodynamic tests
	Other nerve tests (plantar response)
	Miscellaneous tests (respiratory tests, thoracic outlet tests)
Muscle strength	Palpation
Muscle control	Accessory movements and reassessment of each relevant region
Muscle length	

Figure 7.9 *Continued*

jective assessment. An attempt should be made to clear up any misconceptions patients may have regarding their illness or injury.

- Evaluate the findings, formulate a clinical diagnosis and write up a problem list. Clinicians may find the management planning forms shown in Figures 3.53 and 3.54 helpful in guiding them through what is often a complex clinical reasoning process.
- Determine the objectives of treatment.
- Devise an initial treatment plan.

In this way, the clinician will have developed the following hypotheses categories (adapted from Jones & Rivett 2004):

- Function: abilities and restrictions.
- Patients' perspectives on their experience.

- Source of symptoms. This includes the structure or tissue that is thought to be producing the patient's symptoms, the nature of the structure or tissues in relation to the healing process, and the pain mechanisms.
- Contributing factors to the development and maintenance of the problem. There may be environmental, psychosocial, behavioural, physical or heredity factors.
- Precautions/contraindications to treatment and management. This includes the severity and irritability of the patient's symptoms and the nature of the patient's condition.
- Management strategy and treatment plan.
- Prognosis – this can be affected by factors such as the stage and extent of the injury as well as the patient's expectation, personality and lifestyle.

References

Bogduk N 1994 Cervical causes of headache and dizziness. In: Boyling J D, Palastanga N (eds) Grieve's modern manual therapy, 2nd edn. Churchill Livingstone, Edinburgh, ch 22, p 317

Clinical Standards Advisory Report 1994 Report of a CSAG committee on back pain. HMSO, London

Cloward R B 1959 Cervical discography: a contribution to the aetiology and mechanism of neck, shoulder and arm pain. Annals of Surgery 150(6): 1052–1064

Cole J H, Furness A L, Twomey L T 1988 Muscles in action, an approach to manual muscle testing. Churchill Livingstone, Edinburgh

Edwards B C 1999 Manual of combined movements: their use in the examination and treatment of mechanical vertebral column disorders, 2nd edn. Butterworth-Heinemann, Oxford

Grieve G P 1994 Counterfeit clinical presentations. Manipulative Physiotherapist 26: 17–19

Hislop H, Montgomery J 1995 Daniels and Worthingham's muscle testing, techniques of manual examination, 7th edn. W B Saunders, Philadelphia

Janda V 1994 Muscles and motor control in cervicogenic disorders: assessment and management. In: Grant R (ed) Physical therapy of the cervical and thoracic spine, 2nd edn. Churchill Livingstone, New York, ch 10, p 195

Janda V 2002 Muscles and motor control in cervicogenic disorders. In: Grant R (ed) Physical therapy of the cervical and thoracic spine, 3rd edn. Churchill Livingstone, New York, ch 10, p 182

Johnson N M 1990 Respiratory medicine, 2nd edn. Blackwell Scientific Publications, Oxford, ch 3, p 37

Jones M A, Rivett D A 2004 Clinical reasoning for manual therapists. Butterworth-Heinemann, Edinburgh

Jull G A, Janda V 1987 Muscles and motor control in low back pain: assessment and management. In: Twomey L T, Taylor J R (eds) Physical therapy of the low back. Churchill Livingstone, New York, ch 10, p 253

Jull G A, Richardson C A 1994 Rehabilitation of active stabilization of the lumbar spine. In: Twomey L T, Taylor J R (eds) Physical therapy of the low back, 2nd edn. Churchill Livingstone, New York, ch 9, p 251

Kendall F P, McCreary E K, Provance P G 1993 Muscles testing and function, 4th edn. Williams & Wilkins, Baltimore, MD

McKenzie R A 1990 The cervical and thoracic spine mechanical diagnosis and therapy. Spinal Publications, New Zealand

Magee D J 1997 Orthopedic physical assessment, 3rd edn. W B Saunders, Philadelphia

Maitland G D, Hengeveld E, Banks K, English K 2001 Maitland's vertebral manipulation, 6th edn. Butterworth-Heinemann, Oxford

Mulligan B R 1999 Manual therapy 'NAGs', 'SNAGs', 'MWMs' etc., 4th edn. Plane View Services, New Zealand

Sahrmann S A 2002 Diagnosis and treatment of movement impairment syndromes. Mosby, St Louis

Waddell G 2004 The back pain revolution, 2nd edn. Churchill Livingstone, Edinburgh

Walton J H 1989 Essentials of neurology, 6th edn. Churchill Livingstone, Edinburgh

Wilson S H, Cooke N T, Edwards R H T, Spiro S G 1984 Predicted normal values for maximal respiratory pressures in Caucasian adults and children. Thorax 39: 535–538

Chapter 8

Examination of the shoulder region

POSSIBLE CAUSES OF PAIN AND/OR LIMITATION OF MOVEMENT

This region includes the sternoclavicular (SC), acromioclavicular (AC) and glenohumeral (GH) joints and their surrounding soft tissues.

- Trauma:
    - Fracture of the clavicle, humerus or scapula
    - Dislocation of one of the above joints, although this is uncommon for the AC and SC joints
    - Ligamentous sprain
    - Muscular strain
- Calcification of tendons, particularly the rotator cuff
- Spontaneous conditions, e.g. frozen shoulder and rupture of the long head of biceps
- Degenerative conditions: osteoarthrosis
- Inflammatory disorders: rheumatoid arthritis
- Infection, e.g. tuberculosis
- Bursitis
- Muscle-imbalance-related problems, e.g. winged scapula due to weakness of serratus anterior
- Congenital abnormalities, e.g. 'Sprengel's shoulder'
- Snapping scapula (grinding sensation beneath the scapula on movement due to rib prominence)
- Neoplasm
- Thoracic outlet syndrome
- Hypermobility and instability syndromes
- Referral of symptoms from:
    - Viscera, e.g. lungs, heart, diaphragm, gall bladder and spleen (Brown 1983)

 – Joints, e.g. cervical spine, thoracic spine, elbow, wrist or hand.

Further details of the questions asked during the subjective examination and the tests carried out in the physical examination can be found in Chapters 2 and 3, respectively.

The order of the subjective questioning and the physical tests described below can be altered as appropriate for the patient being examined.

SUBJECTIVE EXAMINATION

Body chart

The following information concerning the type and area of current symptoms can be recorded on a body chart (see Fig. 2.3).

Area of current symptoms

Be exact when mapping out the area of the symptoms. Symptoms from the glenohumeral joint are commonly felt at the insertion of deltoid but may be referred proximally to the low cervical spine and/or distally to the forearm and hand. Acromioclavicular and sternoclavicular joint lesions are often felt locally around the joint, although it is not uncommon for the acromioclavicular joint to refer pain proximally over the area of the upper trapezius. Ascertain which is the worst symptom and record where the patient feels the symptoms are coming from.

Areas relevant to the region being examined

All other relevant areas are checked for symptoms; it is important to ask about pain or even stiffness, as this may be relevant to the patient's main symptom. Mark unaffected areas with ticks (✓) on the body chart. Check for symptoms in the cervical spine, thoracic spine, elbow, wrist and hand.

Quality of pain

Establish the quality of the pain. Catching pain or arcs of pain are typical of impingement-related problems around the shoulder.

Intensity of pain

The intensity of pain can be measured using, for example, a visual analogue scale (VAS) as shown in Figure 2.8.

Depth of pain

Establish the depth of the pain. Does the patient feel it is on the surface or deep inside?

Abnormal sensation

Check for any altered sensation locally around the shoulder region as well as over the spine and distally in the arm.

Constant or intermittent symptoms

Ascertain the frequency of the symptoms, whether they are constant or intermittent. If symptoms are constant, check whether there is variation in the intensity of the symptoms, as constant unremitting pain may be indicative of neoplastic disease.

Relationship of symptoms

Determine the relationship between symptomatic areas – do they come together or separately? For example, the patient may have shoulder pain without neck pain, or they may always be present together.

Behaviour of symptoms

Aggravating factors

For each symptomatic area, discover what movements and/or positions aggravate the patient's symptoms, i.e. what brings them on (or makes them worse), are they able to maintain this position or movement (severity), what happens to other symptom(s) when this symptom is produced (or is made worse), and how long does it take for symptoms to ease once the position or movement is stopped (irritability). These questions help to confirm the relationship between the symptoms.

The clinician also asks the patient about theoretically known aggravating factors for structures that could be a source of the symptoms. Common aggravating factors for the shoulder are hand behind back (HBB), above-head activities, lifting and lying on the shoulder. Aggravating factors for other regions, which may need to be queried if they are suspected to be a source of the symptoms, are shown in Table 2.3.

The clinician ascertains how the symptoms affect function, such as: static and active postures, e.g. lying on the affected shoulder, leaning on the forearm or hand, washing, ironing, dusting, driving, lifting, carrying, work, sport and social activities. Note details of training regimen for any sports activities. The clinician finds out whether the patient is left- or right-handed as there may be increased stress on the dominant side.

Detailed information on each of the above activities is useful in order to help determine the structure(s) at fault and identify functional restrictions. This information can be used to determine the aims of treatment and any advice that may be required. The most notable functional restrictions are highlighted with asterisks (*), explored in the physical examination, and reassessed at subsequent treatment sessions to evaluate treatment intervention.

Easing factors

For each symptomatic area, the clinician asks what movements and/or positions ease the patient's symptoms, how long it takes to ease them and what happens to other symptom(s) when this symptom is relieved. These questions help to confirm the relationship between the symptoms.

The clinician asks the patient about theoretically known easing factors for structures that could be a source of the symptoms. For example, symptoms from the shoulder may be relieved by supporting the weight of the arm, whereas symptoms from a cervical rib may be relieved by shoulder girdle elevation. The clinician can then analyse the position or movement that eases the symptoms in order to help determine the structure at fault. Find out what happens to other symptom(s) when one symptom is relieved; this helps to confirm the relationship between symptoms.

Twenty-four-hour behaviour of symptoms

The clinician determines the 24-hour behaviour of symptoms by asking questions about night, morning and evening symptoms.

Night symptoms. The following questions may be asked:

- Do you have any difficulty getting to sleep?
- What position is most comfortable/uncomfortable?
- What is your normal sleeping position?
- What is your present sleeping position?
- Can you lie on the affected shoulder?
- Do your symptom(s) wake you at night? If so,
  - Which symptom(s)?
  - How many times in the past week?
  - How many times in a night?
  - How long does it take to get back to sleep?
- How many and what type of pillows are used?

Morning and evening symptoms. The clinician determines the pattern of the symptoms first thing in the morning, through the day and at the end of the day.

Stage of the condition

In order to determine the stage of the condition, the clinician asks whether the symptoms are getting better, getting worse or remaining unchanged.

Special questions

Special questions must always be asked, as they may identify certain precautions or contraindications to the physical examination and/or treatment (Table 2.4). As mentioned in Chapter 2, the clinician must differentiate between conditions that are suitable for conservative management and systemic, neoplastic and other non-neuromuscu-loskeletal conditions, which require referral to a medical practitioner. The reader is referred to Appendix 2.3 for details of various serious pathological processes that can mimic neuromuscu-loskeletal conditions (Grieve 1994a).

The following information is routinely obtained from patients:

General health. The clinician ascertains the state of the patient's general health, and finds out if the patient suffers from any cough, breathlessness, chest pain, malaise, fatigue, fever, nausea or vomiting, stress, anxiety or depression. Symptoms in the shoulder may be referred from the lungs, pleura, heart, diaphragm, gall bladder and spleen (Brown 1983).

Weight loss. Has the patient noticed any recent unexplained weight loss?

Rheumatoid arthritis. Has the patient (or a member of his/her family) been diagnosed as having rheumatoid arthritis?

Drug therapy. What drugs are being taken by the patient? Has the patient been prescribed long-term (6 months or more) medication/steroids? Has the patient been taking anticoagulants?

X-ray and medical imaging. Has the patient been X-rayed or had any other medical tests recently? Routine spinal X-rays are no longer considered necessary prior to conservative treatment as they only identify the normal age-related degenerative changes, which do not necessarily correlate with the patient's symptoms (Clinical Standards Advisory Report 1994). The medical tests may include blood tests, magnetic resonance imaging, myelography, discography or a bone scan.

Neurological symptoms. Has the patient experienced symptoms of spinal cord compression, which are bilateral tingling in the hands or feet and/or disturbance of gait?

Vertebrobasilar insufficiency. This is relevant where there are symptoms of pain, discomfort and/or altered sensation emanating from the cervical spine, where vertebrobasilar insufficiency (VBI) may be provoked. Further questions about dizziness and testing for vertebrobasilar insufficiency are described more fully in Chapter 6.

History of the present condition (HPC)

For each symptomatic area the clinician needs to know how long the symptom has been present, whether there was a sudden or slow onset and whether there was a known cause that provoked the onset of the symptom. If the onset was slow, the clinician finds out if there has been any change

in the patient's lifestyle, e.g. a new job or hobby or a change in sporting activity; this may have contributed to the patient's condition. To confirm the relationship of the symptoms, the clinician asks what happened to other symptoms when each symptom began.

Past medical history (PMH)

The following information is obtained from the patient and/or the medical notes:

- The details of any relevant medical history.
- The history of any previous attacks: how many episodes, when were they, what was the cause, what was the duration of each episode and did the patient fully recover between episodes? If there have been no previous attacks, has the patient had any episodes of stiffness in the cervical spine, thoracic spine, shoulder or any other relevant region? Check for a history of trauma or recurrent minor trauma.
- Ascertain the results of any past treatment for the same or similar problem. Past treatment records may be obtained for further information.

Social and family history (SH, FH)

Social and family history that is relevant to the onset and progression of the patient's problem is recorded. This includes the patient's perspectives, experience and expectations, their age, employment, home situation, and details of any leisure activities. Factors from this information may indicate direct and/or indirect mechanical influences on the shoulder. In order to treat the patient appropriately, it is important that the condition is managed within the context of the patient's social and work environment.

The clinician may ask the following types of questions to elucidate psychosocial factors:

- Have you had time off work in the past with your pain?
- What do you understand to be the cause of your pain?
- What are you expecting will help you?
- How is your employer/co-workers/family responding to your pain?

- What are you doing to cope with your pain?
- Do you think you will return to work? When?

While these questions are described in relation to psychosocial risk factors for poor outcomes for patients with low back pain (Waddell 2004), they may be relevant to other patients.

Plan of the physical examination

When all this information has been collected, the subjective examination is complete. It is useful at this stage to highlight with asterisks (*), for ease of reference, important findings and particularly one or more functional restrictions. These can then be re-examined at subsequent treatment sessions to evaluate treatment intervention.

In order to plan the physical examination, the following hypotheses need to be developed from the subjective examination:

- The regions and structures that should be examined as a possible cause of the symptoms, e.g. glenohumeral joint, cervical spine, thoracic spine, acromioclavicular joint, sternoclavicular joint, elbow, muscles and nerves. Often it is not possible to examine fully at the first attendance and so examination of the structures must be prioritized over subsequent treatment sessions.
- Other factors that should be examined, e.g. working and everyday postures, muscle weakness and sporting technique, such as service and strokes for tennis, smash for badminton, etc.
- In what way should the physical tests be carried out? Will it be easy or hard to reproduce each symptom? Will it be necessary to use combined movements, repetitive movements, etc. to reproduce the patient's symptoms? Are symptom(s) severe and/or irritable? If symptoms are severe, physical tests may be carried out to just before the onset of symptom production or just to the onset of symptom production; no overpressures will be carried out, as the patient would be unable to tolerate this. If symptoms are irritable, physical tests may be examined to just before symptom production or just to the onset of provocation with less physical tests being examined to allow for rest period between tests.

- Are there any precautions and/or contraindications to elements of the physical examination that need to be explored further, such as vertebrobasilar insufficiency, neurological involvement, cardiac disorder, recent fracture, trauma, steroid therapy or rheumatoid arthritis; there may also be certain contraindications to further examination and treatment, e.g. symptoms of cord compression.

A physical planning form can be useful for clinicians to help guide them through the clinical reasoning process (see Fig. 2.10 and Appendix 2.1).

PHYSICAL EXAMINATION

The information from the subjective examination helps the clinician to plan an appropriate physical examination. The severity, irritability and nature of the condition are the major factors that will influence the choice and priority of physical testing procedures. The first and over-arching question the clinician might ask is: 'is this patient's condition suitable for me to manage as a therapist?' For example, a patient presenting with cauda equina compression symptoms may only need neurological integrity testing, prior to an urgent medical referral. The nature of the patient's condition has had a major impact on the physical examination. The second question the clinician might ask is: 'does this patient have a neuromusculoskeletal dysfunction that I may be able to help?' To answer that, the clinician needs to carry out a full physical examination; however, this may not be possible if the symptoms are severe and/or irritable. If the patient's symptoms are severe and/or irritable, the clinician aims to explore movements as much as possible, within a symptom-free range. If the patient has constant and severe and/or irritable symptoms, then the clinician aims to find physical tests that ease the symptoms. If the patient's symptoms are non-severe and non-irritable, then the clinician aims to find physical tests that reproduce each of the patient's symptoms.

Each significant physical test that either provokes or eases the patient's symptoms is highlighted in the patient's notes by an asterisk (*) for easy reference. The highlighted tests are often referred to as 'asterisks' or 'markers'.

The order and detail of the physical tests described below need to be appropriate to the patient being examined; some tests will be irrelevant, some tests will be carried out briefly, while it will be necessary to investigate others fully. It is important that readers understand that the techniques shown in this chapter are some of many; the choice depends mainly on the relative size of the clinician and patient, as well as the clinician's preference. For this reason, novice clinicians may initially want to copy what is shown, but then quickly adapt to what is best for them.

Observation

Informal observation

The clinician needs to observe the patient in dynamic and static situations; the quality of movement is noted, as are the postural characteristics and facial expression. Informal observation will have begun from the moment the clinician begins the subjective examination and will continue to the end of the physical examination.

Formal observation

Observation of posture. The clinician examines the posture of the patient in sitting and standing, noting the posture of the shoulders, head and neck, thoracic spine and upper limbs. The clinician notes bony and soft tissue contours around the region. The clinician may check the alignment of the head of the humerus with the acromion as this can give clues about possible mechanical insufficiencies. The clinician pinch-grips the anterior and posterior edges of the acromion with one hand and with the other hand pinch-grips the anterior and posterior aspects of the humerus. It is generally thought that normally, no more than one-third of the humeral head lies anterior to the acromion. The clinician passively corrects any asymmetry to determine its relevance to the patient's problem.

A specific abnormal posture relevant to the shoulder region is the shoulder crossed syndrome (Janda 1994, 2002), where there is elevation and protraction of the shoulders, rotation and abduction (winging) of the scapulae and forward head

posture and which has been described in Chapter 3. Other abnormal postures are outlined in Table 6.2.

It is worth noting that pure postural dysfunction rarely influences one region of the body in isolation and it may be necessary to observe the patient more fully for a full postural examination.

Observation of muscle form. The clinician examines the muscle bulk and muscle tone of the patient, comparing left and right sides. It must be remembered that handedness and level and frequency of physical activity may well produce differences in muscle bulk between sides. Some muscles are thought to shorten under stress, while other muscles weaken, producing muscle imbalance (Table 3.2). Patterns of muscle imbalance are thought to produce the postures mentioned above.

Observation of soft tissues. The clinician observes the colour of the patient's skin and notes any swelling over the shoulder region or related areas, taking cues for further examination.

Observation of the patient's attitudes and feelings. The age, gender and ethnicity of patients and their cultural, occupational and social backgrounds will all affect their attitudes and feelings towards themselves, their condition and the clinician. The clinician needs to be aware of and sensitive to these attitudes, and to empathize and communicate appropriately so as to develop a rapport with the patient and thereby enhance the patient's compliance with the treatment.

Joint integrity tests

There are a number of different tests described in the literature (e.g. Magee 1997) and a few of them are described here.

Anterior shoulder instability

Anterior shoulder drawer test (Gerber & Ganz 1984). With the patient supine and the shoulder in abduction (80–120°), forward flexion (0–20°) and lateral rotation (0–30°), the clinician stabilizes the scapula and glides the humerus anteriorly (Fig. 8.1). Excessive movement, a click and/or patient apprehension suggests that there is anterior shoulder instability.

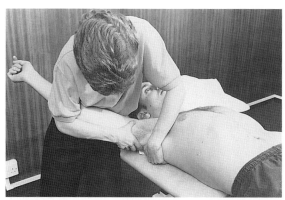

Figure 8.1 Anterior shoulder drawer test. The scapula is stabilized with the left hand and the right hand glides the humerus anteriorly.

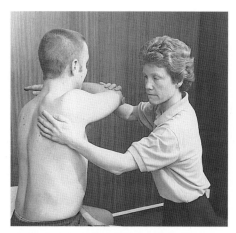

Figure 8.3 Jerk test. The right hand applies a longitudinal cephalad force to the humerus while the left hand stabilizes the trunk.

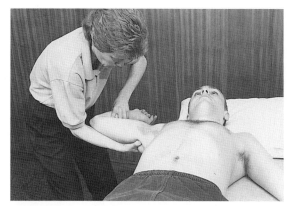

Figure 8.2 Fulcrum test. With the shoulder in 90° abduction, the clinician extends and laterally rotates the humerus.

Fulcrum test (Matsen et al 1990).   With the patient supine, the clinician takes the shoulder into 90° abduction and adds lateral rotation and extension (Fig. 8.2). The test is considered positive – indicating anterior instability – if the patient becomes apprehensive. Further confirmation can be achieved by applying, in this position, an anteroposterior force to the head of the humerus (using the heel of the hand); apprehension is lessened and the clinician is able to take the shoulder further into lateral rotation.

Posterior shoulder instability

Jerk test.   With the patient sitting and the shoulder abducted to 90° and medially rotated, the clin-

ician applies a longitudinal cephalad force to the humerus and moves the arm into horizontal flexion (Fig. 8.3) (Matsen et al 1990). A positive test is indicated if there is a sudden jerk as the arm is moved into horizontal flexion and as it is returned to the start position.

Inferior shoulder instability.   This is tested using the sulcus sign (Matsen et al 1990). The clinician applies a longitudinal caudad force to the humerus with the patient sitting. A positive test is indicated if the patient's pain is reproduced and/or a sulcus appears distal to the acromion, suggesting inferior instability of the shoulder.

Active physiological movements

For active physiological movements, the clinician notes:

- Quality of movement
- Range of movement
- Behaviour of pain through the range of movement
- Resistance through the range of movement and at the end of the range of movement
- Provocation of any muscle spasm.

A movement diagram can be used to depict this information. The active movements with overpressure listed below are shown in Figure 8.4 and

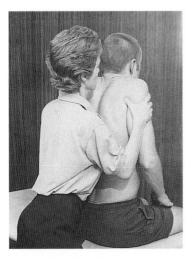

Shoulder (A–D) – **A** Elevation. Both upper arms are grasped and lifted upwards.

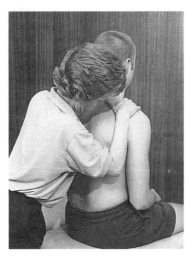

B Depression. Both scapulae are pulled downwards.

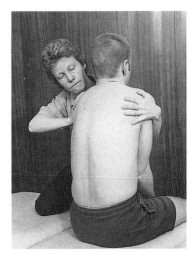

C Protraction. The hands are placed over the scapulae and upper arms and a force is applied to move the scapulae forward around the chest wall.

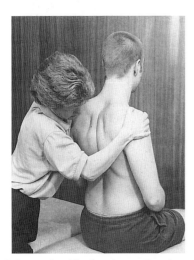

D Retraction. The hands are placed around the upper arms and a force is applied to move the scapulae backward around the chest wall.

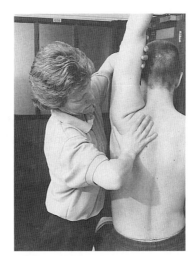

Glenohumeral joint (E–N) – **E** Flexion. The right hand stabilizes the trunk while the left hand applies an overpressure to shoulder flexion.

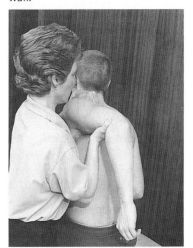

F Extension. The left hand, placed over the top of the scapula and clavicle, stabilizes the trunk while the right hand applies an overpressure to shoulder extension.

Figure 8.4(A–N)   Overpressures applied to the shoulder girdle and glenohumeral joint.

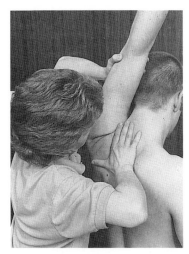

G Abduction. The right hand stabilizes the trunk while the left hand applies an overpressure to shoulder abduction.

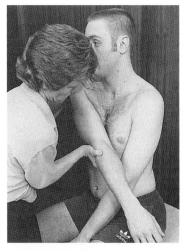

H Adduction. The left hand placed over the top of the scapula and clavicle stabilizes the trunk while the right hand applies an overpressure to shoulder adduction.

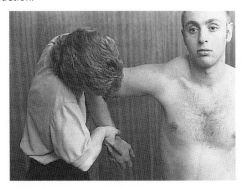

I Medial rotation. The left hand supports the arm in abduction while the right hand moves the forearm to overpress medial rotation of the shoulder.

Figure 8.4 *Continued*

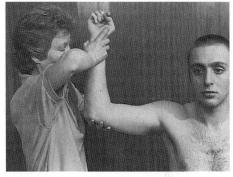

J Lateral rotation. The left hand supports the arm in abduction while the right hand moves the forearm to overpress lateral rotation of the shoulder.

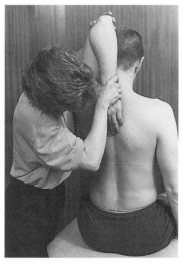

K Hand behind neck (HBN). The left hand pushes down on the elbow as the right hand pulls the forearm downwards.

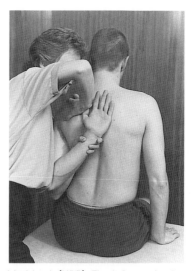

L Hand behind back (HBB). The left arm is placed between the patient's arm and body and holds the wrist. While the right hand stabilizes the trunk, the left arm and hand pulls the wrist upwards.

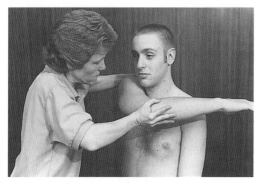

M Horizontal flexion. The left hand stabilizes the trunk while the right hand takes the elbow across the body.

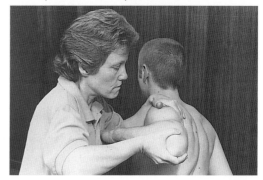

N Horizontal extension. The left hand stabilizes the trunk while the right hand takes the elbow backwards in the horizontal plane.

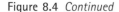

Figure 8.4 *Continued*

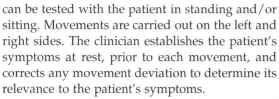

can be tested with the patient in standing and/or sitting. Movements are carried out on the left and right sides. The clinician establishes the patient's symptoms at rest, prior to each movement, and corrects any movement deviation to determine its relevance to the patient's symptoms.

Active movements of the shoulder girdle and glenohumeral joint and possible modifications are shown in Table 8.1. Various differentiation tests (Maitland 1991) can be performed; the choice depends on the patient's signs and symptoms.

For example, when shoulder abduction reproduces the patient's shoulder pain, differentiation between the glenohumeral joint, acromioclavicular joint and subacromial region may be required. The clinician can differentiate between the glenohumeral joint and the subacromial region by adding compression to the glenohumeral joint during the abduction movement; an increase in symptoms implicates the glenohumeral joint. Similarly, a longitudinal cephalad force can be applied to the humerus (to compress the subacromial structures) during the abduction movement; an increase in pain will implicate the subacromial structures. The clinician can implicate the acromioclavicular joint by applying a compression force to the acromioclavicular joint during the abduction movement; if

the pain is increased this suggests the acromioclavicular joint may be the source of pain.

It may be necessary to examine other regions to determine their relevance to the patient's symptoms; they may be the source of the symptoms, or they may be contributing to the symptoms. The most likely regions are the shoulder, sternoclavicular joint, cervical spine, thoracic spine, elbow, wrist and hand. The joints within these regions can be tested fully (see relevant chapter) or partially with the use of clearing tests (Table 8.2).

Some functional ability has already been tested by the general observation of the patient during the subjective and physical examinations, e.g. the postures adopted during the subjective examination and the ease or difficulty of undressing prior to the examination. Any further functional testing can be carried out at this point in the examination and may include various sitting postures or aggravating movements of the upper limb. Clues for appropriate tests can be obtained from the subjective examination findings, particularly aggravating factors.

Capsular pattern. The capsular pattern for the glenohumeral joint is limitation of lateral rotation, abduction and medial rotation (Cyriax 1982).

Passive physiological movements

All the active movements described above can usually be examined passively with the patient in the supine position, comparing left and right sides. In addition, medial and lateral rotation of

Table 8.1 Active physiological movements and possible modifications

Active physiological movements	Modifications
Shoulder girdle	
Elevation	Repeated
Depression	Speed altered
Protraction	Combined, e.g.
Retraction	– abduction with medial
Glenohumeral joint	or lateral rotation
Flexion	– medial/lateral rotation
Extension	with flexion
Abduction	Compression or distraction
Adduction	to scapulothoracic,
Medial rotation	glenohumeral or
Lateral rotation	acromioclavicular joints
Hand behind neck (HBN)	Sustained
Hand behind back (HBB)	Injuring movement
Horizontal flexion	Differentiation tests
Horizontal extension	Functional ability
?Sternoclavicular joint	
?Cervical spine	
?Thoracic spine	
?Elbow	
?Wrist and hand	

Table 8.2 Joint clearing tests

Joint	Physiological movement	Accessory movement
Cervical spine	Quadrants (flexion and extension)	All movements
Thoracic spine	Rotation and quadrants (flexion and extension)	All movements
Shoulder girdle	Elevation, depression, protraction and retraction	
Acromioclavicular joint	All movements (particularly horizontal flexion)	
Sternoclavicular joint	All movements	
Elbow joint	All movements	
Wrist joint	Flexion/extension and radial/ulnar deviation	
Thumb	Extension carpometacarpal and thumb opposition	
Fingers	Flexion at interphalangeal joints and grip	

the scapula can be examined. A comparison of the response of symptoms to the active and passive movements can help to determine whether the structure at fault is non-contractile (articular) or contractile (extra-articular) (Cyriax 1982). If the lesion is non-contractile, such as ligament, then active and passive movements will be painful and/or restricted in the same direction. If the lesion is in a contractile tissue (i.e. muscle), active and passive movements are painful and/or restricted in opposite directions.

The shoulder quadrant and the shoulder lock (Maitland 1991) can be examined; these combine a number of movements and are therefore more stressful tests than the previously examined physiological movements. The tests are therefore particularly useful if the active movements tested previously have not reproduced the patient's symptoms. Both the quadrant and lock stress a number of different structures around the shoulder, including the joint capsule, ligaments, muscles and bursa (Mullen 1989, Slade 1989), and therefore do not in isolation identify the structure at fault.

Shoulder lock. The shoulder lock is an examination of the last few degrees of glenohumeral joint abduction with the joint held in medial rotation (Fig. 8.5). Once in this position, no further abduction is possible and no medial or lateral rotation can occur. The patient lies supine at the edge of the couch and the clinician supports the flexed

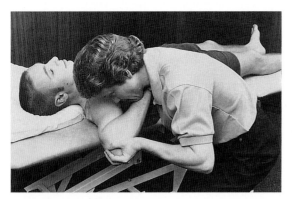

Figure 8.5 Shoulder lock. The right hand grips the superior aspect of the scapula to maintain depression of the scapula. The left hand takes the arm into abduction while the chin maintains full medial rotation.

elbow and forearm with one hand and with the other hand depresses the scapula. The clinician medially rotates the humerus and then passively abducts the humerus in the coronal plane as far as possible. The lock position is where the abduction movement is stopped and it is at this point that the humerus is unable to rotate medially or laterally. A small amount of movement up and down is possible, however, and can be examined by the clinician. Maitland (1991) compares the feel of a normal lock to a rock-lined cave and that of an abnormal lock to a muddy or moss-lined cave. In order to carry out this test effectively, the clinician must prevent any scapular elevation, maintain medial rotation of the humerus and maintain the abduction in the coronal plane – a false soft tissue lock will be felt if the humerus is allowed to fall into horizontal extension.

Shoulder quadrant. The shoulder quadrant is essentially an examination of the resistance to horizontal extension during an arc of shoulder abduction from the point at which the humerus moves from medial rotation to lateral rotation. The patient lies supine at the edge of the couch and the clinician supports the flexed elbow and forearm with one hand, with the other hand resting underneath the scapula. The examination is divided into two phases: the first phase identifies the point in abduction range where the humerus moves from medial to lateral rotation and indicates the beginning of the quadrant; the second phase involves the examination of horizontal extension within the quadrant:

- *First phase*. The clinician passively moves the humerus into medial rotation and then takes the arm from by the patient's side to full elevation through abduction (Fig. 8.6A). During this movement, the clinician allows the humerus to freely rotate laterally, and the point at which this occurs is noted. In addition, the quality of the movement and the plane in which movement occurs are noted; normally the humerus would move in the coronal plane but frequently with dysfunction it moves in a degree of horizontal flexion.
- *Second phase*. With the hands in the same position, the clinician now takes the patient's humerus into flexion (90°) and lateral rotation

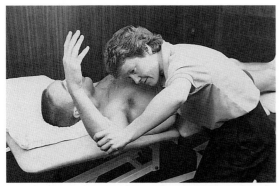 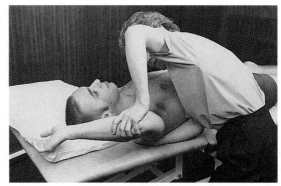

A   B

Figure 8.6   Shoulder quadrant. **A** First phase. The right hand and forearm are placed underneath the patient's scapula. The left hand holds the elbow to support the forearm and moves the arm from the patient's side into abduction, allowing the humerus to move freely from medial to lateral rotation. **B** Second phase. With the right hand in the same position, the left hand now takes the patient's arm down into horizontal extension at various points within the quadrant.

with the elbow flexed 90°. From this position, the clinician takes the humerus down into horizontal extension at various points within the quadrant (Fig. 8.6B) and notes the following:

- The quality of movement
- The range of movement
- The behaviour of pain through the range of movement
- The resistance through the range of movement and at the end of the range of movement
- Any provocation of muscle spasm.

A description of these two tests can be found in Maitland (1991).

It may be necessary to examine other regions to determine their relevance to the patient's symptoms; they may be the source of the symptoms, or they may be contributing to the symptoms. The regions most likely are the shoulder, sternoclavicular joint, cervical spine, thoracic spine, elbow, wrist and hand.

Muscle tests

Muscle tests include examining muscle strength, control, length, isometric muscle testing and some other muscle tests.

Muscle strength

The clinician tests the shoulder girdle elevators, depressors, protractors and retractors as well as the shoulder joint flexors, extensors, abductors, adductors, medial rotators and lateral rotators. For details of these general tests readers are directed to Cole et al (1988), Hislop & Montgomery (1995) and Kendall et al (1993). Greater detail may be required to test the strength of muscles, in particular those thought prone to become weak (Table 3.2); that is, serratus anterior, middle and lower fibres of trapezius and the deep neck flexors (Janda 1994). Testing the strength of these muscles is described in Chapter 3.

Muscle control

The relative strength of muscles is considered to be more important than the overall strength of a muscle group (Janda 1994, 2002, Sahrmann 2002). Relative strength is assessed indirectly by observing posture, as already mentioned, by the quality of active movement, noting any changes in muscle recruitment patterns, and by palpating muscle activity in various positions.

Muscle imbalance around the scapula has been described by a number of workers (Janda 1994, 2002, Jull & Janda 1987, Sahrmann 2002). It is important that the clinician assesses the control of the scapula during the patient's functional activities, particularly sporting activities. In addition to functional activities, abduction of the shoulder is useful to observe and analyse muscle control at the scapulothoracic complex. Winging of the scapula (medial border moving away from the thorax) during the abduction movement indicates weakness of serratus anterior. Increased lateral rotation and elevation of the scapula during the abduction movement may indicate overactivity/ tight upper fibres of trapezius and underactivity/ long lower fibres of trapezius; increased medial rotation and elevation of the scapula may indicate overactivity/tight levator scapula and/or rhomboids (see force couples around the scapula in Fig. 8.7).

Muscle length

The clinician tests the length of muscles, in particular those thought prone to shorten (Janda 1994); that is, latissimus dorsi, pectoralis major and minor, upper trapezius, levator scapula and sternocleidomastoid. Testing the length of these muscles is described in Chapter 3.

Isometric muscle testing

Test the shoulder girdle elevators, depressors, protractors and retractors, as well as the shoulder joint flexors, extensors, abductors, adductors, medial rotators and lateral rotators in resting position and, if indicated, in different parts of the physiological range. In addition the clinician observes the quality of the muscle contraction to hold this position (this can be done with the patient's eyes shut). The patient may, for example, be unable to prevent the joint from moving or may hold with excessive muscle activity; either of these circumstances would suggest a neuromuscular dysfunction.

Other muscle tests

Speed's test for bicipital tendinitis. Tenderness in the bicipital groove when shoulder forward flexion is resisted (with forearm supination and elbow joint extension) suggests bicipital tendinitis.

Impingement of supraspinatus tendon. The clinician passively flexes the patient's shoulder to 90° and then medially rotates the shoulder (Fig. 8.8A). Reproduction of the patient's pain is a positive test, suggesting impingement of the

supraspinatus tendon against the coracoacromial ligament (Hawkins & Bokor 1990). Another test has been named the 'empty can test' (Fig. 8.8B). The patient abducts the arm to 90°, horizontally flexes 30° (so that the humerus is in the scapular plane) and then fully medially rotates the glenohumeral joint. The clinician then applies a force downwards towards the floor and the patient is asked to hold

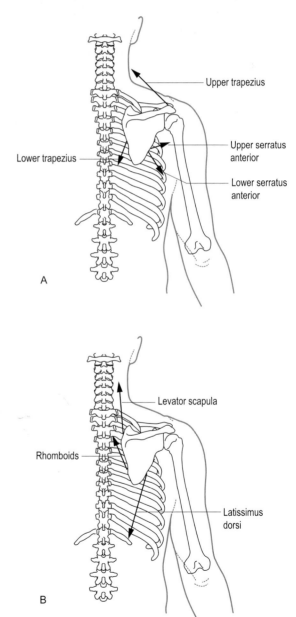

Figure 8.7   Force couples around the scapula.

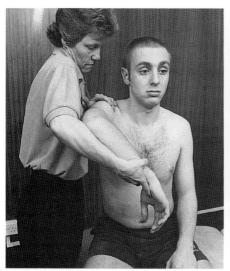

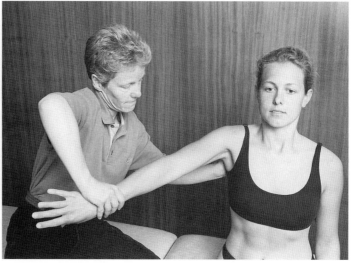

A   B

Figure 8.8   Impingement of supraspinatus tendon. **A** The left hand supports the trunk and palpates over the supraspinatus tendon. The right hand supports the arm in 90° flexion and moves the shoulder into medial rotation. **B** The clinician applies a force downwards towards the floor and the patient is asked to hold the arm in the position of 90° abduction, 30° horizontal flexion (so that the humerus is in the scapula plane) and full medial rotation.

this position. The test is positive if there is reproduction of the patient's pain or there is weakness (Comerford & Kinetic Control 2000).

Neurological tests

Neurological examination includes neurological integrity testing, neurodynamic tests and some other nerve tests.

Integrity of nervous system

The integrity of the nervous system is tested if the clinician suspects that the symptoms are emanating from the spine or from a peripheral nerve.

Dermatomes/peripheral nerves.   Light touch and pain sensation of the upper limb are tested using cotton wool and pinprick respectively, as described in Chapter 3. Knowledge of the cutaneous distribution of nerve roots (dermatomes) and peripheral nerves enables the clinician to distinguish the sensory loss due to a root lesion from that due to a peripheral nerve lesion. The cutaneous nerve distribution and dermatome areas are shown in Figure 3.20.

Myotomes/peripheral nerves.   The following myotomes are tested and are shown in Figure 3.26:

- C4: shoulder girdle elevation
- C5: shoulder abduction
- C6: elbow flexion
- C7: elbow extension
- C8: thumb extension
- T1: finger adduction.

A working knowledge of the muscular distribution of nerve roots (myotomes) and peripheral nerves enables the clinician to distinguish the motor loss due to a root lesion from that due to a peripheral nerve lesion. The peripheral nerve distributions are shown in Figures 3.23 and 3.24.

Reflex testing.   The following deep tendon reflexes are tested (see Fig. 3.28):

- C5–C6: biceps
- C7: triceps and brachioradialis.

Neurodynamic tests

The upper limb tension tests (ULTT) may be carried out in order to ascertain the degree to which neural tissue is responsible for producing

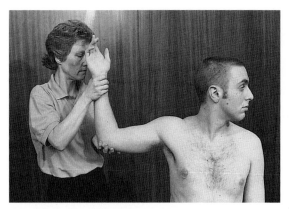

Figure 8.9   The Allen test.

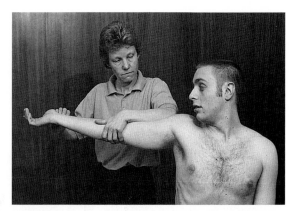

Figure 8.10   Adson's manoeuvre. The left hand supports and moves the arm while the right hand palpates the radial pulse.

the patient's symptom(s). These tests are described in detail in Chapter 3.

Other nerve tests

Tinel's sign determines the distal point of sensory nerve regeneration. The brachial plexus is tapped by the clinician and reproduction of distal pain or paraesthesia indicates the point of recovery of the sensory nerve.

Miscellaneous tests

Vertebral artery test.   The clinician should carry out this test if vertebrobasilar insufficiency is suspected. See Chapter 6 for further details.

Tests for thoracic outlet syndrome.   This syndrome is far from clear; readers are referred to a useful chapter to gain further understanding (Grieve 1994b, Phillips & Grieve 1986).

Allen test.   With the patient sitting and the arm abducted to 90°, the clinician horizontally extends and laterally rotates the arm (Magee 1997). Disappearance of the radial pulse on contralateral cervical rotation is indicative of thoracic outlet syndrome (Fig. 8.9).

Adson's manoeuvre.   In sitting, the patient's head is rotated towards the tested arm (Magee 1997). The patient then extends the head while the clinician extends and laterally rotates the shoulder (Fig. 8.10). The patient then takes a deep breath

and disappearance of the radial pulse indicates a positive test. It should be noted that disappearance of the pulse has been found to occur in a large percentage of asymptomatic subjects (Swift & Nichols 1984, Young & Hardy 1983).

Provocative elevation test (Hawkins & Bokor 1990).   The patient elevates both arms and opens and closes the hands 15 times. Fatigue, cramping and/or tingling indicates a positive test for thoracic outlet syndrome.

Palpation of pulses

If it is suspected that the circulation is compromised, the brachial pulse is palpated on the medial aspect of the humerus in the axilla.

Palpation

The shoulder region is palpated, as well as the cervical spine and thoracic spine and upper limbs as appropriate. It is useful to record palpation findings on a body chart (see Fig. 2.3) and/or palpation chart (see Fig. 3.38).

The clinician notes the following:

- The temperature of the area
- Localized increased skin moisture
- The presence of oedema or effusion
- Mobility and feel of superficial tissues, e.g. ganglions, nodules and scar tissue
- The presence or elicitation of any muscle spasm

- Tenderness of bone, bursae (subacromial and subdeltoid), ligaments, muscle, tendon (long head of biceps, subscapularis, infraspinatus, teres minor, supraspinatus, pectoralis major and long head of triceps), tendon sheath, trigger points (shown in Fig. 3.39) and nerve. Palpable nerves in the upper limb are as follows:
  - The suprascapular nerve can be palpated along the superior border of the scapula in the suprascapular notch
  - The brachial plexus can be palpated in the posterior triangle of the neck; it emerges at the lower third of sternocleidomastoid
  - The suprascapular nerve can be palpated along the superior border of the scapula in the suprascapular notch
  - The dorsal scapular nerve can be palpated medial to the medial border of the scapula
  - The median nerve can be palpated over the anterior elbow joint crease, medial to the biceps tendon, also at the wrist between palmaris longus and flexor carpi radialis
  - The radial nerve can be palpated around the spiral groove of the humerus, between brachioradialis and flexor carpi radialis, in the forearm and also at the wrist in the snuffbox
- Increased or decreased prominence of bones
- Pain provoked or reduced on palpation.

Accessory movements

It is useful to use the palpation chart and movement diagrams (or joint pictures) to record findings. These are explained in detail in Chapter 3.
The clinician notes the:

- Quality of movement
- Range of movement
- Resistance through the range and at the end of the range of movement
- Behaviour of pain through the range
- Provocation of any muscle spasm.

Glenohumeral joint, acromioclavicular joint and sternoclavicular joint accessory movements are shown in Figures 8.11–8.13 and listed in Table 8.3. Following accessory movements to the shoulder region, the clinician reassesses all the physical

asterisks (movements or tests that have been found to reproduce the patient's symptoms) in order to establish the effect of the accessory movements on the patient's signs and symptoms. Accessory movements can then be tested for other regions suspected to be a source of, or contributing to, the patient's symptoms. Again, following accessory movements to any one region, the clinician reassesses all the asterisks. Regions likely to be examined are the cervical spine, thoracic spine, elbow, wrist and hand.

Mobilizations with movement (MWMs) (Mulligan 1999)

For shoulder abduction, the clinician applies an anteroposterior glide to the head of the humerus during active shoulder abduction, with the patient in sitting (Fig. 8.14). An increase in range and no pain or reduced pain are positive examination findings; this may be indicative of anterior instability.

For shoulder medial rotation, the patient stands or sits with the hand behind the back. The clinician stabilizes the scapula and adducts the upper arm while applying a longitudinal caudad glide to the humerus, and at the same time the patient actively rotates the shoulder medially (Fig. 8.15).

COMPLETION OF THE EXAMINATION

Having carried out the above tests, the examination of the shoulder region is now complete. The subjective and physical examinations produce a large amount of information, which must be recorded accurately and quickly. An outline examination chart may be useful for some clinicians and one is suggested in Figure 8.16. It is important, however, that the clinician does not examine in a rigid manner, simply following the suggested sequence outlined in the chart. Each patient presents differently and this should be reflected in the examination process. It is vital at this stage to highlight with an asterisk (*) important findings from the examination. These findings must be reassessed at, and within, subsequent treatment sessions to evaluate the effects of treatment on the patient's condition.

The physical testing procedures which specifically indicate joint, nerve or muscle tissues, as a

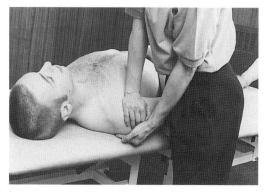

A Anteroposterior. The patient is positioned diagonally on the couch so that the head of the humerus lies over the edge of the couch. The heel of the right hand glides down on the head of the humerus and the left hand feels the movement.

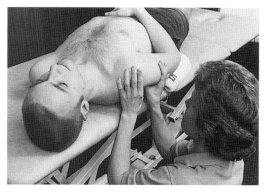

B Posteroanterior. The patient is positioned diagonally on the couch so that the head of the humerus lies over the edge of the couch. The thumbs are used to glide the head of the humerus upwards.

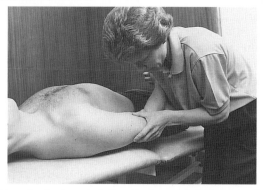

C Longitudinal caudad. The distal end of the humerus is grasped and the humerus is pulled down towards the patient's feet.

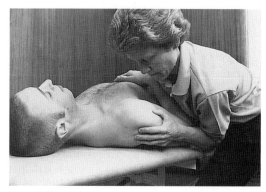

D Lateral. The right hand is placed in the patient's axilla and glides the head of the humerus laterally while the left hand supports and feels the movement.

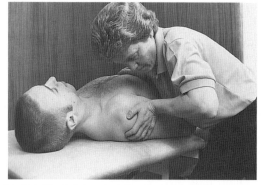

E Medial. The left hand glides the head of the humerus medially.

Figure 8.11   Glenohumeral joint accessory movements. These movements are demonstrated here in neutral; the clinician may need to carry these movements out within a physiological range.

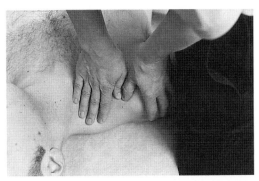

A Anteroposterior. The thumbs push down on the lateral end of the clavicle.

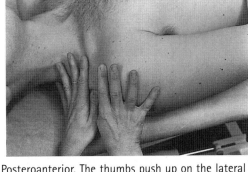

B Posteroanterior. The thumbs push up on the lateral end of the clavicle.

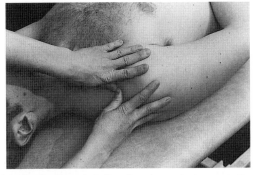

C Longitudinal caudad. The thumbs push down on the superior surface of the clavicle.

Figure 8.12   Acromioclavicular joint accessory movements. Pressure may be applied to the clavicle, to the joint line or over the acromion.

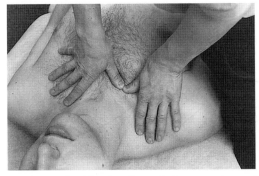

A Anteroposterior. The thumbs push down on the medial end of the clavicle.

Figure 8.13(A–D)   Sternoclavicular joint accessory movements.

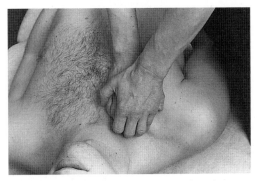

B Posteroanterior. The fingers grip around to the posterior surface of the clavicle and pull anteriorly.

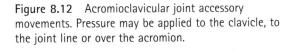

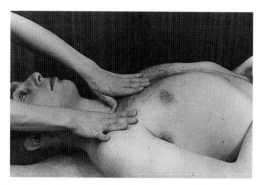

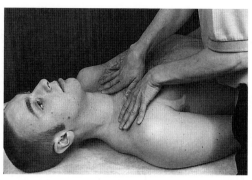

C Longitudinal caudad. The thumbs push inferiorly on the superior surface of the clavicle.

D Longitudinal cephalad. The thumbs push superiorly on the inferior surface of the clavicle.

Figure 8.13 *Continued*

Table 8.3   Accessory movements, choice of application and reassessment of the patient's asterisks

Accessory movements	Choice of application	Identify any effect of accessory movements on patient's signs and symptoms
GH joint (Fig. 8.11) ↑ anteroposterior ↓ posteroanterior ↔ Caud longitudinal caudad ↔ Ceph longitudinal cephalad → Lat lateral → Med medial AC joint (Fig. 8.12) ↑ anteroposterior ↓ posteroanterior ↔ Caud longitudinal caudad SC joint (Fig. 8.13) ↑ anteroposterior ↓ posteroanterior ↔ Caud longitudinal caudad ↔ Ceph longitudinal cephalad	Start position, e.g. – GH joint in flexion, abduction, etc. – AC joint accessory movements carried out with GHJ in horizontal flexion Speed of force application Direction of the applied force Point of application of applied force	Reassess all asterisks
Cervical spine	As above	Reassess all asterisks
Thoracic spine	As above	Reassess all asterisks
Elbow	As above	Reassess all asterisks
Wrist and hand	As above	Reassess all asterisks

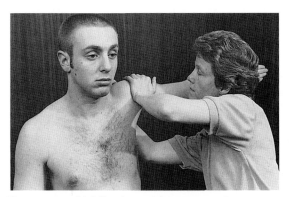

Figure 8.14   Mobilizations with movement for glenohumeral abduction. The right hand stabilizes the trunk while the left hand applies an anteroposterior glide to the head of the humerus as the patient actively abducts the shoulder.

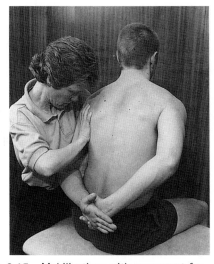

Figure 8.15   Mobilizations with movement for glenohumeral medial rotation. The right hand stabilizes the scapula while the left hand pulls the lower end of the humerus inferiorly as the patient medially rotates the shoulder.

source of the patient's symptoms, are summarized in Table 3.10. The strongest evidence that a joint is the source of the patient's symptoms is that active and passive physiological movements, passive accessory movements and joint palpation all reproduce the patient's symptoms, and that following a treatment dose, reassessment identifies an improvement in the patient's signs and symptoms. Weaker evidence includes an alteration in

range, resistance or quality of physiological and/or accessory movements and tenderness over the joint, with no alteration in signs and symptoms after treatment. One or more of these findings may indicate a dysfunction of a joint, which may or may not be contributing to the patient's condition.

The strongest evidence that a muscle is the source of a patient's symptoms is if active movements, an isometric contraction, passive lengthening and palpation of a muscle all reproduce the patient's symptoms, and that following a treatment dose, reassessment identifies an improvement in the patient's signs and symptoms. Further evidence of muscle dysfunction may be suggested by reduced strength or poor quality during the active physiological movement and the isometric contraction, reduced range, and/or increased/decreased resistance, during the passive lengthening of the muscle, and tenderness on palpation, with no alteration in signs and symptoms after treatment. One or more of these findings may indicate a dysfunction of a muscle, which may or may not be contributing to the patient's condition.

The strongest evidence that a nerve is the source of the patient's symptoms is when active and/or passive physiological movements reproduce the symptoms, which are then increased or decreased with an additional sensitizing movement, at a distance from the symptoms. In addition, there is reproduction of the patient's symptoms on palpation of the nerve and following neurodynamic testing, and that following a treatment dose, reassessment identifies an improvement in the patient's signs and symptoms. Further evidence of nerve dysfunction may be suggested by reduced range (compared to the asymptomatic side) and/or increased resistance to the various arm movements, and tenderness on nerve palpation.

On completion of the physical examination the clinician:

- Warns the patient of possible exacerbation up to 24–48 hours following the examination.
- Requests the patient to report details on the behaviour of the symptoms following examination at the next attendance.
- Explains the findings of the physical examination and how these findings relate to the

Body chart	Name
	Age
	Date

	24-hour behaviour
Relationship of symptoms	Improving static worsening
	Special questions General health Weight loss RA Drugs Steroids Anticoagulants X-ray Cord symptoms Cauda equina symptoms VBI symptoms
Aggravating factors and function	HPC
	PMH
Severe Irritable	
Easing factors	SH & FH (Patient's perspective, experience, expectations. Yellow, blue, black flags)

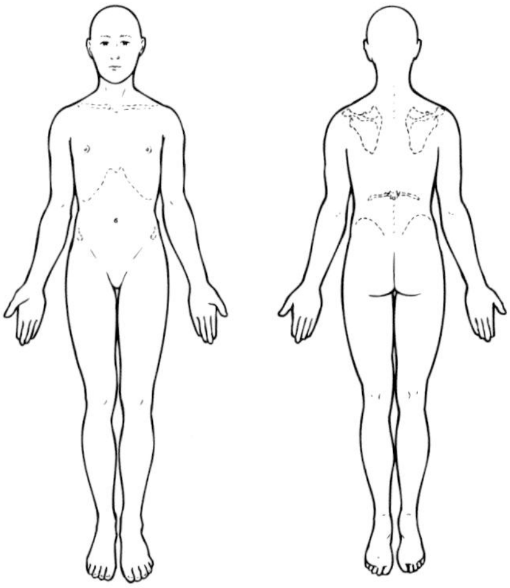

Figure 8.16   Shoulder examination chart.

Physical examination Observation	Muscle length
Joint integrity tests (anterior drawer, fulcrum, jerk, and sulcus sign)	Isometric muscle testing
Active and passive physiological movements of shoulder and other relevant regions	Other muscle tests (Speed's, impingement test)
	Neurological integrity tests
	Neurodynamic tests
	Other nerve tests (Tinel's sign)
Capsular pattern yes/no	Miscellaneous tests (thoracic outlet, pulses, oedema)
Muscle strength	
	Palpation
Muscle control	Accessory movements and reassessment of each relevant region

Figure 8.16 *Continued*

subjective assessment. It is helpful for the patient to clear up any misconceptions they may have regarding their illness or injury.

- Evaluates the findings, formulates a clinical hypothesis and writes up a problem list. Clinicians may find the management planning forms shown in Figures 3.53 and 3.54 helpful in guiding them through what is often a complex clinical reasoning process.
- Determines the objectives of treatment.
- Devises an initial treatment plan.

In this way, the clinician will have developed the following hypotheses categories (adapted from Jones & Rivett 2004):

- Function: abilities and restrictions.
- Patients' perspectives on their experience.

- Source of symptoms. This includes the structure or tissue that is thought to be producing the patients' symptoms, the nature of the structure or tissues in relation to the healing process, and the pain mechanisms.
- Contributing factors to the development and maintenance of the problem. There may be environmental, psychosocial, behavioural, physical or heredity factors.
- Precautions/contraindications to treatment and management. This includes the severity and irritability of the patient's symptoms and the nature of the patient's condition.
- Management strategy and treatment plan.
- Prognosis – this can be affected by factors such as the stage and extent of the injury as well as the patient's expectation, personality and lifestyle.

References

Brown C 1983 Compressive, invasive referred pain to the shoulder. Clinical Orthopaedics and Related Research 173: 55–62

Clinical Standards Advisory Report 1994 Report of a CSAG committee on back pain. HMSO, London

Cole J H, Furness A L, Twomey L T 1988 Muscles in action, an approach to manual muscle testing. Churchill Livingstone, Edinburgh

Comerford M & Kinetic Control 2000 Dynamic stability and muscle balance of the cervical spine and upper quadrant. Course notes.

Cyriax J 1982 Textbook of orthopaedic medicine – diagnosis of soft tissue lesions, 8th edn. Baillière Tindall, London

Gerber C, Ganz R 1984 Clinical assessment of instability of the shoulder. Journal of Bone and Joint Surgery 66B(4): 551–556

Grieve G P 1994a Counterfeit clinical presentations. Manipulative Physiotherapist 26: 17–19

Grieve G P 1994b Thoracic musculoskeletal problems. In: Grieve G P (ed) Modern manual therapy of the vertebral column, Churchill Livingstone, Edinburgh, ch 29, pp 401–428

Hawkins R J, Bokor D J 1990 Clinical evaluation of shoulder problems. In: Rockwood C A, Matsen F A (eds) The shoulder. W B Saunders, Philadelphia, PA, ch 4, p 149

Hislop H, Montgomery J 1995 Daniels and Worthingham's muscle testing, techniques of manual examination, 7th edn. W B Saunders, Philadelphia

Janda V 1994 Muscles and motor control in cervicogenic disorders: assessment and management. In: Grant R (ed) Physical therapy of the cervical and thoracic spine, 2nd edn. Churchill Livingstone, New York, ch 10, p 195

Janda V 2002 Muscles and motor control in cervicogenic disorders. In: Grant R (ed) Physical therapy of the cervical and thoracic spine, 3rd edn. Churchill Livingstone, New York, ch 10, p 182

Jones M A, Rivett D A 2004 Clinical reasoning for manual therapists. Butterworth-Heinemann, Edinburgh

Jull G A, Janda V 1987 Muscles and motor control in low back pain: assessment and management. In: Twomey L T, Taylor J R (eds) Physical therapy of the low back. Churchill Livingstone, New York, ch 10, p 253

Kendall F P, McCreary E K, Provance P G 1993 Muscles testing and function, 4th edn. Williams & Wilkins, Baltimore, MD

Magee D J 1997 Orthopedic physical assessment, 3rd edn. W B Saunders, Philadelphia

Maitland G D 1991 Peripheral manipulation, 3rd edn. Butterworth-Heinemann, London

Matsen F A, Thomas S C, Rockwood C A 1990 Anterior glenohumeral instability. In: Rockwood C A, Matsen F A (eds) The shoulder. W B Saunders, Philadelphia, PA, ch 14, p 526

Mullen F 1989 Locking and quadrant of the shoulder; relationships of the humerus and scapula during locking and quadrant. In: Jones H M, Jones M A, Milde M R (eds) Proceedings of the Manipulative Therapists Association of Australia, 6th biennial conference proceedings, Adelaide, pp 130–137

Mulligan B R 1999 Manual therapy 'NAGs', 'SNAGs', 'MWMs' etc., 4th edn. Plane View Services, New Zealand

Phillips H, Grieve G P 1986 The thoracic outlet syndrome. In: Grieve G P (ed) Modern manual therapy of the vertebral column, Churchill Livingstone, Edinburgh, ch 35, pp 359–369

Sahrmann S A 2002 Diagnosis and treatment of movement impairment syndromes. Mosby, St Louis

Slade S 1989 The glenohumeral joint capsule: its role in the quadrant test. In: Jones H M, Jones M A, Milde M R (eds) Proceedings of the Manipulative Therapists Association of Australia, 6th biennial conference proceedings, Adelaide, pp 178–182

Swift T R, Nichols F T 1984 The droopy shoulder syndrome. Neurology 34: 212–215

Waddell G 2004 The back pain revolution, 2nd edn. Churchill Livingstone, Edinburgh

Young H A, Hardy D G 1983 Thoracic outlet syndrome. British Journal of Hospital Medicine 29: 459–461

Chapter **9**

Examination of the elbow region

POSSIBLE CAUSES OF PAIN AND/OR LIMITATION OF MOVEMENT

This region includes the humeroulnar joint, the radiohumeral joint and the superior radioulnar joints with their surrounding soft tissues.

- Trauma
  - Fracture of humerus, radius or ulna
  - Dislocation of the head of the radius (most commonly seen in young children)
  - Ligamentous sprain
  - Muscular strain
  - Volkmann's ischaemic contracture
  - Tennis elbow/golfer's elbow
- Degenerative conditions: osteoarthrosis
- Calcification of tendons or muscles, e.g. myositis ossificans
- Inflammatory disorders: rheumatoid arthritis
- Infection, e.g. tuberculosis
- Compression of, or injury to, the ulnar nerve
- Bursitis (of subcutaneous olecranon, subtendinous olecranon, radioulnar or bicipitoradial bursa)
- Cubital varus or cubital valgus
- Neoplasm: rare
- Hypermobility syndrome
- Referral of symptoms from the cervical spine, thoracic spine, shoulder, wrist or hand.

Further details of the questions asked during the subjective examination and the tests carried out in the physical examination can be found in Chapters 2 and 3 respectively.

The order of the subjective questioning and the physical tests described below can be altered as appropriate for the patient being examined.

SUBJECTIVE EXAMINATION

Body chart

The following information concerning the type and area of current symptoms can be recorded on a body chart (see Fig. 2.3).

Area of current symptoms

Be exact when mapping out the area of the symptoms. A lesion in the elbow joint complex may refer symptoms distally to the forearm and hand, particularly if the common flexor or extensor tendons of the forearm are affected at the elbow. Ascertain which is the worst symptom and record where the patient feels the symptoms are coming from.

Areas relevant to the region being examined

All other relevant areas are checked for symptoms; it is important to ask about pain or even stiffness, as this may be relevant to the patient's main symptom. Mark unaffected areas with ticks (✓) on the body chart. Check for symptoms in the cervical spine, thoracic spine, shoulder, wrist and hand.

Quality of pain

Establish the quality of the pain.

Intensity of pain

The intensity of pain can be measured using, for example, a visual analogue scale (VAS) as shown in Figure 2.8.

Depth of pain

Establish the depth of the pain. Does the patient feel it is on the surface or deep inside?

Abnormal sensation

Check for any altered sensation (such as paraesthesia or numbness) locally around the elbow region as well as over the shoulder and spine and distally in the arm.

Constant or intermittent symptoms

Ascertain the frequency of the symptoms, whether they are constant or intermittent. If symptoms are constant, check whether there is variation in the intensity of the symptoms, as constant unremitting pain may be indicative of neoplastic disease.

Relationship of symptoms

Determine the relationship between the symptomatic areas – do they come together or separately? For example, the patient could have the elbow pain without the shoulder pain, or they may always be present together.

Behaviour of symptoms

Aggravating factors

For each symptomatic area, discover what movements and/or positions aggravate the patient's symptoms, i.e. what brings them on (or makes them worse), whether they are able to maintain this position or movement (severity), what happens to other symptom(s) when this symptom is produced (or is made worse), and how long does it take for symptoms to ease once the position or movement is stopped (irritability). These questions help to confirm the relationship between the symptoms.

The clinician also asks the patient about theoretically known aggravating factors for structures that could be a source of the symptoms. Common aggravating factors for the elbow are gripping, pronation and supination of the forearm, and leaning on the elbow. Aggravating factors for other regions, which may need to be queried if they are suspected to be a source of the symptoms, are shown in Table 2.3.

The clinician ascertains how the symptoms affect function, such as static and active postures, e.g. leaning on the forearm or hand, writing, turning a key in a lock, opening a bottle, ironing, gripping, lifting, carrying, work, sport and social activities. Note details of training regimen for any sports activities. The clinician finds out if the patient is left- or right-handed as there may be increased stress on the dominant side.

Detailed information on each of the above activities is useful in order to help determine the structure(s) at fault and identify functional restrictions. This information can be used to determine the aims of treatment and any advice that may be required. The most notable functional restrictions are highlighted with asterisks (*), explored in the physical examination, and reassessed at subsequent treatment sessions to evaluate treatment intervention.

Easing factors

For each symptomatic area, the clinician asks what movements and/or positions ease the patient's symptoms, how long it takes to ease them and what happens to other symptoms when this symptom is relieved. These questions help to confirm the relationship between the symptoms.

The clinician asks the patient about theoretically known easing factors for structures that could be a source of the symptoms. For example, symptoms from the elbow joint may be relieved by pulling the forearm away from the upper arm, whereas symptoms from neural tissues may be relieved by shoulder girdle elevation, which reduces tension on the brachial plexus. The clinician can then analyse the position or movement that eases the symptoms to help determine the structure at fault. Find out what happens to other symptom(s) when one symptom is relieved; this helps confirm the relationship of symptoms.

Twenty-four-hour behaviour of symptoms

The clinician determines the 24-hour behaviour of symptoms by asking questions about night, morning and evening symptoms.

Night symptoms. The following questions may be asked:

- Do you have any difficulty getting to sleep?
- What position is most comfortable/uncomfortable?

- What is your normal sleeping position?
- What is your present sleeping position?
- Do your symptom(s) wake you at night? If so,
  - Which symptom(s)?
  - How many times in the past week?
  - How many times in a night?
  - How long does it take to get back to sleep?
- How many and what type of pillows are used?

Morning and evening symptoms. The clinician determines the pattern of the symptoms first thing in the morning, through the day and at the end of the day.

Stage of the condition

In order to determine the stage of the condition the clinician asks whether the symptoms are getting better, getting worse or remaining unchanged.

Special questions

Special questions must always be asked, as they may identify certain precautions or contraindications to the physical examination and/or treatment (Table 2.4). As mentioned in Chapter 2, the clinician must differentiate between conditions that are suitable for conservative management and systemic, neoplastic and other non-neuromusculoskeletal conditions, which require referral to a medical practitioner.

The following information is routinely obtained from patients:

General health. The clinician ascertains the state of the patient's general health, and finds out if the patient suffers from any malaise, fatigue, fever, nausea or vomiting, stress, anxiety or depression.

Weight loss. Has the patient noticed any recent unexplained weight loss?

Rheumatoid arthritis. Has the patient (or a member of his/her family) been diagnosed as having rheumatoid arthritis?

Drug therapy. What drugs are being taken by the patient? Has the patient been prescribed long-term (6 months or more) medication/steroids? Has the patient been taking anticoagulants recently?

X-ray and medical imaging. Has the patient been X-rayed or had any other medical tests recently? Routine spinal X-rays are no longer considered necessary prior to conservative treatment as they only identify the normal age-related degenerative changes, which do not necessarily correlate with the patient's symptoms (Clinical Standards Advisory Report 1994). The medical tests may include blood tests, magnetic resonance imaging, myelography, discography or a bone scan. For further information on these tests, readers are referred to Refshauge & Gass (2004).

Neurological symptoms if a spinal lesion is suspected. Has the patient experienced symptoms of spinal cord compression, which are bilateral tingling in the hands or feet and/or disturbance of gait?

Vertebrobasilar insufficiency. This is relevant where there are symptoms of pain, discomfort and/or altered sensation emanating from the cervical spine, where vertebrobasilar insufficiency (VBI) may be provoked. Further questions about dizziness and testing for vertebrobasilar insufficiency are described more fully in Chapter 6.

History of the present condition (HPC)

For each symptomatic area, the clinician needs to know how long the symptom has been present, whether there was a sudden or slow onset and whether there was a known cause that provoked the onset of the symptom. If the onset was slow, the clinician needs to find out if there has been any change in the patient's lifestyle, e.g. a new job or hobby or a change in sporting activity, that may have contributed to the patient's condition. To confirm the relationship between the symptoms, the clinician asks what happened to other symptoms when each symptom began.

Past medical history (PMH)

The following information is obtained from the patient and/or the medical notes:

- The details of any relevant medical history.
- The history of any previous attacks: how many episodes, when were they, what was the cause, what was the duration of each episode and did the patient fully recover between episodes? If there have been no previous attacks, has the patient had any episodes of stiffness in the cervical spine, thoracic spine, shoulder, elbow, wrist, hand or any other relevant region? Check for a history of trauma or recurrent minor trauma.
- Ascertain the results of any past treatment for the same or similar problem. Past treatment records may be obtained for further information.

Social and family history (SH, FH)

Social and family history that is relevant to the onset and progression of the patient's problem is recorded. This includes the patient's perspectives, experience and expectations, their age, employment, home situation, and details of any leisure activities. Factors from this information may indicate direct and/or indirect mechanical influences on the elbow. In order to treat the patient appropriately, it is important that the condition is managed within the context of the patient's social and work environment.

The clinician may ask the following types of questions to elucidate psychosocial factors:

- Have you had time off work in the past with your pain?
- What do you understand to be the cause of your pain?
- What are you expecting will help you?
- How is your employer/co-workers/family responding to your pain?
- What are you doing to cope with your pain?
- Do you think you will return to work? When?

While these questions are described in relation to psychosocial risk factors for poor outcomes for patients with low back pain (Waddell 2004), they may be relevant to other patients.

Plan of the physical examination

When all this information has been collected, the subjective examination is complete. It is useful at this stage to highlight with asterisks (*), for ease of reference, important findings and particularly one or more functional restrictions. These can then be re-examined at subsequent treatment sessions to evaluate treatment intervention.

In order to plan the physical examination, the following hypotheses should be developed from the subjective examination:

- The regions and structures that need to be examined as a possible cause of the symptoms, e.g. elbow, cervical spine, thoracic spine, shoulder, wrist, hand, muscles and nerves. Often, it is not possible to examine fully at the first attendance and so examination of the structures must be prioritized over subsequent treatment sessions.
- Other factors that need to be examined, e.g. working and everyday postures, muscle weakness, grip on tennis racket and sporting technique, such as service and strokes for tennis, smash for badminton, etc.
- In what way should the physical tests be carried out? Will it be easy or hard to reproduce each symptom? Will it be necessary to use combined movements, repetitive movements, etc. to reproduce the patient's symptoms? Are symptom(s) severe and/or irritable? If symptoms are severe, physical tests may be carried out to just before the onset of symptom production or just to the onset of symptom production; no overpressures will be carried out, as the patient would be unable to tolerate this. If symptoms are irritable, physical tests may be examined to just before symptom production or just to the onset of provocation with less physical tests being examined to allow for rest period between tests.
- Are there any precautions and/or contraindications to elements of the physical examination that need to be explored further, such neurological involvement, recent fracture, trauma, steroid therapy or rheumatoid arthritis; there may also be certain contraindications to further examination and treatment, e.g. symptoms of cord compression.

A physical planning form can be useful for clinicians to help guide them through the clinical reasoning process (see Fig. 2.10 and Appendix 2.1).

PHYSICAL EXAMINATION

The information from the subjective examination helps the clinician to plan an appropriate physical examination. The severity, irritability and nature of the condition are the major factors that will influence the choice and priority of physical testing procedures. The first and over-arching question the clinician might ask is: 'is this patient's condition suitable for me to manage as a therapist?' For example, a patient presenting with cauda equina compression symptoms may only need neurological integrity testing, prior to an urgent medical referral. The nature of the patient's condition has had a major impact on the physical examination. The second question the clinician might ask is: 'does this patient have a neuromusculoskeletal dysfunction that I may be able to help?' To answer that, the clinician needs to carry out a full physical examination; however, this may not be possible if the symptoms are severe and/or irritable. If the patient's symptoms are severe and/or irritable, the clinician aims to explore movements as much as possible, within a symptom-free range. If the patient has constant and severe and/or irritable symptoms, then the clinician aims to find physical tests that ease the symptoms. If the patient's symptoms are non-severe and non-irritable, then the clinician aims to find physical tests that reproduce each of the patient's symptoms.

Each significant physical test that either provokes or eases the patient's symptoms is highlighted in the patient's notes by an asterisk (*) for easy reference. The highlighted tests are often referred to as 'asterisks' or 'markers'.

The order and detail of the physical tests described below need to be appropriate to the patient being examined; some tests will be irrelevant, some tests will be carried out briefly, while it will be necessary to investigate others fully. It is important that readers understand that the techniques shown in this chapter are some of many; the choice depends mainly on the relative size of the clinician and patient, as well as the clinician's preference. For this reason, novice clinicians may initially want to copy what is shown, but then quickly adapt to what is best for them.

Observation

Informal observation

The clinician needs to observe the patient in dynamic and static situations; the quality of movement is noted, as are the postural characteristics and facial expression. Informal observation will have begun from the moment the clinician begins the subjective examination and will continue to the end of the physical examination.

Formal observation

Observation of posture. The clinician observes the bony and soft tissue contours of the elbow region, as well as the patient's posture in sitting and standing, noting the posture of the head and neck, thoracic spine and upper limbs. Any asymmetry can be corrected passively to determine its relevance to the patient's problem. The normal carrying angle is 5–10° in males and 10–15° in females (Magee 1997).

Observation of muscle form. The clinician examines the muscle bulk and muscle tone of the patient, comparing left and right sides. It must be remembered that handedness and level and frequency of physical activity may well produce differences in muscle bulk between sides.

Observation of soft tissues. The clinician observes the colour of the patient's skin and notes any swelling over the elbow region or related areas, taking cues for further examination.

Observation of the patient's attitudes and feelings. The age, gender and ethnicity of patients and their cultural, occupational and social backgrounds will all affect their attitudes and feelings towards themselves, their condition and the clinician. The clinician needs to be aware of and sensitive to these attitudes, and to empathize and communicate appropriately so as to develop a rapport with the patient and thereby enhance the patient's compliance with the treatment.

Joint integrity tests

The clinician observes the relative position of the olecranon and the medial and lateral epicondyles. They should form a straight line with the elbow in extension and an isosceles triangle with the elbow in 90° flexion (Fig. 9.1) (Magee 1997). Alteration in this positioning may indicate a fracture or dislocation.

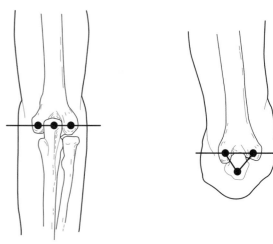

Figure 9.1 The position of the olecranon and medial and lateral epicondyles should form a straight line with the elbow in extension and an isosceles triangle with the elbow flexed to 90°. (From Magee 1992, with permission.)

Ligamentous instability test

The medial collateral ligament is tested by applying an abduction force to the forearm with the elbow in slight flexion; the lateral collateral ligament is tested by applying an adduction force to the forearm with the elbow in slight flexion. These tests are more fully described under passive physiological movements and are shown in Figure 9.2A and B. Excessive movement or reproduction of the patient's symptoms is a positive test and suggests instability of the elbow joint (Volz & Morrey 1993).

Active physiological movements

For active physiological movements, the clinician makes a note of the following:

- Quality of movement
- Range of movement
- Behaviour of pain through the range of movement
- Resistance through the range of movement and at the end of the range of movement
- Provocation of any muscle spasm.

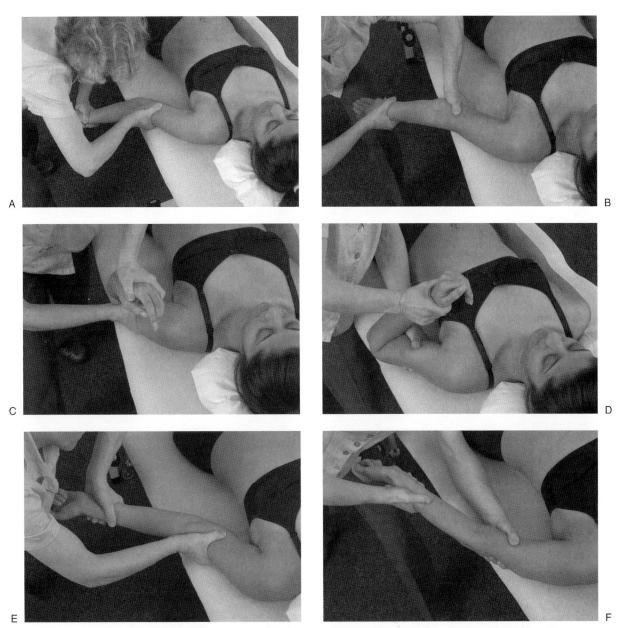

Figure 9.2 Passive physiological movements to the elbow complex. **A** Abduction. The right hand stabilizes the humerus while the left hand abducts the forearm. **B** Adduction. The left hand stabilizes the humerus while the right hand adducts the forearm. **C** Flexion/abduction. The right hand supports underneath the upper arm while the left hand takes the arm into flexion and abduction. **D** Flexion/adduction. The left hand supports underneath the upper arm while the right hand takes the arm into flexion and adduction. **E** Extension/abduction. The right hand supports underneath the upper arm while the left hand takes the arm into extension and abduction. **F** Extension/adduction. The left hand supports underneath the upper arm while the right hand takes the forearm into extension and adduction.

A movement diagram can be used to depict this information. The active movements with overpressure listed below and shown in Figure 9.3 are tested with the patient lying supine or sitting. Movements are carried out on the left and right sides. The clinician establishes symptoms at rest, prior to each movement, and corrects any movement deviation to determine its relevance to the patient's symptoms.

Active physiological movements of the elbow and forearm and possible modifications are shown in Table 9.1. Various differentiation tests (Maitland 1991) can be performed; the choice depends on the patient's signs and symptoms. For example, when elbow flexion reproduces the patient's elbow pain, differentiation between the radiohumeral and humeroulnar joint may be required. In this case, the clinician takes the elbow into flexion to produce the symptoms and then in turn adds a compression force through the radius and then through the ulna by radial and ulnar deviation of the wrist and compares the pain response in each case (Fig. 9.4). If symptoms are from the radioulnar joint, for example, then the patient may feel an increase in pain when compression is applied to the radiohumeral joint but not when compression is applied to the humeroulnar joint. The converse would occur for the humeroulnar joint.

It may be necessary to examine other regions to determine their relevance to the patient's symptoms; they may be the source of the symptoms, or they may be contributing to the symptoms. The regions most likely are the shoulder, cervical spine, thoracic spine, wrist and hand. The joints within these regions can be tested fully (see rele-

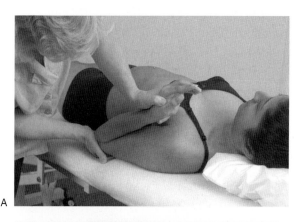

A

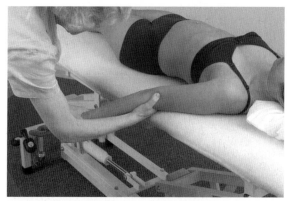

B

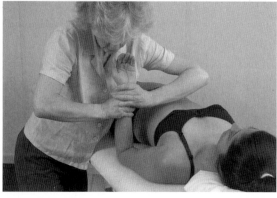

C

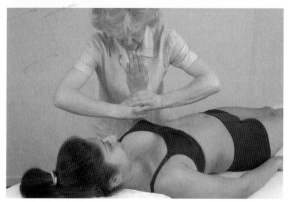

D

Figure 9.3 Overpressures to the elbow complex. **A** Flexion. The right hand supports underneath the elbow while the left hand flexes the elbow. **B** Extension. The right hand supports underneath the elbow while the left hand extends the elbow. **C** Supination. **D** Pronation.

Table 9.1   Active physiological movements and possible modifications

Active physiological movements	Modifications
Elbow flexion	Repeated
Elbow extension	Speed altered
Forearm pronation	Combined, e.g.
Forearm supination	– flexion with pronation or
?Shoulder	supination
?Cervical spine	– pronation with elbow flexion or
?Thoracic spine	extension
?Wrist and hand	Compression or distraction, e.g.
	– compression to humeroulnar
	joint in flexion
	Sustained
	Injuring movement
	Differentiation tests
	Function

vant chapter) or partially with the use of clearing tests (Table 9.2).

Some functional ability has already been tested by the general observation of the patient during the subjective and physical examinations, e.g. the postures adopted during the subjective examination and the ease or difficulty of undressing prior to the examination. Any further functional testing can be carried out at this point in the examination and may include sitting postures, aggravating movements of the upper limb, etc. Clues for appropriate tests can be obtained from the subjective examination findings, particularly aggravating factors. An elbow evaluation chart such as the one devised by Morrey et al (1993) may be useful to document elbow function.

Capsular pattern.   The capsular pattern for the elbow joint is greater limitation of flexion than

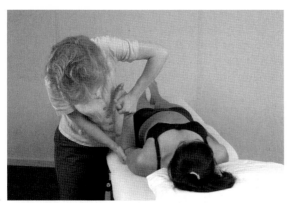 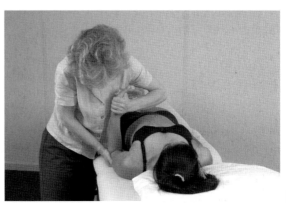

A   B

Figure 9.4   Differentiation test between the radiohumeral and humeroulnar joint. The clinician takes the elbow into flexion to produce the symptoms and then in turn adds a compression force through the radius (**A**) and then the ulna (**B**) by taking the wrist into radial and ulnar deviation respectively.

Table 9.2   Joint clearing tests

Joint	Physiological movement	Accessory movement
Cervical spine	Quadrants (flexion and extension)	All movements
Thoracic spine	Rotation and quadrants (flexion and extension)	All movements
Shoulder girdle	Elevation, depression, protraction and retraction	
Shoulder joint	Flexion and hand behind back	
Acromioclavicular joint	All movements (particularly horizontal flexion)	
Sternoclavicular joint	All movements	
Wrist joint	Flexion/extension and radial/ulnar deviation	
Thumb	Extension carpometacarpal and thumb opposition	
Fingers	Flexion at interphalangeal joints and grip	

extension, and the pattern for the inferior radio-ulnar joint is full range with pain at extremes of range (Cyriax 1982).

Passive physiological joint movement

All the active movements described above can be examined passively with the patient usually in supine, comparing left and right sides. A comparison of the response of symptoms to the active and passive movements can help to determine whether the structure at fault is non-contractile (articular) or contractile (extra-articular) (Cyriax 1982). If the lesion is non-contractile, such as would occur in ligaments, then active and passive movements will be painful and/or restricted in the same direction. If the lesion is in a contractile tissue (i.e. muscle), then active and passive movements are painful and/or restricted in opposite directions.

Additional movement (Fig. 9.2) can be tested passively (Maitland 1991), including:

- Abduction
- Adduction
- Flexion/abduction
- Flexion/adduction
- Extension/abduction
- Extension/adduction.

It may be necessary to examine other regions to determine their relevance to the patient's symptoms; they may be the source of the symptoms, or they may be contributing to the symptoms. The regions most likely are the shoulder, cervical spine, thoracic spine, wrist and hand.

Muscle tests

Muscle tests include examining muscle strength, length and isometric muscle testing.

Muscle strength

The clinician tests the elbow flexors, extensors, forearm pronators, supinators and wrist flexors, extensors, radial deviators and ulnar deviators and any other relevant muscle groups. For details of these general tests, readers are directed to Cole et al (1988), Hislop & Mongtomery (1995) or Kendall et al (1993). Greater detail may be required to test the strength of muscles, in particular those thought prone to weakness (Janda 1994, 2002). These muscles and a description of the tests for muscle strength are given in Chapter 3.

Muscle length

The clinician tests for tennis elbow by stretching the extensor muscles of the wrist and hand, by extending the elbow, pronating the forearm and then flexing the wrist and fingers. A positive test (i.e. muscle shortening) is indicated if the patient's symptoms are reproduced or if range of movement is limited compared to the other side.

The clinician tests for golfer's elbow by stretching the flexor muscles of the wrist and hand, by extending the elbow, supinating the forearm and then extending the wrist and fingers. A positive test is indicated if the patient's symptoms are reproduced or if the range of movement is limited compared to the other side.

The clinician may test the length of other muscles, in particular those thought prone to shorten (Janda 1994, 2002). Descriptions of the tests for muscle length are given in Chapter 3.

Isometric muscle testing

The clinician tests the elbow flexors, extensors, forearm pronators, supinators and wrist flexors, extensors, radial deviators and ulnar deviators (and any other relevant muscle group) in resting position and, if indicated, in different parts of the physiological range. In addition the clinician observes the quality of the muscle contraction to hold this position (this can be done with the patient's eyes shut). The patient may, for example, be unable to prevent the joint from moving or may hold with excessive muscle activity; either of these circumstances would suggest a neuromuscular dysfunction.

An additional test for tennis elbow is an isometric contraction of extension of the third digit – reproduction of pain or weakness over the lateral epicondyle indicates a positive test. In the same way, isometric contraction of the flexor muscles of the wrist and hand can be examined for golfer's elbow.

Neurological tests

Neurological examination includes neurological integrity testing, neurodynamic tests and some other nerve tests.

Integrity of the nervous system

The integrity of the nervous system is tested if the clinician suspects that the symptoms are emanating from the spine or from a peripheral nerve.

Dermatomes/peripheral nerves. Light touch and pain sensation of the upper limb are tested using cotton wool and pinprick respectively, as described in Chapter 3. Knowledge of the cutaneous distribution of nerve roots (dermatomes) and peripheral nerves enables the clinician to distinguish the sensory loss due to a root lesion from that due to a peripheral nerve lesion. The cutaneous nerve distribution and dermatome areas are shown in Figure 3.20.

Myotomes/peripheral nerves. The following myotomes are tested (see Fig. 3.26):

- C4: shoulder girdle elevation
- C5: shoulder abduction
- C6: elbow flexion
- C7: elbow extension
- C8: thumb extension
- T1: finger adduction.

A working knowledge of the muscular distribution of nerve roots (myotomes) and peripheral nerves enables the clinician to distinguish the motor loss due to a root lesion from that due to a peripheral nerve lesion. The peripheral nerve distributions are shown in Figures 3.23 and 3.24.

Reflex testing. The following deep tendon reflexes are tested (see Fig. 3.28):

- C5–C6: biceps
- C7: triceps and brachioradialis.

Neurodynamic tests

The upper limb tension tests (ULTT) may be carried out in order to ascertain the degree to which neural tissue is responsible for producing the patient's symptom(s). These tests are described in detail in Chapter 3.

Other nerve tests

Ulnar nerve

Tinel's sign. This is used to determine the distal point of sensory nerve regeneration. The ulnar nerve is tapped by the clinician where it lies in the groove between the olecranon and the medial epicondyle and the most distal point that produces abnormal sensation in the distribution of the ulnar nerve indicates the point of recovery of the sensory nerve (Magee 1997).

Sustained elbow flexion for 3–5 minutes producing paraesthesia in the distribution of the ulnar nerve is a positive test for cubital tunnel syndrome (Magee 1997).

Median nerve

Pinch-grip test. This tests for anterior interosseous nerve entrapment (anterior interosseous syndrome) between the two heads of pronator teres muscle (Magee 1997). The test is considered positive if the patient is unable to pinch tip-to-tip the index and thumb, which is caused by impairment of flexor pollicis longus, the lateral half of flexor digitorum profundus and pronator quadratus.

Test for pronator syndrome. This involves compression of the median nerve just proximal to the formation of the anterior interosseous nerve (Magee 1997). In addition to the anterior interosseous syndrome described above, the flexor carpi radialis, palmaris longus and flexor digitorum muscles are affected, thus weakening grip strength; in addition, there is sensory loss in the distribution of the median nerve. With the elbow flexed to 90°, the clinician resists pronation as the elbow is extended. Tingling in the distribution of the median nerve is a positive test.

Test for humerus supracondylar process syndrome. This test involves compression of the median nerve as it passes under the ligament of Struthers (found in 1% of the population) running from the shaft of the humerus to the medial epicondyle (Magee 1997). In addition to pronator syndrome described above, the pronator teres muscle is affected, thus weakening the strength of forearm pronation.

Test for radial tunnel syndrome. This involves compression of the posterior interosseous nerve between the two supinator heads in the canal of Frohse (found in 30% of the population) (Magee 1997). Forearm extensor muscles are affected, weakening the strength of wrist and finger extension; there are no sensory symptoms. This syndrome can mimic tennis elbow.

Miscellaneous tests

Thoracic outlet syndrome. These tests are described in Chapter 8.

Palpation of pulses. If the circulation is suspected of being compromised, the brachial artery pulse is palpated on the medial aspect of humerus in the axilla and the radial artery at the wrist.

Palpation

The elbow region is palpated, as well as the cervical spine and thoracic spine, shoulder, wrist and hand as appropriate. It is useful to record palpation findings on a body chart (see Fig. 2.3) and/or palpation chart (see Fig. 3.38).

The clinician notes the following:

- The temperature of the area
- Localized increased skin moisture
- The presence of oedema or effusion. This can be measured using a tape measure and comparing left and right sides
- Mobility and feel of superficial tissues, e.g. ganglions, nodules and scar tissue
- The presence or elicitation of any muscle spasm
- Tenderness of bone, the subcutaneous olecranon bursa, ligaments, muscle, tendon (long head of biceps, forearm flexors and extensors), tendon sheath, trigger points (shown in Fig. 3.39) and nerve. Palpable nerves in the upper limb are as follows:
  - The suprascapular nerve can be palpated along the superior border of the scapula in the suprascapular notch

  - The brachial plexus can be palpated in the posterior triangle of the neck; it emerges at the lower third of sternocleidomastoid
  - The suprascapular nerve can be palpated along the superior border of the scapula in the suprascapular notch
  - The dorsal scapular nerve can be palpated medial to the medial border of the scapula
  - The median nerve can be palpated over the anterior elbow joint crease, medial to the biceps tendon, also at the wrist between palmaris longus and flexor carpi radialis
  - The radial nerve can be palpated around the spiral groove of the humerus, between brachioradialis and flexor carpi radialis, in the forearm and also at the wrist in the snuffbox
- Increased or decreased prominence of bones
- Pain provoked or reduced on palpation.

Accessory movements

It is useful to use the palpation chart and movement diagrams (or joint pictures) to record findings. These are explained in detail in Chapter 3.

The clinician notes the:

- Quality of movement
- Range of movement
- Resistance through the range and at the end of the range of movement
- Behaviour of pain through the range
- Provocation of any muscle spasm.

Humeroulnar joint (Fig. 9.5), radiohumeral joint (Fig. 9.6), superior radioulnar joint (Fig. 9.7) and inferior radioulnar joint accessory movements are listed in Table 9.3. Note that each of these accessory movements will move more than one of the joints in the elbow complex – a medial glide on the olecranon, for example, will cause movement at the superior radioulnar joint as well as the humeroulnar joint.

Following accessory movements to the elbow region, the clinician reassesses all the physical asterisks (movements or tests that have been found to reproduce the patient's symptoms) in order to establish the effect of the accessory movements on the patient's signs and symptoms. Accessory movements can then be tested for other

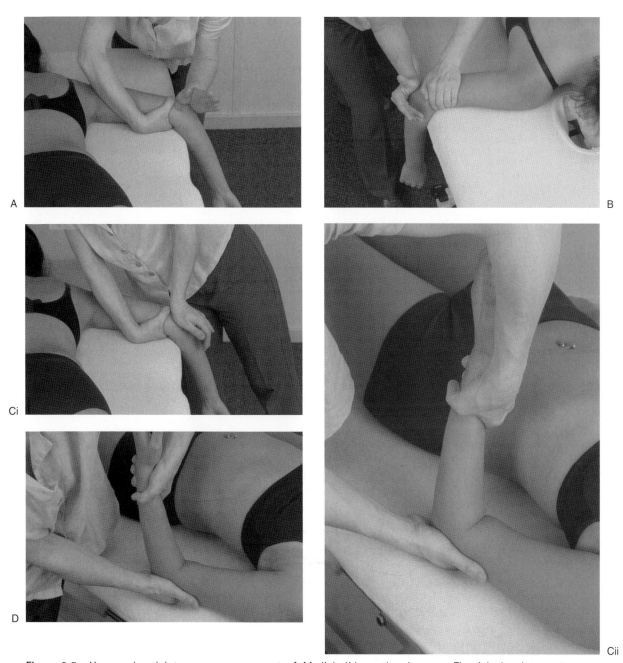

Figure 9.5 Humeroulnar joint accessory movements. **A** Medial glide on the olecranon. The right hand supports underneath the upper arm and the left heel of hand applies a medial glide to the olecranon. **B** Lateral glide on the olecranon. The right hand supports the forearm while the left thumb applies a lateral glide to the olecranon. **C** Longitudinal caudad. Longitudinal caudad can be applied directly on the olecranon; i) the right hand supports underneath the upper arm and the left heel of hand applies a longitudinal caudad glide to the olecranon or ii) right hand supports underneath upper arm and the left hand pulls the forearm upwards to produce a longitudinal caudad movement at the elbow region. **D** Compression. The left hand supports underneath the elbow while the right hand pushes down through the hand and forearm.

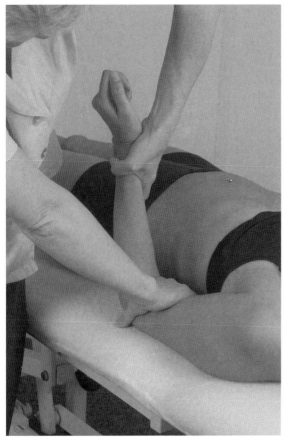 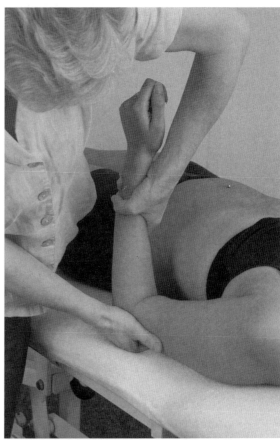

A   B

Figure 9.6   Radiohumeral joint accessory movements. **A** Longitudinal caudad. The right hand blocks the upper arm movement and the left hand pulls the radial side of the forearm. **B** Longitudinal cephalad. The right hand supports underneath the elbow and the left hand pushes the down through the radial side of the forearm.

regions suspected to be a source or contributing to the patient's symptoms. Again, following accessory movements to any one region the clinician reassesses all the asterisks. Regions likely to be examined are the cervical spine, thoracic spine, shoulder, wrist and hand (Table 9.3).

Mobilizations with movement (MWMs) (Mulligan 1999)

With the patient supine, the clinician applies a lateral glide to the ulna (Fig. 9.9). A seat belt can be used to apply the force if preferred. An increase in the range of movement and no pain or reduced

pain on active flexion or extension of the elbow are positive examination findings, indicating a mechanical joint problem.

For patients with suspected tennis elbow, the clinician applies a lateral glide to the ulna while the patient makes a fist. Relief of pain is a positive finding, indicating a tracking or positional fault at the elbow that is contributing to the soft tissue lesion.

COMPLETION OF THE EXAMINATION

Having carried out the above tests, the examination of the elbow region is now complete. The sub-

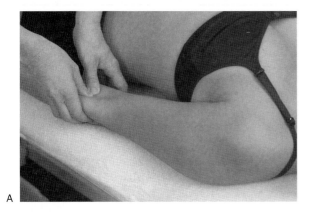

A

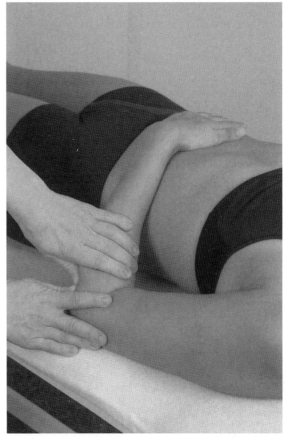

B

Figure 9.7 Superior radioulnar joint accessory movements. **A** Anteroposterior. Thumb pressure is applied slowly through the soft tissue to the anterior aspect of the head of the radius. **B** Posteroanterior. Thumb pressure is applied to the posterior aspect of the head of the radius.

Table 9.3 Accessory movements, choice of application and reassessment of the patient's asterisks

Accessory movements	Choice of application	Identify any effect of accessory movements on patient's signs and symptoms
Humeroulnar joint (Fig. 9.5)	Start position, e.g.	Reassess all asterisks
↦ Med medial glide on olecranon or coronoid	− in flexion	
↦ Lat lateral glide on olecranon or coronoid	− in extension	
↤↦ Caud longitudinal caudad	− in pronation	
Comp compression	− in supination	
Radiohumeral joint (Fig. 9.6)	− in flexion and supination	
↤↦ Caud longitudinal caudad	− in flexion and pronation	
↤↦ Ceph longitudinal cephalad	− in extension and supination	
Superior radioulnar joint (Fig. 9.7)	− in extension and pronation	
↕ anteroposterior	Speed of force application	
↕ posteroanterior	Direction of the applied force	
Inferior radioulnar joint (Fig. 9.8)	Point of application of applied force	
↕ anteroposterior		
↕ posteroanterior		
?Cervical spine	As above	Reassess all asterisks
?Thoracic spine	As above	Reassess all asterisks
?Shoulder	As above	Reassess all asterisks
?Wrist and hand	As above	Reassess all asterisks

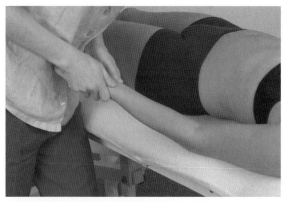

Figure 9.8 Inferior radioulnar joint accessory movements: anteroposterior/posteroanterior glide. The left and right hands each grasp the anterior and posterior aspect of the radius and ulna. The hands then apply a force in opposite directions to produce an anteroposterior posteroanterior glide.

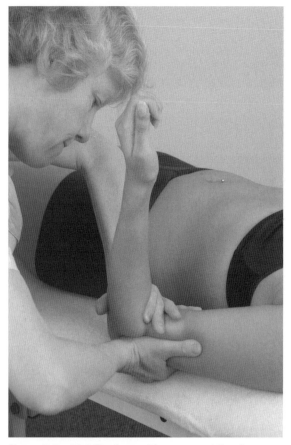

Figure 9.9 Mobilizations with movement for elbow flexion. The right hand supports the upper arm while the left hand applies a lateral glide to the ulna and the patient actively flexes the elbow.

jective and physical examinations produce a large amount of information, which should be recorded accurately and quickly. An outline examination chart may be useful for some clinicians and one is suggested in Figure 9.10. It is important, however, that the clinician does not examine in a rigid manner, simply following the suggested sequence outlined in the chart. Each patient presents differently and this should be reflected in the examination process. It is vital at this stage to highlight with an asterisk (*) important findings from the examination. These findings must be reassessed at, and within, subsequent treatment sessions to evaluate the effects of treatment on the patient's condition.

The physical testing procedures which specifically indicate joint, nerve or muscle tissues, as a source of the patient's symptoms, are summarized in Table 3.10. The strongest evidence that a joint is the source of the patient's symptoms is that active and passive physiological movements, passive accessory movements and joint palpation all reproduce the patient's symptoms, and that following a treatment dose, reassessment identifies an improvement in the patient's signs and symptoms. Weaker evidence includes an alteration in range, resistance or quality of physiological and/or accessory movements and tenderness over the joint, with no alteration in signs and symptoms after treatment. One or more of these findings may indicate a dysfunction of a joint which may, or may not, be contributing to the patient's condition.

The strongest evidence that a muscle is the source of a patient's symptoms is if active movements, an isometric contraction, passive lengthening and palpation of a muscle all reproduce the patient's symptoms, and that following a treatment dose, reassessment identifies an improvement in the patient's signs and symptoms. Further evidence of muscle dysfunction may be suggested by reduced strength or poor quality during the active physiological movement and the isometric contraction, reduced range and/or increased/decreased resistance, during the passive lengthening of the muscle, and tenderness on palpation, with no alteration in signs and symptoms after treatment. One or more of these findings may indicate a dysfunction of a muscle which may, or may not, be contributing to the patient's condition.

Body chart	Name
	Age
	Date
	24-hour behaviour
	Improving static worsening
Relationship of symptoms	Special questions General health Weight loss RA Drugs Steroids Anticoagulants X-ray Cord symptoms Cauda equina symptoms VBI symptoms
Aggravating factors and function	HPC
	PMH
Severe Irritable	
Easing factors	SH & FH (Patient's perspective, experience, expectations. Yellow, blue, black flags)

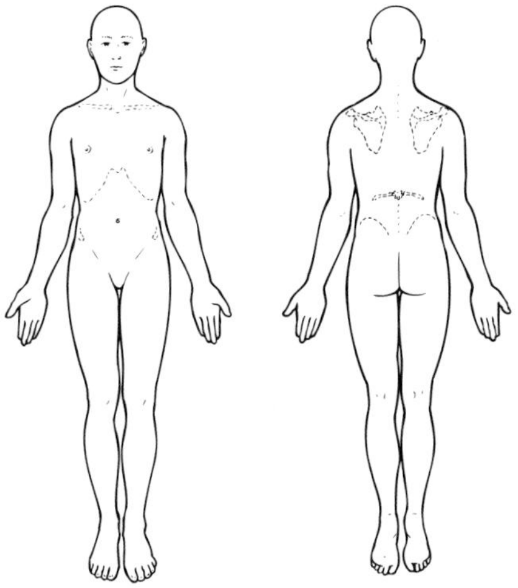

Figure 9.10 Elbow examination chart.

Physical examination Observation	**Isometric muscle testing**
Joint integrity tests (medial and lateral ligament tests)	**Neurological integrity tests**
Active and passive physiological movements of elbow and other relevant regions	**Neurodynamic tests**
	Other nerve tests (ulnar, median, radial)
	Miscellaneous tests (thoracic outlet, pulses, oedema)
	Palpation
Capsular pattern yes/no	
Muscle strength	**Accessory movements and reassessment of each relevant region**
Muscle length	

Figure 9.10 *Continued*

The strongest evidence that a nerve is the source of the patient's symptoms is when active and/or passive physiological movements reproduce the patient's symptoms, which are then increased or decreased with an additional sensitizing movement, at a distance from the patient's symptoms. In addition, there is reproduction of the patient's symptoms on palpation of the nerve and neurodynamic testing, sufficient to be considered a treatment dose, results in an improvement in the above signs and symptoms. Further evidence of nerve dysfunction may be suggested by reduced range (compared to the asymptomatic side) and/or increased resistance to the various arm movements, and tenderness on nerve palpation.

On completion of the physical examination, the clinician:

- Warns the patient of possible exacerbation up to 24–48 hours following the examination.
- Requests the patient to report details on the behaviour of the symptoms following examination at the next attendance.
- Explains the findings of the physical examination and how these findings relate to the subjective assessment. Any misconceptions patients may have regarding their illness or injury should be cleared up here.
- Evaluates the findings, formulates a clinical diagnosis and writes up a problem list. Clini-

cians may find the management planning forms shown in Figures 3.53 and 3.54 helpful in guiding them through what is often a complex clinical reasoning process.

- Determines the objectives of treatment.
- Devises an initial treatment plan.

In this way, the clinician will have developed the following hypotheses categories (adapted from Jones & Rivett 2004):

- Function: abilities and restrictions.
- Patients' perspectives on their experience.
- Source of symptoms. This includes the structure or tissue that is thought to be producing the patients' symptoms, the nature of the structure or tissues in relation to the healing process, and the pain mechanisms.
- Contributing factors to the development and maintenance of the problem. There may be environmental, psychosocial, behavioural, physical or heredity factors.
- Precautions/contraindications to treatment and management. This includes the severity and irritability of the patient's symptoms and the nature of the patient's condition.
- Management strategy and treatment plan.
- Prognosis – this can be affected by factors such as the stage and extent of the injury as well as the patient's expectation, personality and lifestyle.

References

Clinical Standards Advisory Report 1994 Report of a CSAG committee on back pain. HMSO, London

Cole J H, Furness A L, Twomey L T 1988 Muscles in action, an approach to manual muscle testing. Churchill Livingstone, Edinburgh

Cyriax J 1982 Textbook of orthopaedic medicine – diagnosis of soft tissue lesions, 8th edn. Baillière Tindall, London

Hislop H, Montgomery J 1995 Daniels and Worthingham's muscle testing, techniques of manual examination, 7th edn. W B Saunders, Philadelphia

Janda V 1994 Muscles and motor control in cervicogenic disorders: assessment and management. In: Grant R (ed) Physical therapy of the cervical and thoracic spine, 2nd edn. Churchill Livingstone, New York, ch 10, p 195

Janda V 2002 Muscles and motor control in cervicogenic disorders. In: Grant R (ed) Physical therapy of the cervical and thoracic spine, 3rd edn. Churchill Livingstone, New York, ch 10, p 182

Jones M A, Rivett D A 2004 Clinical reasoning for manual therapists. Butterworth-Heinemann, Edinburgh

Kendall F P, McCreary E K, Provance P G 1993 Muscles testing and function, 4th edn. Williams & Wilkins, Baltimore, MD

Magee D J 1997 Orthopedic physical assessment, 3rd edn. W B Saunders, Philadelphia

Maitland G D 1991 Peripheral manipulation, 3rd edn. Butterworth-Heinemann, London

Morrey B F, An K N, Chao E Y S 1993 Functional evaluation of the elbow. In: Morrey B F (ed) The elbow and its disorders, 2nd edn. W B Saunders, Philadelphia, PA, ch 6, p 86

Mulligan B R 1999 Manual therapy 'NAGs', 'SNAGs', 'MWMs' etc., 4th edn. Plane View Services, New Zealand

Refshauge K, Gass E (eds) 2004 Musculoskeletal physiotherapy clinical science and evidence-based practice. Butterworth-Heinemann, Oxford

Volz R C, Morrey B F 1993 The physical examination of the elbow. In: Morrey B F (ed) The elbow and its disorders, 2nd edn. W B Saunders, Philadelphia, PA, ch 5, p 73

Waddell G 2004 The back pain revolution, 2nd edn. Churchill Livingstone, Edinburgh

Chapter **10**

Examination of the wrist and hand

POSSIBLE CAUSES OF PAIN AND/OR LIMITATION OF MOVEMENT

This region includes the superior and inferior radioulnar, radiocarpal, intercarpal, carpometacarpal, intermetacarpal, metacarpophalangeal and interphalangeal joints and their surrounding soft tissues.

- Trauma
  - Fracture of the radius, ulna (e.g. Colles' or Smith fracture), carpal or metacarpal bones or phalanges
  - Dislocation of interphalangeal joints
  - Crush injuries to the hand
  - Ligamentous sprain
  - Muscular strain
  - Tendon and tendon sheath injuries
  - Digital amputations
  - Peripheral nerve injuries
- Degenerative conditions: osteoarthrosis
- Inflammatory conditions: rheumatoid arthritis
- Tenosynovitis, e.g. de Quervain's disease
- Carpal tunnel syndrome
- Guyon's canal compression
- Infections, e.g. animal or human bites
- Dupuytren's disease
- Raynaud's disease
- Complex regional pain syndrome (reflex sympathetic dystrophy)
- Neoplasm
- Hypermobility syndrome
- Referral of symptoms from the cervical spine, thoracic spine, shoulder or elbow.

Further details of the questions asked during the subjective examination and the tests carried out in the physical examination can be found in Chapters 2 and 3 respectively.

The order of the subjective questioning and the physical tests described below can be altered as appropriate for the patient being examined.

SUBJECTIVE EXAMINATION

Body chart

The following information concerning the type and area of current symptoms can be recorded on a body chart (see Fig. 2.3). In order to be specific, it may be necessary to use an enlarged chart of the hand and wrist.

Area of current symptoms

Be exact when mapping out the area of the symptoms. Lesions of the joints in this region usually produce localized symptoms over the affected joint. Ascertain which is the worst symptom and record where the patient feels the symptoms are coming from.

Areas relevant to the region being examined

All other relevant areas are checked for symptoms; it is important to ask about pain or even stiffness, as this may be relevant to the patient's main symptom. Mark unaffected areas with ticks (✓) on the body chart. Check for symptoms in the cervical spine, thoracic spine, shoulder and elbow.

Quality of pain

Establish the quality of the pain.

Intensity of pain

The intensity of pain can be measured using, for example, a visual analogue scale (VAS) as shown in Figure 2.8.

Depth of pain

Establish the depth of the pain. Does the patient feel it is on the surface or deep inside?

Abnormal sensation

Check for any altered sensation (such as paraesthesia or numbness) locally around the wrist and hand, as well as proximally over the elbow, shoulder and spine as appropriate. For a brief assessment, where this is appropriate, sensation can be limited to: index finger and thumb, for median nerve; little finger and hypothenar eminence for ulnar nerve; and first and second metacarpal for radial nerve (dorsal branch).

Constant or intermittent symptoms

Ascertain the frequency of the symptoms; whether they are constant or intermittent. If symptoms are constant, check whether there is variation in the intensity of the symptoms, as constant unremitting pain may be indicative of neoplastic disease.

Relationship of symptoms

Determine the relationship between the symptomatic areas – do they come together or separately? For example, the patient could have the wrist pain without the elbow pain, or they may always be present together.

Behaviour of symptoms

Aggravating factors

For each symptomatic area, discover what movements and/or positions aggravate the patient's symptoms, i.e. what brings them on (or makes them worse), are they able to maintain this position or movement (severity), what happens to other symptom(s) when this symptom is produced (or is made worse), and how long does it take for symptoms to ease once the position or movement is stopped (irritability). These questions help to confirm the relationship between the symptoms.

The clinician also asks the patient about theoretically known aggravating factors for structures that could be a source of the symptoms. Common aggravating factors for the wrist and hand are flexion and extension of the wrist, resisted grips (both pinch and power) and grips with pronation and supination, and weight-bearing. Cold intolerance commonly occurs after nerve injury, causing pain and vascular changes in cold weather. Aggravating factors for other regions, which may need to be queried if they are suspected to be a source of the symptoms, are shown in Table 2.3.

The clinician ascertains how the symptoms affect function, such as: static and active postures, e.g. leaning on the forearm or hand, gripping, turning a key in a lock, ironing, dusting, driving, lifting, carrying, work, sport and social activities. Note details of training regimen for any sports activities. The clinician finds out if the patient is left- or right-handed as there may be increased stress on the dominant side

Detailed information on each of the above activities is useful in order to help determine the structure(s) at fault and identify functional restrictions. This information can be used to determine the aims of treatment and any advice that may be required. The most notable functional restrictions are highlighted with asterisks (*), explored in the physical examination, and reassessed at subsequent treatment sessions to evaluate treatment intervention.

Easing factors

For each symptomatic area, the clinician asks what movements and/or positions ease the patient's symptoms, how long it takes to ease them and what happens to other symptom(s) when this symptom is relieved. These questions help to confirm the relationship between the symptoms.

The clinician asks the patient about theoretically known easing factors for structures that could be a source of the symptoms. For example, symptoms from the wrist may be relieved by pulling the hand away from the forearm (i.e. distraction), whereas symptoms from the neural tissue may be eased by certain cervical positions. The clinician can then analyse the position or movement that eases the symptoms to help determine the structure at fault.

Twenty-four-hour behaviour of symptoms

The clinician determines the 24-hour behaviour of symptoms by asking questions about night, morning and evening symptoms.

Night symptoms.   The following questions may be asked:

- Do you have any difficulty getting to sleep?
- What position is most comfortable/uncomfortable?
- What is your normal sleeping position?
- What is your present sleeping position?
- Do your symptom(s) wake you at night? If so,
  - Which symptom(s)?
  - How many times in the past week?
  - How many times in a night?
  - How long does it take to get back to sleep?
- How many and what type of pillows are used?

Morning and evening symptoms.   The clinician determines the pattern of the symptoms first thing in the morning, through the day and at the end of the day.

Stage of the condition

In order to determine the stage of the condition, the clinician asks whether the symptoms are getting better, getting worse or remaining unchanged.

Special questions

Special questions must always be asked, as they may identify certain precautions or contraindications to the physical examination and/or treatment (see Table 2.4). As mentioned in Chapter 2, the clinician must differentiate between conditions that are suitable for conservative management and systemic, neoplastic and other non-neuromusculoskeletal conditions, which require referral to a medical practitioner.

The following information is routinely obtained from patients:

General health.   The clinician ascertains the state of the patient's general health, and finds out if the patient suffers from malaise, fatigue, fever, nausea or vomiting, stress, anxiety or depression.

Weight loss.   Has the patient noticed any recent unexplained weight loss?

Rheumatoid arthritis.   Has the patient (or a member of his/her family) been diagnosed as having rheumatoid arthritis?

Dupuytren's disease. Has the patient or anyone in the patient's family been diagnosed with Dupuytren's disease? Has the patient noticed nodules in the palm?

Drug therapy. What drugs are being taken by the patient? Has the patient ever been prescribed long-term (6 months or more) medication/steroids? Has the patient been taking anticoagulants recently?

Diabetes. Has the patient been diagnosed as having diabetes? How long ago was it diagnosed? Healing of tissues is likely to be slower in the presence of this disease.

X-ray and medical imaging. Has the patient been X-rayed or had any other medical tests recently? X-rays are vital in hand or joint fractures, dislocations and joint disease. Joint and bone position give information that will help guide rehabilitation and indicate likely prognosis. Imaging in theatre of internal fixation and bone grafts is an excellent method of educating the patient and the medical staff. Routine spinal X-rays are no longer considered necessary prior to conservative treatment as they only identify the normal age-related degenerative changes, which do not necessarily correlate with the patient's symptoms (Clinical Standards Advisory Report 1994). The medical tests may include blood tests, magnetic resonance imaging, myelography, discography or a bone scan. For further information on these tests, the reader is referred to Refshauge & Gass (2004).

Neurological symptoms. Has the patient experienced any tingling, pins and needles, pain or hypersensitivity in the hand? Are these symptoms unilateral or bilateral? Has the patient noticed any weakness in the hand? Has s/he experienced symptoms of spinal cord compression, which are bilateral tingling in the hands or feet and/or disturbance of gait?

History of the present condition (HPC)

For trauma cases, the clinician may ask how (e.g. knife, glass, assault, accidental, self-inflicted) and where the accident occurred. For each symptomatic area, the clinician needs to know how long the symptom has been present, whether there was a sudden or slow onset and whether there was a known cause that provoked the onset of the symptom. If the onset was slow, the clinician finds out if there has been any change in the patient's lifestyle, e.g. a new job or hobby or a change in sporting activity. This may be contributing to the patient's condition. To confirm the relationship of symptoms, the clinician asks what happened to other symptoms when each symptom began.

Past medical history (PMH)

The following information is obtained from the patient and/or the medical notes:

- The details of any relevant medical history.
- The history of any previous attacks: how many episodes, when were they, what was the cause, what was the duration of each episode and did the patient fully recover between episodes? If there have been no previous attacks, has the patient had any episodes of stiffness in the cervical spine, thoracic spine, shoulder, elbow, wrist, hand or any other relevant region? Check for a history of trauma or recurrent minor trauma.
- Ascertain the results of any past treatment for the same or similar problem. Past treatment records may be obtained for further information.

Social and family history (SH, FH)

Social and family history that is relevant to the onset and progression of the patient's problem is recorded. This includes the patient's perspectives, experience and expectations, their age, employment, home situation, and details of any leisure activities. Particularly in trauma cases, check the working situation, financial situation and any potential compensation claims. Factors from this information may indicate direct and/or indirect mechanical influences on the wrist and hand. In order to treat the patient appropriately, it is important that the condition is managed within the context of the patient's social and work environment.

The clinician may ask the following types of questions to elucidate psychosocial factors:

- Have you had time off work in the past with your pain?
- What do you understand to be the cause of your pain?
- What are you expecting will help you?
- How is your employer/co-workers/family responding to your pain?
- What are you doing to cope with your pain?
- Do you think you will return to work? When?

While these questions are described in relation to psychosocial risk factors for poor outcomes for patients with low back pain (Waddell 2004), they may be relevant to other patients.

Plan of the physical examination

When all this information has been collected, the subjective examination is complete. It is useful at this stage to highlight with asterisks (*), for ease of reference, important findings and particularly one or more functional restrictions. These can then be re-examined at subsequent treatment sessions to evaluate treatment intervention.

In order to plan the physical examination, the following hypotheses need to be developed from the subjective examination:

- The regions and structures that need to be examined as a possible cause of the symptoms, e.g. wrist and hand, cervical spine, thoracic spine, shoulder, elbow, radioulnar joints, muscles and nerves. Often it is not possible to examine fully at the first attendance and so examination of the structures must be prioritized over subsequent treatment sessions.
- Other factors that need to be examined, e.g. working and everyday postures, muscle weakness and sporting technique, such as service and strokes for tennis, smash for badminton, etc.
- In what way should the physical tests be carried out? Will it be easy or hard to reproduce each symptom? Will it be necessary to use combined movements, repetitive movements, etc. to reproduce the patient's symptoms? Are symptom(s) severe and/or irritable? If symptoms are severe, physical tests may be carried out to just before the onset of symptom production or just to the onset of symptom production; no overpressures

will be carried out, as the patient would be unable to tolerate this. If symptoms are irritable, physical tests may be examined to just before symptom production or just to the onset of provocation with less physical tests being examined to allow for rest period between tests.

- Are there any precautions and/or contraindications to elements of the physical examination that need to be explored further, such as neurological involvement, recent fracture, trauma, steroid therapy or rheumatoid arthritis; there may also be certain contraindications to further examination and treatment, e.g. symptoms of cord compression.

A physical planning form can be useful for clinicians to help guide them through the clinical reasoning process (see Fig. 2.10 and Appendix 2.1).

PHYSICAL EXAMINATION

The information from the subjective examination helps the clinician to plan an appropriate physical examination. The severity, irritability and nature of the condition are the major factors that will influence the choice and priority of physical testing procedures. The first and over-arching question the clinician might ask is: 'is this patient's condition suitable for me to manage as a therapist?' For example, a patient presenting with cauda equina compression symptoms may only need neurological integrity testing, prior to an urgent medical referral. The nature of the patient's condition has had a major impact on the physical examination. The second question the clinician might ask is: 'does this patient have a neuromusculoskeletal dysfunction that I may be able to help?' To answer that, the clinician needs to carry out a full physical examination; however, this may not be possible if the symptoms are severe and/or irritable. If the patient's symptoms are severe and/or irritable, the clinician aims to explore movements as much as possible, within a symptom-free range. If the patient has constant and severe and/or irritable symptoms, then the clinician aims to find physical tests that ease the symptoms. If the patient's symptoms are non-severe and non-irritable, then the clinician aims to find physical tests that reproduce each of the patient's symptoms.

Each significant physical test that either provokes or eases the patient's symptoms is highlighted in the patient's notes by an asterisk (*) for easy reference. The highlighted tests are often referred to as 'asterisks' or 'markers'.

The order and detail of the physical tests described below need to be appropriate to the patient being examined; some tests will be irrelevant, some tests will be carried out briefly, while it will be necessary to investigate others fully. It is important that readers understand that the techniques shown in this chapter are some of many; the choice depends mainly on the relative size of the clinician and patient, as well as the clinician's preference. For this reason, novice clinicians may initially want to copy what is shown, but then quickly adapt to what is best for them.

Observation

Informal observation

The clinician needs to observe the patient in dynamic and static situations; the quality of movement is noted, as are the postural characteristics and facial expression. Informal observation will have begun from the moment the clinician begins the subjective examination and will continue to the end of the physical examination.

Formal observation

Observation of posture. The clinician observes the bony and soft tissue contours of the elbow, wrist and hand, as well as the patient's posture in sitting and standing, noting the posture of the head and neck, thoracic spine and shoulders. Look for abnormal posture of the hand such as dropped wrist and fingers in radial nerve palsy, clawing of the ulnar two fingers in ulnar nerve palsy, or adducted thumb in median nerve palsy. Any asymmetry can be corrected passively to determine its relevance to the patient's problem.

Observation of muscle form. The clinician examines the muscle bulk and muscle tone of the patient, comparing left and right sides. Check for wasting of specific muscles such as the first dorsal

interosseous muscle supplied by the ulnar nerve, or opponens pollicis supplied by the median nerve. It must be remembered that handedness and level and frequency of physical activity may well produce differences in muscle bulk between sides.

Observation of soft tissues. The clinician observes the colour of the patient's skin, any swelling, increased hair growth on the hand, brittle fingernails, infection of the nail bed, sweating or dry palm, shiny skin, scars and bony deformities, and takes cues for further examination. These changes could be indicative of a peripheral nerve injury, peripheral vascular disease, diabetes mellitus, Raynaud's disease, complex regional pain syndrome (previously reflex sympathetic dystrophy) or shoulder–hand syndrome (Magee 1997).

Common deformities of the hand include the following:

* Swan-neck deformity of fingers or thumb: the proximal interphalangeal joint (PIPJ) is hyperextended and the distal interphalangeal joint (DIPJ) is flexed (Fig. 10.1). It has a variety of causes; see Eckhaus (1993) for further details.
* Boutonnière deformity of fingers or thumb: the PIPJ is flexed and the DIPJ is hyperextended (Fig. 10.2). The central slip of the extensor tendon is damaged and the lateral bands displace volarly (Eddington 1993).

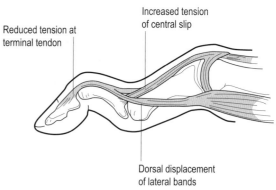

Increased tension of central slip

Reduced tension at terminal tendon

Dorsal displacement of lateral bands

Figure 10.1 Swan-neck deformity. (From Eckhaus 1993, with permission.)

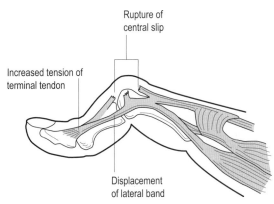

Figure 10.2 Boutonnière deformity. (From Eddington 1993, with permission.)

- Claw hand: the little and ring fingers are hyper-extended at the metacarpophalangeal joint (MCPJ) and flexed at the interphalangeal joints (IPJs). This condition is due to ulnar nerve palsy.
- Mallet finger: rupture of the terminal extensor tendon at the DIPJ.
- Clinodactyly: congenital radial deviation of the distal joints of the fingers, most commonly seen in the little finger.
- Camptodactyly: congenital flexion contracture at the PIPJ and DIPJ, commonly seen in the little finger.
- The presence of Heberden's nodes over the dorsum of the DIPJs is indicative of osteoarthritis, and Bouchard's nodes over the dorsum of the PIPJs are indicative of rheumatoid arthritis. Club nails, where there is excessive soft tissue under the nail, are indicative of respiratory or cardiac disorders.

Observation of the patient's attitudes and feelings. The age, gender and ethnicity of patients and their cultural, occupational and social backgrounds will all affect their attitudes and feelings towards themselves, their condition and the clinician. Hands are particularly visual and are used regularly to show feelings, in conversation and for function. The clinician needs to be aware of and sensitive to these attitudes, and to empathize and communicate appropriately so as to develop a rapport with the patient and thereby enhance the patient's compliance with the treatment.

Joint integrity tests

At the wrist, ligamentous instability can occur between the scaphoid and lunate, the lunate and triquetrum, and the triquetrum and hamate (mid-carpal). These instabilities need to be diagnosed by passive movement tests as routine radiographs appear normal (Taleisnik 1988).

Watson's scaphoid shift test. The clinician applies an anterior glide to the scaphoid while passively moving the wrist from a position of ulnar deviation and slight extension to radial deviation and slight flexion. Posterior subluxation of the scaphoid and/or reproduction of the patient's pain indicate instability of the scaphoid (Watson et al 1988).

Lunotriquetral ballottement test. This tests for instability at the joint between the lunate and triquetral bones. Excessive movement, crepitus or pain with anterior and posterior glide of the lunate on the triquetrum indicates a positive test (Linscheid & Dobyns 1987).

Midcarpal test. The examiner applies an antero-posterior force to the scaphoid while distracting and flexing the wrist (Louis et al 1984). Reproduction of the patient's pain indicates a positive test, suggesting instability between the radius, scaphoid, lunate and capitate.

Ligamentous instability test for the joints of the thumb and fingers. Excessive movement when an abduction or adduction force is applied to the joint is indicative of joint instability due to a laxity of the collateral ligaments.

Active physiological movements

For active physiological movements, the clinician notes the following:

- Quality of movement
- Range of movement
- Behaviour of pain through the range of movement
- Resistance through the range of movement and at the end of the range of movement
- Provocation of any muscle spasm.

A movement diagram can be used to depict this information. The active movements with over-

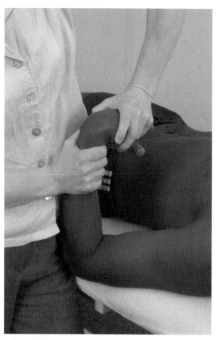

A (i) Flexion. The wrist and hand is grasped by both hands and taken into flexion.

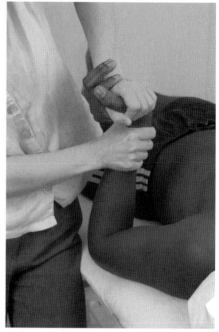

A (ii) Extension. The right hand supports the patient's forearm and the left hand takes the wrist and hand into extension.

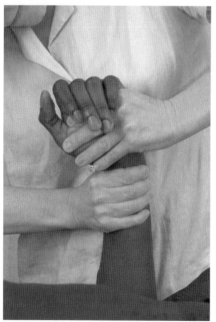

A (iii) Radial deviation. The right hand supports just proximal to the wrist joint while the left hand moves the wrist into radial deviation.

Figure 10.3(A–E)   Overpressures to the wrist and hand.

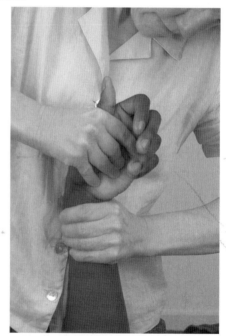

A (iv) Ulnar deviation. The left hand supports just proximal to the wrist joint while the right hand moves the wrist into ulnar deviation.

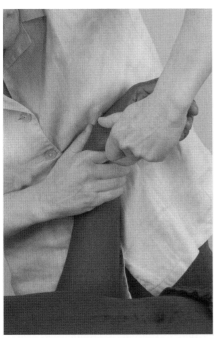

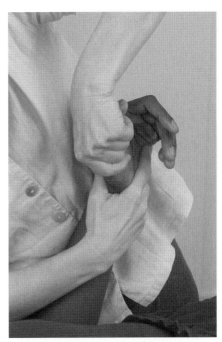

B (i) Flexion. The right hand supports the carpus while the left hand takes the metacarpal into flexion.

B (ii) Extension. The right hand supports the carpus while the left hand takes the metacarpal into extension.

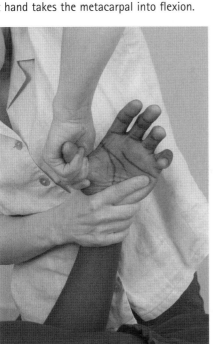

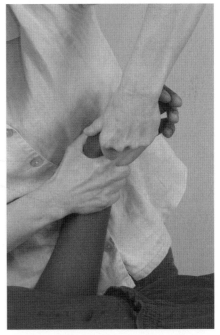

B (iii) Abduction and adduction. The right hand supports the carpus while the left hand takes the metacarpal into abduction and adduction.

B (iv) Opposition. The right hand supports the carpus while the left hand takes the metacarpal across the palm into opposition.

Figure 10.3 *Continued*   B Carpometacarpal joint of thumb. For all these movements, the hands are placed immediately proximal and distal to the joint line.

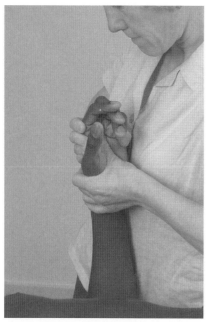

C (i) Horizontal flexion. The left thumb is placed in the centre of the palm at the level of the metacarpal heads. The right hand cups around the back of the metacarpal heads and moves them into horizontal flexion.

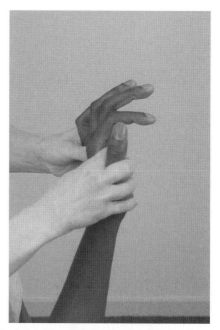

C (ii) Horizontal extension. The thumbs are placed in the centre of the dorsum of the palm at the level of the metacarpal heads. The fingers wrap around the anterior aspect of the hand and pull the metacarpal heads into horizontal extension.

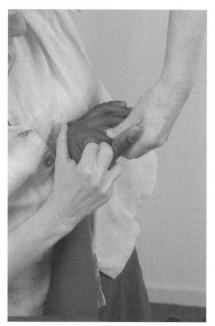

D (i) Flexion. The right hand supports the metacarpal while the left hand takes the proximal phalanx into flexion.

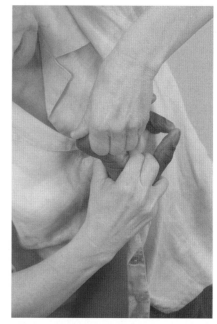

D (ii) Extension. The right hand supports the metacarpal while the left hand takes the proximal phalanx into extension.

Figure 10.3 *Continued* **C** Distal intermetacarpal joints **D** Metacarpophalangeal joints.

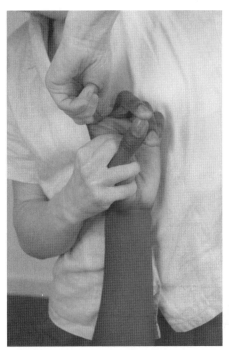

D (iii) Abduction and adduction. The right hand supports the metacarpal while the left hand takes the proximal phalanx into abduction and adduction.

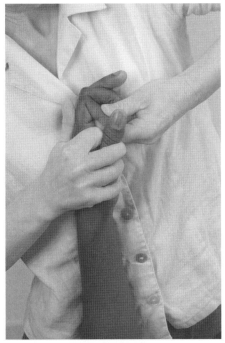

E (i) Flexion. The right hand supports the metacarpophalangeal joint in extension while the left hand takes the proximal interphalangeal joint into flexion.

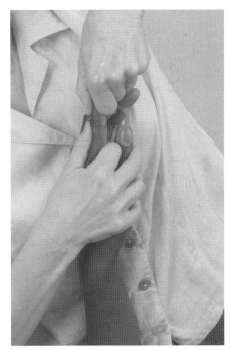

E (ii) Extension. The right hand supports the metacarpophalangeal joint in extension while the left hand takes the proximal interphalangeal joint into extension.

Figure 10.3 *Continued*   D Metacarpophalangeal joints.   E Proximal and distal interphalangeal joints.

Table 10.1 Active physiological movements and possible modifications

Active physiological movements	Modifications
Forearm pronation	Repeated
Forearm supination	Speed altered
Wrist flexion	Combined, eg.
Wrist extension	– Wrist flexion in supination
Radial deviation	– Wrist ulnar deviation with flexion
Ulnar deviation	Compression or distraction, e.g.
Carpometacarpal (CMC) and metacarpophalangeal joints of thumb (Fig. 10.4)	– Wrist extension with distraction
– Flexion	– MCP flexion with compression
– Extension	Sustained
– Abduction	Injuring movement
– Adduction	Differentiation tests
– Opposition	Function includes:
Distal intermetacarpal joints	– Power grips: hook, cylinder, fist and spherical span
– Horizontal flexion	– Precision (or pinch) grips: pulp pinch, tip-to-tip pinch,
– Horizontal extension	tripod pinch and lateral key grip, fastening a button,
Metacarpophalangeal joints (of the fingers) (MCPJs)	tying a shoelace, writing, etc.
– Flexion	– Purdue pegboard test
– Extension	– Nine-hole peg test
– Adduction	– Minnesota rate of manipulation test
– Abduction	– Moberg pick-up test
Proximal and distal interphalangeal joints (PIPJs and DIPJs)	– Jebson–Taylor hand function test
– Flexion	
– Extension	
?Cervical spine	
?Thoracic spine	
?Shoulder	
?Elbow	

pressure listed in Figure 10.3 are tested with the patient in supine or sitting. Movements are carried out on the left and right sides. The clinician establishes the patient's symptoms at rest, prior to each movement, and corrects any movement deviation to determine its relevance to the patient's symptoms.

The active physiological movements of the forearm, wrist and hand, and possible modifications are shown in Table 10.1. Various differentiation tests (Maitland 1991) can be performed; the choice depends on the patient's signs and symptoms. For example, when supination reproduces the patient's wrist symptoms, differentiation between the inferior radioulnar joint and the radiocarpal joint may be required. The patient actively moves the forearm into supination just to

the point where symptoms are produced. The clinician applies a supination force to the radius and ulna; if the symptoms are coming from the inferior radioulnar joint, then pain may increase. The radiocarpal joint is then isolated: a supination force around the scaphoid and lunate is applied, while maintaining the supination position of the forearm; if the symptoms are coming from the radiocarpal joint, then pain may increase. A pronation force to the scaphoid and lunate might then be expected to reduce symptoms (Fig. 10.5).

It may be necessary to examine other regions to determine their relevance to the patient's symptoms; they may be the source of the symptoms, or they may be contributing to the symptoms. The regions most likely are the cervical spine, thoracic spine, shoulder and elbow. The joints within these

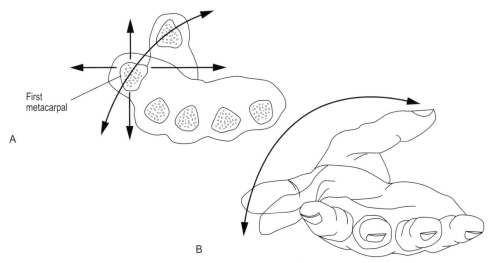

First
metacarpal

A

B

Figure 10.4 Movement at the carpometacarpal joint of the thumb. (From Fess & Philips 1987, with permission.)
A The arrows illustrate the multiple planes of movement that occur at the carpometacarpal joint of the thumb.
B The arrow illustrates the movement of the thumb from a position of adduction against the second metacarpal
to a position of extension and abduction away from the hand and fingers. It can then be rotated into positions
of opposition and flexion.

regions can be tested fully (see relevant chapter) or partially with the use of clearing tests (Table 10.2).

Some functional ability has already been tested by the general observation of the patient during the subjective and physical examinations, e.g. the postures adopted during the subjective examination and the ease or difficulty of undressing prior to the examination. Any further functional testing can be carried out at this point in the examination and may include various activities of the upper limb such as using a computer, handling tools, writing, etc. Clues for appropriate tests can be obtained from the subjective examination findings, particularly aggravating factors. Functional testing of the hand is very important and can include the ability to perform various power and precision (or pinch) grips, as well as more general activities, such as fastening a button, tying a shoelace, writing, etc.

It is also important to measure hand dexterity and function as two different aspects. Dexterity relates to fine manipulative tasks carried out at speed, whereas function is the combination of all aspects of the hand, including sensibility, move-

Table 10.2   Joint clearing tests

Joint	Physiological movement	Accessory movement
Cervical spine	Quadrants (flexion and extension)	All movements
Thoracic spine	Rotation and quadrants (flexion and extension)	All movements
Shoulder joint	Flexion and hand behind back	
Elbow joint	All movements	
Wrist joint	Flexion/extension and radial/ulnar deviation	

ment and cognitive ability. Common documented dexterity tests are as follows:

The Purdue pegboard test (Blair et al 1987).   A timed test measuring fine coordination of the hand with a series of unilateral and bilateral standardized tests using pegs and washers.

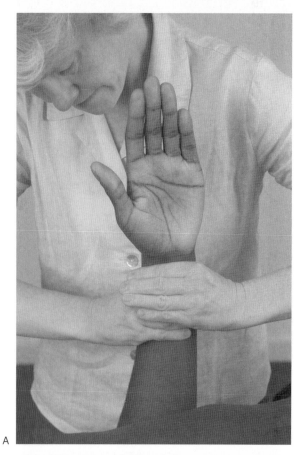

A

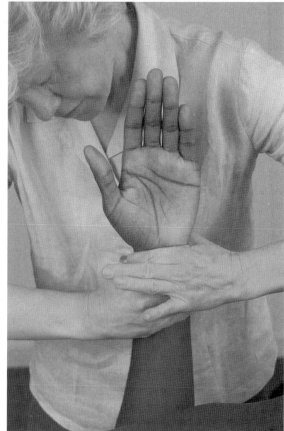

B

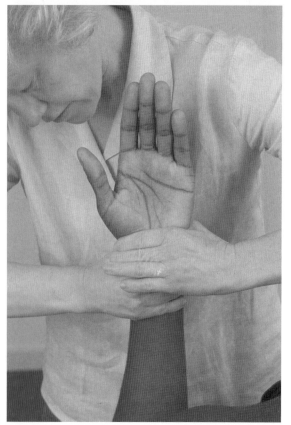

C

Figure 10.5 Differentiation between the superior/ inferior radioulnar joint with radiocarpal joint and mid-carpal joints. The patient supinates the forearm to the onset of their symptoms. The clinician then applies: **A** a supination force to the radius and ulna; **B** holds the radius and ulna and applies a supination force around the proximal row of carpal bones to affect the radiocarpal joint; **C** fixes the proximal row of carpal bones and applies a supination force of the distal carpal bones. The clinician determines the effect of each overpressure on the symptoms. The symptoms would be expected to increase when the supination force is applied to the symptomatic level; further examination of accessory movements of individual bones may then identify a symptomatic joint. This is a somewhat crude attempt to differentiate between joints and so it may only be a helpful test on some patients.

Nine-hole peg test (Totten & Flinn-Wagner 1992). A simple timed test placing nine pegs in nine holes. Excellent for children or those with cognitive difficulties.

Minnesota rate of manipulation test (Totten & Flinn-Wagner 1992). Measures gross coordination and dexterity. Used in work assessment for arm-hand dexterity.

Moberg pick-up test (Moberg 1958). The test uses nine standardized everyday objects. Each is picked up as quickly as possible and placed in a pot, first with the eyes open and then with eyes closed. This tests both dexterity and functional sensation.

Function tests may be developed and standardized within each clinical unit so long as they are repeatable and measurable. Other tests include:

Jebson–Taylor hand function test (Jebson et al 1969). Requires limited upper extremity coordination. There are seven functional subtests such as turning over a card, writing and simulated eating.

Capsular pattern. Capsular patterns for these joints (Cyriax 1982) are as follows:

- Inferior radioulnar joint: full range but pain at extremes of range
- Wrist: flexion and extension equally limited
- Carpometacarpal (CMC) joint of the thumb: full flexion, more limited abduction than extension
- Thumb and finger joints: more limitation of flexion than of extension.

Passive physiological movements

All the active movements described above can be examined passively with the patient usually in sitting or supine, comparing left and right sides. A comparison of the response of symptoms to the active and passive movements can help to determine whether the structure at fault is non-contractile (articular) or contractile (extra-articular) (Cyriax 1982). If the lesion is non-contractile, such as ligament, then active and passive movements will be painful and/or restricted in the same direction. If the lesion is in a contractile tissue (i.e. muscle), active and passive movements are painful and/or restricted in opposite directions.

Other regions may need to be examined to determine their relevance to the patient's symptoms; they may be the source of the symptoms, or they may be contributing to the symptoms. The regions most likely are the cervical spine, thoracic spine, shoulder and elbow.

Muscle tests

Muscle tests include examining muscle strength, length, isometric muscle testing and some other muscle tests.

Muscle strength

Grip strength, comparing left and right sides, can be measured using a dynamometer. The second handle position is recommended and three trials are carried out recording the mean value (American Society for Surgery of the Hand 1990) with the wrist between 0° and 15° of extension (Pryce 1980). Pinch strength can be measured using a pinch meter, again repeating the test three times and taking the mean value. Measure and record pure pinch, lateral key pinch and tripod grip separately.

Manual muscle testing may be carried out for the following muscle groups:

- Elbow: flexors and extensors
- Forearm: pronators and supinators
- Wrist joint: flexors, extensors, radial deviators and ulnar deviators
- Thenar eminence: flexors, extensors, adductors, abductors and opposition
- Hypothenar eminence: flexors, extensors, adductors, abductors and opposition
- Finger: flexors, extensors, abductors and adductors.

For details of these general tests the reader is directed to Cole et al (1988), Hislop & Montgomery (1995) or Kendall et al (1993).

Greater detail may be required to test the strength of muscles, in particular those thought prone to become weak (Janda 1994, 2002). These muscles and a description of the test for muscle strength are given in Chapter 3.

Muscle length

Tenodesis effect. Tests the balance in the extrinsic flexor and extensor muscle length. With the wrist flexed, the fingers and thumb will extend and with the wrist extended, the fingers will flex towards the palm and the thumb oppose towards the index finger.

Intrinsic muscle tightness. In a normal hand, the clinician is able to passively maintain MCPJ in extension and then passively flex the IPJs. Intrinsic muscle tightness is where there is increased range of passive IPJ flexion when the MCPJs are positioned in flexion. Further details on intrinsic muscle tightness can be found in Aulicino (1995).

Extrinsic muscle tightness. Extensor tightness: the clinician compares the range of passive IPJ flexion with the MCPJs positioned in flexion and then in extension. Extrinsic tightness is when there is greater range of IPJ flexion with the MCPJs in extension. Flexor tightness: the clinician compares the range of passive IPJ extension with the MCPJs positioned in flexion and then in extension. Extrinsic tightness is where there is a greater range of extension with the MCPJs in flexion.

The clinician may test the length of other muscles, in particular those thought prone to shorten (Janda 1994, 2002). Descriptions of the tests for muscle length are given in Chapter 3.

Isometric muscle testing

Manual muscle testing can be useful in differential diagnosis of nerve compression trauma. Following carpal tunnel compression, for example, damage to the median nerve can be checked by testing the isometric strength of opponens pollicis and abductor pollicis brevis. Test forearm pronation and supination, wrist flexion, extension, radial and ulnar deviation, finger and thumb flexion, extension, abduction and adduction and thumb opposition in resting position and, if indicated, in different parts of the physiological range. In addition the clinician observes the quality of the muscle contraction to hold this position (this can be done with the patient's eyes shut). The patient may, for example, be unable to prevent the joint from moving or may hold with excessive muscle activity; either of these circumstances would suggest a neuromuscular dysfunction.

Other muscle tests

Sweater finger sign test. Loss of distal interphalangeal joint flexion when a fist is made is a positive test indicating a ruptured flexor digitorum profundus tendon (Magee 1997).

Finkelstein test for de Quervain's disease. The patient makes a fist with the thumb inside the fingers, and passive ulnar deviation of the wrist is added by the clinician (Fig. 10.6) (Magee 1997). Reproduction of the patient's pain is indicative of

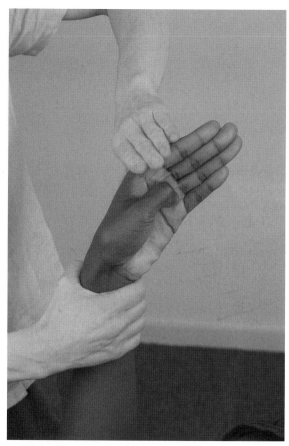

Figure 10.6 Finkelstein test. The patient flexes the thumb and the clinician guides the patient into ulnar deviation of the wrist.

de Quervain's disease (tenosynovitis of the abductor pollicis longus and extensor pollicis brevis tendons).

Linburg's sign. This tests for tendinitis at the interconnection between flexor pollicis longus and the flexor indices (Magee 1997). The thumb is flexed on to the hypothenar eminence and the index finger is extended. Limited range of index finger extension is a positive test.

Test for flexor digitorum superficialis (FDS). The clinician holds all of any three fingers in extension and asks the patient to actively flex the MCPJ and PIPJ of the remaining finger. The DIPJ should be flail as the FDP has been immobilized. If the FDS is inactive, the finger will flex strongly at the DIPJ as well as at the PIPJ and MCPJ, indicating activity of FDP. If the finger does not flex at all, neither flexor is active. Be aware that a proportion of the population do not have an effective FDS to the little finger, so the test is then invalidated for this digit (Austin et al 1989).

Tennis/golfer's elbow. The clinician may need to test for these (described in Ch. 9).

Neurological tests

Neurological examination includes neurological integrity testing, neurodynamic tests and some other nerve tests.

Integrity of the nervous system

The integrity of the nervous system is tested if the clinician suspects that the symptoms are emanating from the spine or from a peripheral nerve.

Dermatomes/peripheral nerves. Light touch and pain sensation of the upper limb are tested using cotton wool and pinprick respectively, as described in Chapter 3. Following trauma or compression to peripheral nerves, it is vital to assess the cutaneous sensation, looking at temperature sense, vibration, protective sensation, deep pressure to light touch, proprioception and stereognosis. The use of monofilaments and other tests are described in Chapter 3. Knowledge of the cutaneous distribution of nerve roots (dermatomes) and peripheral nerves enables the clinician to distinguish the

sensory loss due to a root lesion from that due to a peripheral nerve lesion. The cutaneous nerve distribution and dermatome areas are shown in Figure 3.20.

Myotomes/peripheral nerves. The following myotomes are tested (see Fig. 3.26):

- C5: shoulder abduction
- C6: elbow flexion
- C7: elbow extension
- C8: thumb extension
- T1: finger adduction.

A working knowledge of the muscular distribution of nerve roots (myotomes) and peripheral nerves enables the clinician to distinguish the motor loss due to a root lesion from that due to a peripheral nerve lesion. The peripheral nerve distributions are shown in Figures 3.23 and 3.24.

Reflex testing. The following deep tendon reflexes are tested (see Fig. 3.28):

- C5–C6: biceps
- C7: triceps and brachioradialis.

Neurodynamic tests

The upper limb tension tests (ULTT) may be carried out in order to ascertain the degree to which neural tissue is responsible for the production of the patient's symptom(s). These tests are described in detail in Chapter 3.

Other nerve tests

Tinel's sign (Tubiana et al 1998). This is used to determine the first detectable sign of nerve regeneration or of nerve damage. The clinician taps from distal to proximal along the line of the nerve, until the patient feels a 'pins and needles' sensation peripherally in the nerve distribution. The most distal point of pins and needles sensation indicates the furthest point of axonal regeneration, or of compression of a nerve. Tinel's sign is not always accurate (Tubiana et al 1998) and so needs to be used in conjunction with other tests, such as pain, temperature, vibration and, at a later stage of regeneration, monofilaments, EMG and two-point discrimination.

Median nerve. A common condition affecting the median nerve is carpal tunnel syndrome and this can be tested as follows:

Phalen's wrist flexion test (American Society for Surgery of the Hand 1990). One-minute sustained bilateral wrist flexion producing paraesthesia in the distribution of the median nerve indicates a positive test.

Reverse Phalen's test (Linscheid & Dobyns 1987). The patient makes a fist with the wrist in extension and the clinician applies pressure over the carpal tunnel for 1 minute. Paraesthesia in the distribution of the median nerve indicates a positive test.

Ulnar nerve

Froment's sign for ulnar nerve paralysis (Magee 1997). The patient holds a piece of paper between the index finger and thumb in a lateral key grip, and the clinician attempts to pull it away. In ulnar nerve paralysis, flexion at the IPJ of the thumb due to paralysis of adductor pollicis (Froment's sign) and clawing of the little and ring fingers is apparent as a result of paralysis of the interossei and lumbrical muscles and the unopposed action of the extrinsic extensors and flexors.

Miscellaneous tests

In the case of the wrist and hand, these are *vascular tests*.

If it is suspected that the circulation is compromised, the pulses of the radial and ulnar arteries are palpated at the wrist.

Allen test for the radial and ulnar arteries at the wrist (American Society for Surgery of the Hand 1990). The clinician applies pressure to the radial and ulnar arteries at the wrist and the patient is then asked to open and close the hand a few times and then to keep it open. The patency of each artery is tested by releasing the pressure over the radial and then the ulnar arteries. The hand should flush within 5 seconds on release of the pressure.

Tests for thoracic outlet syndrome. These have been described in Chapter 8.

Hand volume test. This can be used to measure swelling of the hand. A volumeter is used and a difference of 30–50 ml between one measurement and the next indicates significant hand swelling (Bell-Krotoski et al 1995). The clinician may also measure oedema at each joint or in the forearm using a tape measure and comparing affected and unaffected sides.

Palpation

The elbow region is palpated, as well as the cervical spine and thoracic spine, shoulder, wrist and hand as appropriate. It is useful to record palpation findings on a body chart (see Fig. 2.3) and/or palpation chart (see Fig. 3.38).

The clinician notes the following:

- The temperature of the area
- Localized increased skin moisture
- The presence of oedema or effusion. This can be measured with a tape measure comparing left and right sides
- Mobility and feel of superficial tissues, e.g. ganglions, nodules and scar tissue
- The presence or elicitation of any muscle spasm
- Tenderness of bone, ligaments, muscle, tendon (forearm flexors and extensors and superficial tendons around the wrist), tendon sheath, trigger points (shown in Fig. 3.39) and nerve. Palpable nerves in the upper limb are as follows:
  - The suprascapular nerve can be palpated along the superior border of the scapula in the suprascapular notch
  - The brachial plexus can be palpated in the posterior triangle of the neck; it emerges at the lower third of sternocleidomastoid
  - The suprascapular nerve can be palpated along the superior border of the scapula in the suprascapular notch
  - The dorsal scapular nerve can be palpated medial to the medial border of the scapula
  - The median nerve can be palpated over the anterior elbow joint crease, medial to the biceps tendon, also at the wrist between palmaris longus and flexor carpi radialis
  - The radial nerve can be palpated around the spiral groove of the humerus, between

brachioradialis and flexor carpi radialis, in the forearm and also at the wrist in the snuffbox
- Increased or decreased prominence of bones
- Pain provoked or reduced on palpation.

Accessory movements

It is useful to use the palpation chart and movement diagrams (or joint pictures) to record findings. These are explained in detail in Chapter 3. The clinician notes the following:

- The quality of movement
- The range of movement
- The resistance through the range and at the end of the range of movement
- The behaviour of pain through the range
- Any provocation of muscle spasm.

Wrist and hand (Fig. 10.7) accessory movements are listed in Table 10.3. Following accessory movements to the wrist and hand, the clinician reassesses all the physical asterisks (movements or tests that have been found to reproduce the

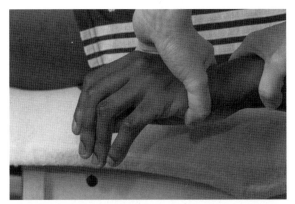

A (i) Anteroposterior and posteroanterior. The right hand grasps around the distal end of the radius and ulna and the left grasps the hand at the level of the proximal end of the metacarpals. The left hand then glides the patient's hand anteriorly and then posteriorly.

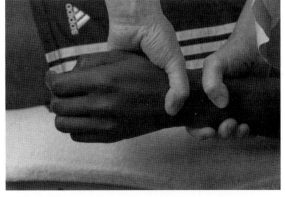

A (ii) Medial and lateral transverse. The hands grasp around the distal radius and ulna and proximal end of the metacarpals. The left hand then glides the patient's hand medially and laterally.

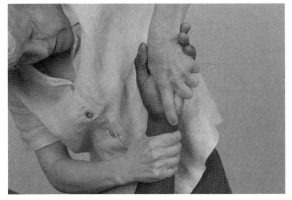

A (iii) Longitudinal cephalad. The right hand grasps around the distal radius and ulna and the left hand applies a longitudinal force to the wrist through the heel of the hand.

Figure 10.7(A–F)   Wrist and hand accessory movements.

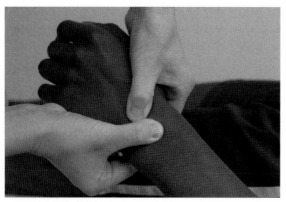

B (i) Anteroposterior and posteroanterior. Thumb pressure can be applied to the anterior or posterior aspect of each carpal bone to produce an anteroposterior or posteroanterior movement respectively. A posteroanterior pressure to the lunate is shown here.

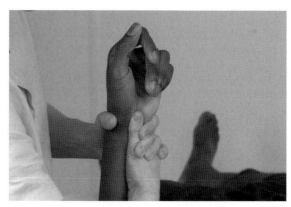

B (ii) Horizontal flexion. The left thumb is placed in the centre of the anterior aspect of the wrist and the right hand cups around the carpus to produce horizontal flexion.

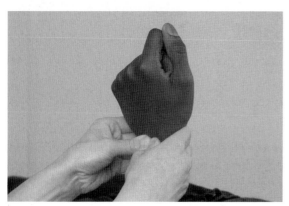

B (iii) Horizontal extension. The thumbs are placed in the centre of the posterior aspect of the wrist and the fingers wrap around the anterior aspect of the carpus to produce horizontal extension.

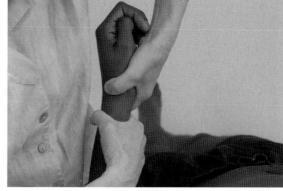

B (iv) Longitudinal cephalad and caudad. The right hand grasps around the distal end of the radius and ulna and the left grasps the hand at the level of the proximal end of the metacarpals. The right hand then pushes the hand towards the wrist (longitudinal cephalad) and away from the wrist (longitudinal caudad).

Figure 10.7 *Continued*   B Intercarpal joints.

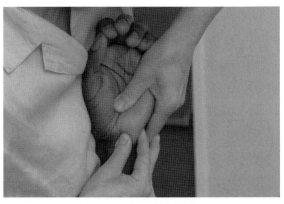

C Pisotriquetral joint. Medial and lateral transverse, longitudinal caudad and cephalad and distraction. Shown here the left hand stabilizes the hand and the right hand grasps the triquetral bone and applies a medial and lateral transverse force to the bone.

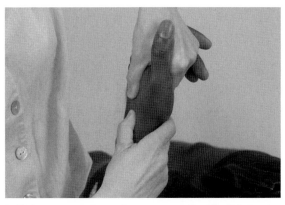

D (i) Anteroposterior and posteroanterior. The left hand glides the metacarpal forwards and backwards.

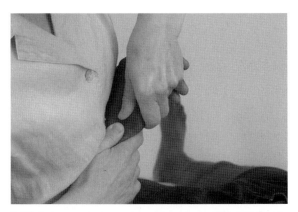

D (ii) Anteroposterior and posteroanterior. The left hand glides the thumb metacarpal forwards and backwards.

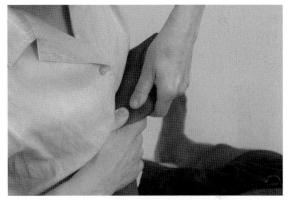

D (iii) Medial and lateral rotation. The left hand rotates the thumb metacarpal medially and laterally.

Figure 10.7 *Continued*   D Carpometacarpal joints. *Fingers* – the left hand grasps around the relevant distal carpal bone while the right hand grasps the proximal end of the metacarpal.

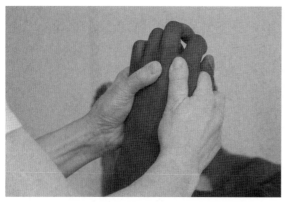

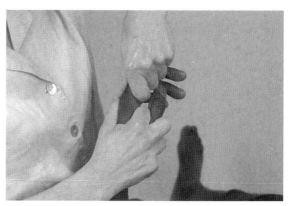

E Proximal and distal intermetacarpal joints of the fingers – anteroposterior and posteroanterior. The finger and thumb of each hand gently pinch the anterior and posterior aspects of adjacent metacarpal heads and apply a force in opposite directions to glide the heads anteriorly and posteriorly.

Figure 10.7 *Continued*

F Anteroposterior and posteroanterior. The left hand glides the proximal phalanx anteriorly and posteriorly.

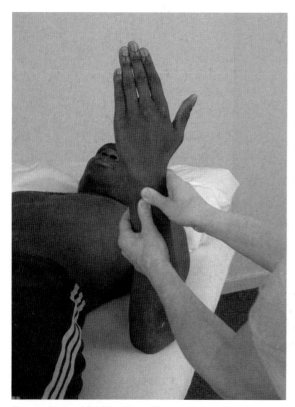

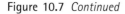

Figure 10.8 Mobilization with movement for supination. A posteroanterior force is applied to the ulna as the patient actively supinates.

patient's symptoms) in order to establish the effect of the accessory movements on the patient's signs and symptoms. Accessory movements can then be tested for other regions suspected to be a source of, or contributing to, the patient's symptoms. Again, following accessory movements to any one region, the clinician reassesses all the asterisks. Regions likely to be examined are the cervical spine, thoracic spine, shoulder and elbow.

Mobilizations with movement (MWMs)
(Mulligan 1999)

Forearm pronation and supination. The patient actively supinates or pronates the forearm while the clinician applies a sustained anterior or posterior force to the distal end of the ulna at the wrist. Figure 10.8 demonstrates a posteroanterior force to distal ulna as the patient actively supinates. An increase in range and no pain or reduced pain on active supination or pronation are positive examination findings, indicating a mechanical joint problem.

Wrist. The patient actively flexes or extends the wrist while the clinician applies a sustained medial or lateral glide to the carpal bones. Figure 10.9 demonstrates a lateral glide to the carpal

Table 10.3 Accessory movements, choice of application and reassessment of the patient's asterisks

Accessory movements	Choice of application	Identify any effect of accessory movements on patient's signs and symptoms
Radiocarpal joint	Start position, e.g. in wrist flexion,	Reassess all asterisks
↕ anteroposterior	extension, radial or ulnar	
↕ posteroanterior	deviation fingers or thumb in	
→→ Med medial transverse	flexion, extension, abduction	
→→ Lat lateral transverse	Speed of force application	
←→ Ceph longitudinal cephalad	Direction of the applied force	
←→ Caud longitudinal caudad	Point of application of applied force	
Intercarpal joints		
↕ anteroposterior		
↕ posteroanterior		
↕↕ AP/PA gliding		
HF horizontal flexion		
HE horizontal extension		
←→ Ceph longitudinal cephalad		
←→ Caud longitudinal caudad		
Pisotriquetral joint		
→→ Med medial transverse		
→→ Lat lateral transverse		
←→ Ceph longitudinal cephalad		
←→ Caud longitudinal caudad		
Dist distraction		
Carpometacarpal joints		
– Fingers		
↕ anteroposterior		
↕ posteroanterior		
→→ Med medial transverse		
→→ Lat lateral transverse		
∩ medial rotation		
lateral rotation		
– Thumb		
↕ anteroposterior		
↕ posteroanterior		
→→ Med medial transverse		
→→ Lat lateral transverse		
←→ Ceph longitudinal cephalad		
←→ Caud longitudinal caudad		
∩ Med medial rotation		
∩ Lat lateral rotation		
Proximal and distal intermetacarpal joints		
↕ anteroposterior		
↕ posteroanterior		
HF horizontal flexion		
HE horizontal extension		

Continued

Table 10.3 *Continued*

Accessory movements	Choice of application	Identify any effect of accessory movements on patient's signs and symptoms
RMCP, PIP and DIP joints of fingers and thumb		
↕ anteroposterior		
↕ posteroanterior		
→• Med medial transverse		
→• Lat lasteral transverse		
←•→ Ceph longitudinal cephalad		
←•→ Caud longitudinal caudad		
↻ Med medial rotation		
↺ Lat lateral rotation		
Ten movement test for the carpal bones (Kaltenborn 2002)		
Movements around the capitate		
– Fix the capitate and move the trapezoid		
– Fix the capitate and move the scaphoid		
– Fix the capitate and move the lunate		
– Fix the capitate and move the hamate		
Movement on the radial side of the wrist		
– Fix the scaphoid and move the trapezoid and trapezium		
Movements in the radiocarpal joint		
– Fix the radius and move the scaphoid		
– Fix the radius and move the lunate		
– Fix the ulna and move the triquetrum		
Movements on the ulnar side of the wrist		
– Fix the triquetrum and move the hamate		
– Fix the triquetrum and move the pisiform		
?Cervical spine	As above	Reassess all asterisks
?Thoracic spine	As above	Reassess all asterisks
?Shoulder	As above	Reassess all asterisks
?Elbow	As above	Reassess all asterisks

bones as the patient actively flexes the wrist. An increase in range and no pain or reduced pain are positive examination findings.

Interphalangeal joints. The patient actively flexes or extends the finger while the clinician applies a sustained medial or lateral glide just distal to the affected joint. Figure 10.10 demonstrates a medial glide to the distal interphalangeal joint as the patient actively extends the joint. An increase in range and no pain or reduced pain are positive examination findings.

COMPLETION OF THE EXAMINATION

Having carried out the above tests, the examination of the wrist and hand is now complete. The subjective and physical examinations produce a large amount of information, which needs to be recorded accurately and quickly. An outline examination chart may be useful for some clinicians and one is suggested in Figure 10.11. It is important, however, that the clinician does not examine in a rigid manner, simply following the suggested

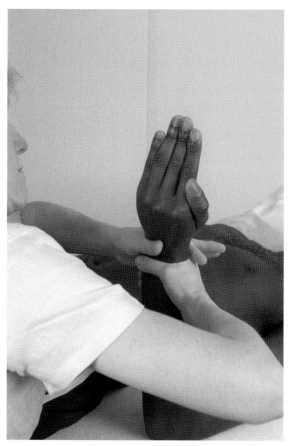

Figure 10.9 Mobilization with movement for wrist flexion. The right hand supports the forearm while the left hand cups around the ulnar aspect of the wrist and applies a lateral glide as the patient actively extends the wrist.

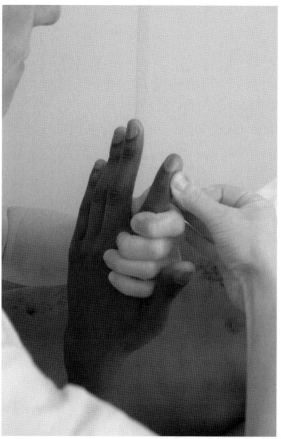

Figure 10.10 Mobilization with movement for finger extension. The left hand supports the finger joint. The right hand applies a medial glide just distal to the distal interphalangeal joint as the patient actively extends the joint.

sequence outlined in the chart. Each patient presents differently and this needs to be reflected in the examination process. It is vital at this stage to highlight important findings from the examination with an asterisk (*). These findings must be reassessed at, and within, subsequent treatment sessions to evaluate the effects of treatment on the patient's condition.

The physical testing procedures which specifically indicate joint, nerve or muscle tissues, as a source of the patient's symptoms, are summarized in Table 3.10. The strongest evidence that a joint is the source of the patient's symptoms is that active and passive physiological movements, passive accessory movements and joint palpation all reproduce the patient's symptoms, and that following a treatment dose, reassessment identifies an improvement in the patient's signs and symptoms. Weaker evidence includes an alteration in range, resistance or quality of physiological and/or accessory movements and tenderness over the joint, with no alteration in signs and symptoms after treatment. One or more of these findings may indicate a dysfunction of a joint, which may or may not be contributing to the patient's condition.

The strongest evidence that a muscle is the source of a patient's symptoms is if active move-

Body chart	Name
	Age
	Date
	24-hour behaviour
	Improving static worsening
	Special questions General health Weight loss RA Drugs Steroids Anticoagulants X-ray Cord symptoms Cauda equina symptoms VBI symptoms
Relationship of symptoms	
Aggravating factors and function	**HPC**
	PMH
Severe Irritable	
Easing factors	**SH & FH** (Patient's perspective, experience, expectations. Yellow, blue, black flags)

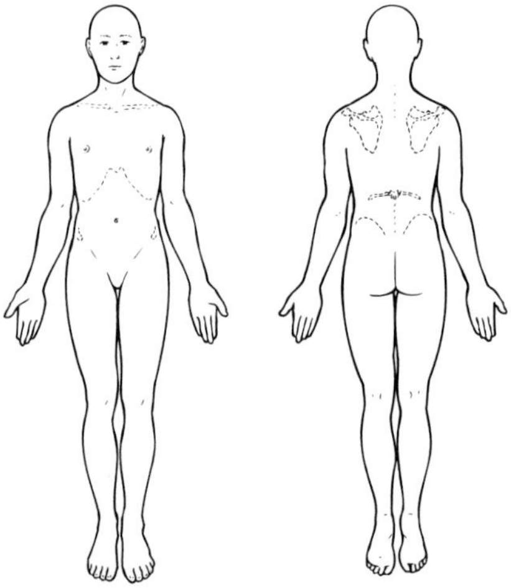

Figure 10.11   Wrist and hand examination chart.

Physical examination Observation	Other muscle tests (sweater finger, Finkelstein, Linburg's sign, FDS, tennis/golfer elbow)
Joint integrity tests (Watson's scaphoid shift, lunotriquetral ballottmement, midcarpal, thumb and finger instability test)	Neurological integrity tests
Active and passive physiological movements of wrist and hand and other relevant regions	Neurodynamic tests
	Other nerve tests (Tinel's sign, median, ulnar)
	Miscellaneous tests (pulses, Allen, thoracic outlet, hand volume)
Capsular pattern yes/no	
Muscle strength	Palpation
Muscle length (tendodesis, intrinsic and extrinsic muscle tightness)	Accessory movements and reassessment of each relevant region
Isometric muscle testing	

Figure 10.11 *Continued*

ments, an isometric contraction, passive lengthening and palpation of a muscle all reproduce the patient's symptoms, and that following a treatment dose, reassessment identifies an improvement in the patient's signs and symptoms. Further evidence of muscle dysfunction may be suggested by reduced strength or poor quality during the active physiological movement and the isometric contraction, reduced range, and/or increased/decreased resistance, during the passive lengthening of the muscle, and tenderness on palpation, with no alteration in signs and symptoms after treatment. One or more of these findings may indicate a dysfunction of a muscle which may, or may not, be contributing to the patient's condition.

The strongest evidence that a nerve is the source of the patient's symptoms is when active and/or passive physiological movements reproduce the patient's symptoms, which are then increased or decreased with an additional sensitizing movement, at a distance from the patient's symptoms. In addition, there is reproduction of the patient's symptoms on palpation of the nerve, and neurodynamic testing, sufficient to be considered a treatment dose, results in an improvement in the above signs and symptoms. Further evidence of nerve dysfunction may be suggested by reduced range (compared to the asymptomatic side) and/or increased resistance to the various arm movements, and tenderness on nerve palpation.

On completion of the physical examination, the clinician:

- Warns the patient of possible exacerbation up to 24–48 hours following the examination.
- Requests the patient to report details on the behaviour of the symptoms following examination at the next attendance.

- Explains the findings of the physical examination and how these findings relate to the subjective assessment. Any misconceptions patients may have regarding their illness or injury are cleared up.
- Evaluates the findings, formulates a clinical diagnosis and writes up a problem list. Clinicians may find the management planning forms shown in Figures 3.53 and 3.54 helpful in guiding them through what is often a complex clinical reasoning process.
- Determines the objectives of treatment.
- Devises an initial treatment plan.

In this way, the clinician will have developed the following hypotheses categories (adapted from Jones & Rivett 2004):

- Function: abilities and restrictions.
- Patients' perspectives on their experience.
- Source of symptoms. This includes the structure or tissue that is thought to be producing the patients' symptoms, the nature of the structure or tissues in relation to the healing process, and the pain mechanisms.
- Contributing factors to the development and maintenance of the problem. There may be environmental, psychosocial, behavioural, physical or heredity factors.
- Precautions/contraindications to treatment and management. This includes the severity and irritability of the patient's symptoms and the nature of the patient's condition.
- Management strategy and treatment plan.
- Prognosis – this can be affected by factors such as the stage and extent of the injury as well as the patient's expectation, personality and lifestyle.

References

American Society for Surgery of the Hand 1990 The hand – examination and diagnosis, 3rd edn. Churchill Livingstone, New York

Aulicino P 1995 Clinical examination of the hand. In: Hunter J M, Mackin E J, Callahan A D (eds) Rehabilitation of the hand: surgery and therapy, 4th edn. Mosby, St Louis, MO, ch 5, p 53

Austin G J, Leslie B M, Ruby L K 1989 Variations of the flexor digitorum superficialis of the small finger. Journal of Hand Surgery 14A: 262

Bell-Krotoski J A, Breger-Lee D E, Beach R B 1995 Biomechanics and evaluation of the hand. In: Hunter J M, Mackin E J, Callahan A D (eds) Rehabilitation of the hand: surgery and therapy, 4th edn. Mosby, St Louis, MO, ch 11, p 153

Blair S J, McCormick E, Bear-Lehman J, Fess E E, Rader E 1987 Evaluation of impairment of the upper extremity. Clinical Orthopaedics and Related Research 221: 42–58

Clinical Standards Advisory Report 1994 Report of a CSAG committee on back pain. HMSO, London

Cole J H, Furness A L, Twomey L T 1988 Muscles in action, an approach to manual muscle testing. Churchill Livingstone, Edinburgh

Cyriax J 1982 Textbook of orthopaedic medicine – diagnosis of soft tissue lesions, 8th edn. Baillière Tindall, London

Eckhaus D 1993 Swan-neck deformity. In: Clark G L, Wilgis E F S, Aiello B (eds) Hand rehabilitation, a practical guide. Churchill Livingstone, Edinburgh, ch 16

Eddington L V 1993 Boutonnière deformity. In: Clark G L, Wilgis E F S, Aiello B (eds) Hand rehabilitation, a practical guide. Churchill Livingstone, Edinburgh, ch 17

Fess E, Philips C 1987 Hand splinting, principles and methods. C V Mosby, St Louis, MO

Hislop H, Montgomery J 1995 Daniels and Worthingham's muscle testing, techniques of manual examination, 7th edn. W B Saunders, Philadelphia

Janda V 1994 Muscles and motor control in cervicogenic disorders: assessment and management. In: Grant R (ed) Physical therapy of the cervical and thoracic spine, 2nd edn. Churchill Livingstone, New York, ch 10, p 195

Janda V 2002 Muscles and motor control in cervicogenic disorders. In: Grant R (ed) Physical therapy of the cervical and thoracic spine, 3rd edn. Churchill Livingstone, New York, ch 10, p 182

Jebson R H, Taylor N, Trieschmann R B, Trotter M J, Howard L A 1969 An objective and standardized test of hand function. Archives of Physical Medicine and Rehabilitation 50: 311–319

Jones M A, Rivett D A 2004 Clinical reasoning for manual therapists. Butterworth-Heinemann, Edinburgh

Kaltenborn F M 2002 Manual mobilization of the joints, vol I, The extremities, 6th edn. Norli, Oslo

Kendall F P, McCreary E K, Provance P G 1993 Muscles, testing and function, 4th edn. Williams & Wilkins, Baltimore, MD

Linscheid R L, Dobyns J H 1987 Physical examination of the wrist. In: Post M (ed) Physical examination of the musculoskeletal system. Year Book Medical Publishers, Chicago, IL, ch 4, p 80

Louis D S, Hankin F M, Greene T L, Braunstein E M, White S J 1984 Central carpal instability – capitate lunate instability pattern. Diagnosis by dynamic placement. Orthopedics 7(11): 1693–1696

Magee D J 1997 Orthopedic physical assessment, 3rd edn. W B Saunders, Philadelphia

Maitland G D 1991 Peripheral manipulation, 3rd edn. Butterworth-Heinemann, London

Moberg E 1958 Objective methods for determining the functional value of sensibility in the hand. Journal of Bone and Joint Surgery 40B(3): 454–476

Mulligan B R 1999 Manual therapy 'NAGs', 'SNAGs', 'MWMs' etc., 4th edn. Plane View Services, New Zealand

Pryce J C 1980 The wrist position between neutral and ulnar deviation that facilitates the maximum power grip strength. Journal of Biomechanics 13: 505–511

Refshauge K, Gass E (eds) 2004 Musculoskeletal physiotherapy clinical science and evidence-based practice. Butterworth-Heinemann, Oxford

Taleisnik J 1988 Carpal instability. Journal of Bone and Joint Surgery 70A(8): 1262–1268

Totten P, Flinn-Wagner S 1992 Functional evaluation of the hand. In: Stanely B, Tribuzi S (eds) Concepts in hand rehabilitation. F A Davies, New York, ch 5, p 128

Tubiana R, Thomine J M, Mackin E 1998 Examination of the hand and wrist. Martin Dunitz, Boston, MA

Waddell G 2004 The back pain revolution, 2nd edn. Churchill Livingstone, Edinburgh

Watson H K, Ashmead D I V, Makhlouf M V 1988 Examination of the scaphoid. Journal of Hand Surgery 13A(5): 657–660

Chapter 11

Examination of the lumbar spine

POSSIBLE CAUSES OF PAIN AND/OR LIMITATION OF MOVEMENT

This region includes T12 to the sacrum and coccyx.

- Trauma and degeneration:
  - Fracture of spinous process, transverse process, vertebral arch or vertebral body; fracture dislocation
  - Spondylolysis and spondylolisthesis
  - Ankylosing vertebral hyperostosis
  - Scheuermann's disease
  - Syndromes: arthrosis of the zygapophyseal joints, spondylosis (intervertebral disc degeneration), intervertebral disc lesions, prolapsed intervertebral disc, osteitis condensans ilii, coccydynia, hypermobility
  - Ligamentous sprain
  - Muscular strain
- Inflammatory:
  - Ankylosing spondylitis
  - Rheumatoid arthritis
- Metabolic:
  - Osteoporosis
  - Paget's disease
  - Osteomalacia
- Infections:
  - Tuberculosis of the spine
  - Pyogenic osteitis of the spine
- Tumours, benign and malignant
- Postural low back pain
- Piriformis syndrome.

Further details of the questions asked during the subjective examination and the tests carried out in the physical examination can be found in Chapters 2 and 3 respectively.

The order of the subjective questioning and the physical tests described below can be altered as appropriate for the patient being examined.

SUBJECTIVE EXAMINATION

Body chart

The following information concerning the type and area of the current symptoms can be recorded on a body chart (see Fig. 2.3).

Area of current symptoms

Be exact when mapping out the area of the symptoms. Lesions in the lumbar spine can refer symptoms over a large area – symptoms are commonly felt around the spine, abdomen, groin and lower limbs. Occasionally, symptoms may be felt in the head, cervical and thoracic spine. Ascertain which is the worst symptom and record the patient's interpretation of where s/he feels the symptom(s) are coming from.

The area of symptoms may, alongside other signs and symptoms, indicate illness behaviour (Table 11.1).

Areas relevant to the region being examined

All other relevant areas are checked for symptoms; it is important to ask about pain or even stiffness, as this may be relevant to the patient's main symptom. Mark unaffected areas with ticks (✓) on the body chart. Check for symptoms in the cervical spine, thoracic spine, abdomen, groin and lower limbs.

Quality of pain

Establish the quality of the pain.

Intensity of pain

The intensity of pain can be measured using, for example, a visual analogue scale (VAS) as shown in Figure 2.8. A pain diary may be useful for

Table 11.1 Indications of illness behaviour (Waddell 2004)

Signs and symptoms	Illness behaviour	Physical disease
Pain		
Pain drawing	Non-anatomical, regional, magnified	Localized, anatomical
Pain adjectives	Emotional	Sensory
Symptoms		
Pain	Whole leg pain	Musculoskeletal or neurological distribution
	Pain at the tip of the coccyx	
Numbness	Whole leg numbness	Dermatomal
Weakness	Whole leg giving way	Myotomal
Behaviour of pain	Constant pain	Varies with time and activity
Response to treatment	Intolerance of treatments	Variable benefit
	Emergency hospitalization	
Signs		
Tenderness	Superficial, non-anatomical	Musculoskeletal distribution
Axial loading	Low back pain	Neck pain
Simulated rotation	Low back pain	Nerve root pain
Straight leg raise	Marked improvement with distraction	Limited on formal examination
		No improvement with distraction
Motor	Regional jerky, giving way	Myotomal
Sensory	Regional	Dermatomal

patients with chronic low back pain to determine the pain patterns and triggering factors over a period of time.

Depth of pain

Establish the depth of the pain. Does the patient feel it is on the surface or deep inside?

Abnormal sensation

Check for any altered sensation over the lumbar spine and other relevant areas. Common abnormalities are paraesthesia and numbness.

Constant or intermittent symptoms

Ascertain the frequency of the symptoms and whether they are constant or intermittent. If symptoms are constant, check whether there is variation in the intensity of the symptoms, as constant unremitting pain may be indicative of neoplastic disease.

Relationship of symptoms

Determine the relationship between symptomatic areas – do they come together or separately? For example, the patient could have thigh pain without lumbar spine pain, or they may always be present together.

Behaviour of symptoms

Aggravating factors

For each symptomatic area, discover what movements and/or positions aggravate the patient's symptoms, i.e. what brings them on (or makes them worse), are they able to maintain this position or movement (severity), what happens to other symptom(s) when this symptom is produced (or is made worse), and how long does it take for symptoms to ease once the position or movement is stopped (irritability). These questions help to confirm the relationship between the symptoms.

The clinician also asks the patient about theoretically known aggravating factors for structures

that could be a source of the symptoms. Common aggravating factors for the lumbar spine are flexion (e.g. when putting shoes and socks on), sitting, standing, walking, standing up from the sitting position, driving and coughing/sneezing. These movements and positions can increase symptoms because they stress various structures in the lumbar spine (Table 11.2). Aggravating factors for other regions, which may need to be queried if they are suspected to be a source of the symptoms, are shown in Table 2.3.

The clinician ascertains how the symptoms affect function, such as: static and active postures, e.g. sitting, standing, lying, bending, walking, running, walking on uneven ground and up and down stairs, washing, driving, lifting and digging, work, sport and social activities. Note details of training regimen for any sports activities. The clinician finds out if the patient is left- or right-handed as there may be increased stress on the dominant side.

Detailed information on each of the above activities is useful in order to help determine the structure(s) at fault and identify functional restrictions. This information can be used to determine the aims of treatment and any advice that may be required. The most notable functional restrictions are highlighted with asterisks (*), explored in the physical examination, and reassessed at subsequent treatment sessions to evaluate treatment intervention.

Easing factors

For each symptomatic area, the clinician asks what movements and/or positions ease the patient's symptoms, how long it takes to ease them and what happens to other symptom(s) when this symptom is relieved. These questions help to confirm the relationship between the symptoms.

The clinician asks the patient about theoretically known easing factors for structures that could be a source of the symptoms. Commonly found easing factors for the lumbar spine are shown in Table 11.2. The clinician can then analyse the position or movement that eases the symptoms to help determine the structure at fault. A patient who is never free of pain or who needs

Table 11.2   Effect of position and movement on pain-sensitive structures of the lumbar spine (Jull 1986)

Activity	Symptoms	Possible structural and pathological implications
Sitting		Compressive forces (White & Panjabi 1990)
		High intradiscal pressure (Nachemson 1992)
Sitting with extension	Decreased	Intradiscal pressure reduced
		Decreased paraspinal muscle activity (Andersson et al 1977)
	Increased	Greater compromise of structures of lateral and central canals
		Compressive forces on lower zygapophyseal joints
Sitting with flexion	Decreased	Little compressive load on lower zygapophyseal joints
		Greater volume lateral and central canals
		Reduced disc bulge posteriorly
	Increased	Very high intradiscal pressure
		Increased compressive loads upper and mid zygapophyseal joints
Prolonged sitting	Increased	Gradual creep of tissues (Kazarian 1975)
Sit to stand	Increased	Creep, time for reversal, difficulty in straightening up
		Extension of spine, increase in disc bulge posteriorly
Standing	Increased	Creep into extension
Walking	Increased	Shock loads greater than body weight
		Compressive load (vertical creep) (Kirkaldy-Willis & Farfan 1982)
		Leg pain – neurogenic claudication, intermittent claudication
Driving	Increased	Sitting: compressive forces
		Vibration: muscle fatigue, increased intradiscal pressure, creep (Pope & Hansson 1992)
		Increased dural tension sitting with legs extended
		Short hamstrings: pulls lumbar spine into greater flexion
Coughing/sneezing/straining	Increased	Increased pressure subarachnoid space
		Increased intradiscal pressure
		Mechanical 'jarring' of sudden uncontrolled movement

long periods of lying down during the day may be exhibiting illness behaviour.

Twenty-four-hour behaviour of symptoms

The clinician determines the 24-hour behaviour of symptoms by asking questions about night, morning and evening symptoms.

Night symptoms.   The following questions may be asked:

- Do you have any difficulty getting to sleep?
- What position is most comfortable/uncomfortable?
- What is your normal sleeping position?
- What is your present sleeping position?
- Do your symptom(s) wake you at night? If so,
  - Which symptom(s)?
  - How many times in the past week?

- How many times in a night?
- How long does it take to get back to sleep?
- How many and what type of pillows are used?
- Is the mattress firm or soft?
- Has the mattress been changed recently?

Morning and evening symptoms.   The clinician determines the pattern of the symptoms first thing in the morning, through the day and at the end of the day. Stiffness in the morning for the first few minutes might suggest spondylosis; stiffness and pain for a few hours are suggestive of an inflammatory process such as ankylosing spondylitis.

Stage of the condition

In order to determine the stage of the condition, the clinician asks whether the symptoms are getting better, getting worse or remaining unchanged.

Special questions

Special questions must always be asked, as they may identify certain precautions or contraindications to the physical examination and/or treatment (see Table 2.4). As mentioned in Chapter 2, the clinician must differentiate between conditions that are suitable for conservative management and systemic, neoplastic and other non-neuromusculoskeletal conditions, which require referral to a medical practitioner. The reader is referred to Appendix 2.2 for details of various serious pathological processes which can mimic neuromusculoskeletal conditions (Grieve 1994).

The following information is routinely obtained from patients.

General health. Ascertain the general health of the patient – find out if the patient suffers from any malaise, fatigue, fever, nausea or vomiting, stress, anxiety or depression.

Weight loss. Has the patient noticed any recent unexplained weight loss?

Rheumatoid arthritis. Has the patient (or a member of his/her family) been diagnosed as having rheumatoid arthritis?

Drug therapy. What drugs are being taken by the patient? Has the patient ever been prescribed long-term (6 months or more) medication/steroids? Has the patient been taking anticoagulants recently?

X-ray and medical imaging. Has the patient been X-rayed or had any other medical tests recently? Routine spinal X-rays are no longer considered necessary prior to conservative treatment as they only identify the normal age-related degenerative changes, which do not necessarily correlate with the patient's symptoms (Clinical Standards Advisory Report 1994). The medical tests may include blood tests, magnetic resonance imaging, myelography, discography or a bone scan.

Neurological symptoms. Has the patient experienced symptoms of spinal cord compression (i.e. compression to L1 level) such as bilateral tingling in hands or feet and/or disturbance of gait?

Has the patient experienced symptoms of cauda equina compression (i.e. compression below L1), which are saddle anaesthesia/paraesthesia and bladder and/or bowel sphincter disturbance (loss of control, retention, hesitancy, urgency or a sense of incomplete evacuation) (Grieve 1991)? These symptoms may be due to interference of S3 and S4 (Grieve 1981). Prompt surgical attention is required to prevent permanent sphincter paralysis.

History of the present condition (HPC)

For each symptomatic area, the clinician needs to know how long the symptom has been present, whether there was a sudden or slow onset and whether there was a known cause that provoked the onset of the symptom. If the onset was slow, the clinician finds out if there has been any change in the patient's lifestyle, e.g. a new job or hobby or a change in sporting activity. To confirm the relationship between the symptoms, the clinician asks what happened to other symptoms when each symptom began.

Past medical history (PMH)

The following information is obtained from the patient and/or the medical notes:

- The details of any relevant medical history.
- The history of any previous attacks: how many episodes, when were they, what was the cause, what was the duration of each episode and did the patient fully recover between episodes? If there have been no previous attacks, has the patient had any episodes of stiffness in the lumbar spine, thoracic spine or any other relevant region? Check for a history of trauma or recurrent minor trauma. Emergency admission for non-specific low back pain and intolerance of several past management programmes may indicate illness behaviour.
- Ascertain the results of any past treatment for the same or similar problem. Past treatment records may be obtained for further information.

Social and family history (SH, FH)

Social and family history that is relevant to the onset and progression of the patient's problem is recorded. This includes the patient's perspectives, experience and expectations, their age, employment, home situation, and details of any leisure activities. Factors from this information may indicate direct and/or indirect mechanical influences on the lumbar spine. Frequent and wide-ranging help with personal care may be part of illness behaviour. In order to treat the patient appropriately, it is important to manage within the context of the patient's social and work environment.

The following questions may be asked to evaluate the psychosocial risk factors, or 'yellow flags' for poor treatment outcome (Waddell 2004):

- Have you had time off work in the past with back pain?
- What do you understand to be the cause of your back pain?
- What are you expecting will help you?
- How is your employer/co-workers/family responding to your back pain?
- What are you doing to cope with your back pain?
- Do you think you will return to work? When?

Readers are referred to the excellent text by Waddell (2004) for further details on the management of patients demonstrating psychosocial risk factors.

Plan of the physical examination

When all this information has been collected, the subjective examination is complete. It is useful at this stage to highlight with asterisks (*), for ease of reference, important findings and particularly one or more functional restrictions. These can then be re-examined at subsequent treatment sessions to evaluate treatment intervention.

In order to plan the physical examination, the following hypotheses need to be developed from the subjective examination:

- The regions and structures that need to be examined as a possible cause of the symptoms, e.g. lumbar spine, thoracic spine, cervical spine, sacroiliac joint, pubic symphysis, hip, knee, ankle and foot, muscles and nerves. Often it is not possible to examine fully at the first attendance and so examination of the structures

must be prioritized over subsequent treatment sessions.
- Other factors that need to be examined, e.g. working and everyday postures, leg length, muscle weakness.
- In what way should the physical tests be carried out? Will it be easy or hard to reproduce each symptom? Will it be necessary to use combined movements, repetitive movements, etc. to reproduce the patient's symptoms? Are symptom(s) severe and/or irritable? If symptoms are severe, physical tests may be carried out to just before the onset of symptom production or just to the onset of symptom production; no overpressures will be carried out, as the patient would be unable to tolerate this. If symptoms are irritable, physical tests may be examined to just before symptom production or just to the onset of provocation with less physical tests being examined to allow for rest period between tests.
- Are there any precautions and/or contraindications to elements of the physical examination that need to be explored further, such neurological involvement, recent fracture, trauma, steroid therapy or rheumatoid arthritis; there may also be certain contraindications to further examination and treatment, e.g. symptoms of cord compression.

A physical planning form can be useful for clinicians to help guide them through the clinical reasoning process (see Fig. 2.10 and Appendix 2.1).

PHYSICAL EXAMINATION

The information from the subjective examination helps the clinician to plan an appropriate physical examination. The severity, irritability and nature of the condition are the major factors that will influence the choice and priority of physical testing procedures. The first and over-arching question the clinician might ask is: 'is this patient's condition suitable for me to manage as a therapist?' For example, a patient presenting with cauda equina compression symptoms may only need neurological integrity testing, prior to an urgent medical referral. The nature of the patient's condition has had a major impact on the physical examination. The second question the clinician might ask is: 'does this patient have a neuromusculoskeletal dysfunction that I may be able to help?' To answer that, the clinician needs to carry out a full physical examination; however, this may not be possible if the symptoms are severe and/or irritable. If the patient's symptoms are severe and/or irritable, the clinician aims to explore movements as much as possible, within a symptom-free range. If the patient has constant and severe and/or irritable symptoms, then the clinician aims to find physical tests that ease the symptoms. If the patient's symptoms are non-severe and non-irritable, then the clinician aims to find physical tests that reproduce each of the patient's symptoms.

Each significant physical test that either provokes or eases the patient's symptoms is highlighted in the patient's notes by an asterisk (*) for easy reference. The highlighted tests are often referred to as 'asterisks' or 'markers'.

The order and detail of the physical tests described below need to be appropriate to the patient being examined; some tests will be irrelevant, some tests will be carried out briefly, while it will be necessary to investigate others fully. It is important that readers understand that the techniques shown in this chapter are some of many; the choice depends mainly on the relative size of the clinician and patient, as well as the clinician's preference. For this reason, novice clinicians may initially want to copy what is shown, but then quickly adapt to what is best for them.

Observation

Informal observation

The clinician needs to observe the patient in dynamic and static situations; the quality of movement is noted, as are the postural characteristics and facial expression. Informal observation will have begun from the moment the clinician begins the subjective examination and will continue to the end of the physical examination.

Formal observation

Observation of posture. The clinician observes the patient's spinal, pelvic and lower limb posture in standing, from anterior, lateral and posterior views. The presence of a lateral shift, scoliosis, kyphosis or lordosis is noted. A lateral shift indicates a displacement of the position of the upper trunk relative to the pelvis (McKenzie 1981). A left lateral shift means that the shoulders are displaced to the left of the pelvis; a right lateral shift is displacement of the shoulders to the right. The patient may stand with unequal weight through the legs because of a short leg or in order to obtain pain relief. The clinician passively corrects any asymmetry to determine its relevance to the patient's problem.

Typical postures include the following, which are shown in Figures 3.3–3.8:

- Lower (or pelvic) crossed syndrome (Jull & Janda 1987), otherwise known as the kyphosis–lordosis posture (Kendall et al 1993)
- Layer syndrome (Jull & Janda 1987)
- Flat back (Kendall et al 1993)
- Sway back (Kendall et al 1993)
- Handedness pattern (Kendall et al 1993).

A step deformity of the spinous processes may indicate a spondylolisthesis.

Observation of muscle form. The clinician observes the muscle bulk and muscle tone of the patient, comparing left and right sides. It must be remembered that the level and frequency of physical activity, as well as the dominant side, may well produce differences in muscle bulk between sides. Some muscles are thought to shorten under stress, while other muscles weaken, producing muscle imbalance (see Table 3.2). Patterns of muscle imbalance are thought to produce the postures mentioned above.

Observation of soft tissues. The clinician observes the quality and colour of the patient's skin and any area of swelling or presence of scarring, and takes cues for further examination. A tuft of hair over the low lumbar spine may indicate spina bifida occulta.

Observation of gait. The typical gait patterns that might be expected in patients with low back pain are the gluteus maximus gait, the Trendelenburg gait and the short leg gait (see Ch. 3 for further details).

Observation of the patient's attitudes and feelings. The age, gender and ethnicity of patients and their cultural, occupational and social backgrounds will all affect their attitudes and feelings towards themselves, their condition and the clinician. Guarding, bracing, rubbing, grimacing and sighing are noted for possible signs of illness behaviour (see Box 2.2 for further information).

After 2–4 weeks of symptoms, the risk of long-term disability and loss of work has to be assessed. Most of the following risk factors are psychosocial and can be established by careful questioning or by using questionnaires (Kendall et al 1997):

- The belief that back pain is associated with damage and possible disability
- Avoidance of movement or activity because of fear of pain and its consequences
- Low mood and social withdrawal
- Reliance on passive treatment rather than active participation.

The clinician needs to be aware of and sensitive to these attitudes, and to empathize and communicate appropriately so as to develop a rapport with the patient and thereby enhance the patient's compliance with the treatment.

Joint integrity tests

In side lying with the lumbar spine in extension and hips flexed to 90°, the clinician pushes along the femoral shafts while palpating the interspinous spaces between adjacent lumbar vertebrae to feel for any excessive movement (Fig. 11.1). In the same position but with the lumbar spine in flexion, the clinician pulls along the shaft of the femur and again palpates the interspinous spaces to feel for any excessive movement. Observation of the quality of active flexion and extension can also indicate instability of the lumbar spine (see below). This test is described more fully by Maitland et al (2001).

Active physiological movements

For active physiological movements, the clinician notes the:

- Quality of movement
- Range of movement

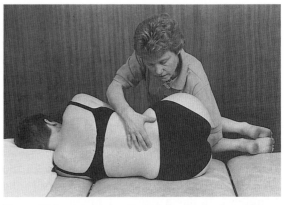

Figure 11.1   Joint integrity test for the lumbar spine. The fingers are placed in the interspinous space to feel the relative movement of the spinous processes as the clinician passively pushes and then pulls along the femoral shafts.

- Behaviour of pain through the range of movement
- Resistance through the range of movement and at the end of the range of movement
- Provocation of any muscle spasm.

A movement diagram can be used to depict this information. The active movements with overpressure listed below (Fig. 11.2) are tested with the patient in standing. The clinician establishes the patient's symptoms at rest prior to each movement and passively corrects any movement deviation to determine its relevance to the patient's symptoms. A typical observation suggesting lumbar instability is seen when patients require the support of their hands on their legs as they move into flexion and return from flexion. Active physiological movements of the lumbar spine and possible modifications are shown in Table 11.3. Side gliding movements can be useful when a lateral shift is present. A left side glide is when the hips are taken to the left, and would attempt to correct a left lateral shift. A right side glide is when the hips are taken to the right, and would attempt to correct a right lateral shift.

It is worth noting here the work of Robin McKenzie, who has described three syndromes for patients with spinal pain. If all the active movements are full-range and symptom-free on overpressure and symptoms are aggravated by certain postures, the condition is categorized as a postural

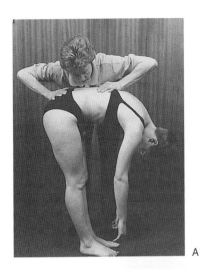

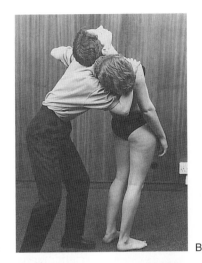

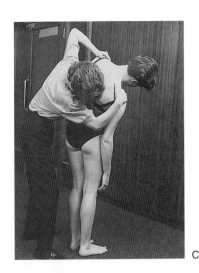

A   B   C

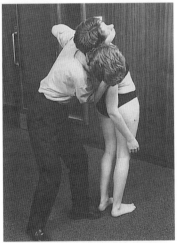

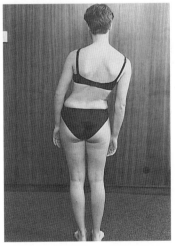

D   E

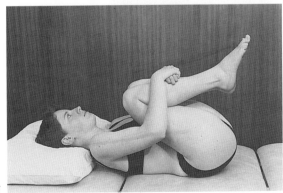

F

Figure 11.2(A–G) Overpressures to the lumbar spine.
A Flexion. The hands are placed proximally over the lower
thoracic spine and distally over the sacrum. Pressure is
then applied through both hands to increase lumbar spine
flexion. B Extension. Both hands are placed over the
shoulders, which are then pulled down in order to
increase lumbar spine extension. The clinician observes the
spinal movement. C Lateral flexion. Both hands are placed
over the shoulders and a force is applied that increases
lumbar lateral flexion. D Right extension quadrant. This
movement is a combination of extension, right rotation
and right lateral flexion. The hand hold is the same as
extension. The patient actively extends and the clinician
maintains this position and passively rotates the spine
and then adds lateral flexion overpressure. E Left side
gliding in standing (SGIS). F Flexion in lying (FIL).

syndrome (McKenzie 1981). If on repeated movement there is no change in the area of the symptoms then the condition is categorized as a dysfunction syndrome. However, if on repeated movement peripheralization and centralization phenomena are manifested then the condition is

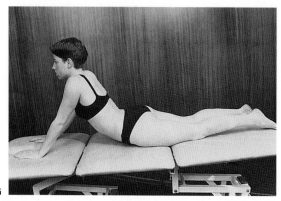

G

Figure 11.2 *Continued* **G** Extension in lying (EIL).

categorized as a derangement syndrome. A lateral shift is usually associated with a derangement syndrome (see Ch. 3 for further details). There are seven derangement syndromes described and these are shown in Table 11.4.

In the lumbar spine, flexion and extension are repeated in both standing and lying supine, as they have different effects on the spine (McKenzie 1981). In standing, the movements take place from above downwards, body weight is taken through the spine and lumbar spine flexion will stretch the sciatic nerve. In supine, the movements occur from below upwards, there is virtually no body weight through the spine and with lumbar spine flexion there is comparatively less stretch on the sciatic nerve. The point in range at which symptoms are provoked may, therefore, differ in the positions of standing and lying. For example, a problem at the L5/S1 joint may produce symptoms at the end of range when flexion occurs in standing, but as soon as the patient flexes when

Table 11.3 Active physiological movements and possible modifications

Active physiological movements	Modifications
Lumbar spine	Repeated movements
Flexion	Speed altered
Extension	Combined movements (Edwards 1994, 1999), e.g.
L lateral flexion	– flexion then lateral flexion (Fig. 11.3)
R lateral flexion	– extension then lateral flexion
L rotation (see Fig. 7.3D)	– lateral flexion then flexion
R rotation (see Fig. 7.3D)	– lateral flexion then extension
Repetitive flexion in standing (RFIS)	Compression or distraction
Repetitive extension in standing (REIS)	Sustained
L side gliding in standing (SGIS)	Injuring movement
L repetitive side gliding in standing (RSGIS)	Differentiation tests
R side gliding in standing (SGIS)	Function
R repetitive side gliding in standing (RSGIS)	
Flexion in lying (FIL)	
Repetitive flexion in lying (RFIL)	
Extension in lying (EIL)	
Repetitive extension in lying (REIL)	
?Sacroiliac joint	
?Hip	
?Knee	
?Foot and ankle	

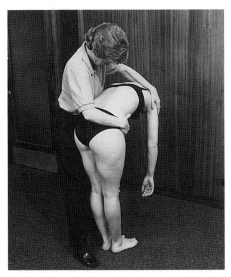

Figure 11.3 Combined movement of the lumbar spine. The patient moves into lumbar spine flexion and the clinician then maintains this position and passively adds left lateral flexion.

Table 11.4 Derangement syndromes of the lumbar spine (McKenzie 1981)

Derangement	Clinical presentation
1	Central or symmetrical pain across L4/5 Rarely buttock or thigh pain No deformity
2	Central or symmetrical pain across L4/5 With or without buttock and/or thigh pain Lumbar kyphosis
3	Unilateral or asymmetrical pain across L4/5 With or without buttock and/or thigh pain No deformity
4	Unilateral or asymmetrical pain across L4/5 With or without buttock and/or thigh pain Lumbar scoliosis
5	Unilateral or asymmetrical pain across L4/5 With or without buttock and/or thigh pain With leg pain extending below the knee No deformity
6	Unilateral or asymmetrical pain across L4/5 With or without buttock and/or thigh pain With leg pain extending below the knee Sciatic scoliosis
7	Symmetrical or asymmetrical pain across L4/5 With or without buttock and/or thigh pain Increased lumbar lordosis

carried out in supine. If there is a neurodynamic component, flexion in standing may provoke symptoms, whereas flexion in lying may be symptom-free.

Numerous differentiation tests (Maitland et al 2001) can be performed; the choice depends on the patient's signs and symptoms. For example, when trunk rotation in standing on one leg (causing rotation in the lumbar spine and hip joint) reproduces the patient's buttock pain, differentiation between the lumbar spine and hip joint may be required. The clinician can increase and decrease the lumbar spine rotation and the pelvic rotation in turn, to find out what effect each has on the buttock pain. If the pain is emanating from the hip then the lumbar movements will have no effect, but pelvic movements will alter the pain; conversely, if the pain is emanating from the lumbar spine, then lumbar spine movements will alter the pain, but pelvic movement will have no effect.

It may be necessary to examine other regions to determine their relevance to the patient's symptoms; they may be the source of the symptoms, or they may be contributing to the symptoms. The regions most likely are the sacroiliac joint, hip, knee, foot and ankle. The joints within these regions can be tested fully (see relevant chapter) or partially with the use of clearing tests (Table 11.5).

Some functional ability has already been tested by the general observation of the patient during the subjective and physical examinations, e.g. the postures adopted during the subjective examination and the ease or difficulty of undressing and changing position prior to the examination. Any further functional testing can be carried out at this point in the examination and may include lifting, sitting postures, dressing, etc. Clues for appropriate tests can be obtained from the subjective examination findings, particularly aggravating factors.

Table 11.5 Joint clearing tests

Joint	Physiological movement	Accessory movement
Thoracic spine	Rotation and flexion/extension quadrants	All movements
Sacroiliac joint	Compression, distraction and sacral rock caudad and cephalad	
Hip joint	Squat and hip quadrant	
Knee joint	All movements and squat	
Ankle joint	Plantarflexion/dorsiflexion and inversion/eversion	
Patellofemoral joint	Medial/lateral glide and cephalad/caudad glide	

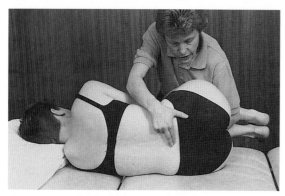

Figure 11.4 Flexion/extension PPIVMs of the lumbar spine. The clinician palpates the gap between the spinous processes of L4 and L5 to feel the range of intervertebral movement during flexion and extension.

Capsular pattern. There are no clear capsular patterns apparent in the lumbar spine.

Passive physiological movements

This can take the form of passive physiological intervertebral movements (PPIVMs), which examine the movement at each segmental level. PPIVMs may be a useful adjunct to passive accessory intervertebral movements (PAIVMs, described later in this chapter) to identify segmental hypomobility and hypermobility. They can be performed with the patient in side lying with the hips and knees flexed (Fig. 11.4) or in standing. The clinician palpates the gap between adjacent spinous processes to feel the range of intervertebral movement during flexion, extension, lateral flexion and rotation.

It may be necessary to examine other regions to determine their relevance to the patient's symptoms; they may be the source of the symptoms, or they may be contributing to the symptoms. The regions most likely are the sacroiliac joint, hip, knee, foot and ankle.

Muscle tests

The muscle tests include examining muscle strength, control, length and isometric muscle testing.

Muscle strength

The clinician tests the trunk flexors, extensors, lateral flexors and rotators and any other relevant muscle groups. For details of these general tests readers are directed to Cole et al (1988), Hislop & Montgomery (1995) or Kendall et al (1993).

Greater detail may be required to test the strength of muscles, in particular those thought prone to become weak; that is: gluteus maximus, medius and minimus, vastus lateralis, medialis and intermedius, tibialis anterior and the peronei (Jull & Janda 1987, Sahrmann 2002). Testing the strength of these muscles is described in Chapter 3.

In addition, lumbar multifidus has been found to atrophy in patients with low back pain and so may need to be tested (Hides et al 1994). The patient lies prone and the clinician applies fairly deep pressure on either side of the lumbar spinous processes (Fig. 11.5). The patient attempts to contract the muscle under the clinician's hands. Normal function is when the contraction can be held for 10 seconds and repeated 10 times (Hodges, personal communication, 1996).

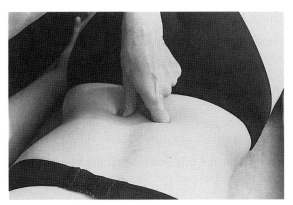

Figure 11.5 Testing active contraction of multifidus. The clinician applies fairly deep pressure on either side of the lumbar spinous processes and the patient attempts to contract the muscle under the clinician's hand.

Muscle control

The relative strength of muscles is considered to be more important than the overall strength of a muscle group (Sahrmann 2002, White & Sahrmann 1994). Relative strength is assessed indirectly by observing posture, as already mentioned, by the quality of active movement, noting any changes in muscle recruitment patterns, and by palpating muscle activity in various positions.

A method of measuring isometric muscle contraction of the lateral abdominal muscles has been described by Hodges & Richardson (1999). A pressure sensor (set at a baseline pressure of 70 mmHg) is placed between the lower abdomen and the couch with the patient in prone lying. Abdominal hollowing, i.e. drawing in the stomach and 'tightening the waist' (Kendall et al 1993), is then attempted by the patient, which normally would cause a decrease in pressure of 6–10 mmHg. An increase in pressure (of the order of 20 mmHg) indicates the incorrect contraction of rectus abdominis. The clinician observes for excessive activity of external oblique by noticing whether the patient can breathe normally during the abdominal hollowing exercise. The clinician can also observe whether any pelvic movement may be causing the reduction in pressure. The time during which the correct activation is sustained gives an indication of muscle endurance. Normal function is achieved if the patient is able to sustain the correct contraction for 10 seconds and repeat the contraction 10 times.

Active lumbar stabilization can be tested further by determining the ability of the patient to control the same position of the lumbar spine (using abdominal hollowing) while it is indirectly loaded via the upper or lower limbs, e.g. hip or shoulder flexion. Testing of lumbar stabilization can be progressed still further by more functional postures, such as sitting or standing, during exercises such as curl-ups and pelvic rotation, and while using isokinetic exercise equipment. Further information can be found in Richardson et al (2004).

Muscle length

The clinician tests the length of muscles, in particular those thought prone to shorten (Janda 1994); that is: erector spinae, quadratus lumborum, piriformis, iliopsoas, rectus femoris, tensor fasciae latae, hamstrings, tibialis posterior, gastrocnemius and soleus (Jull & Janda 1987). Testing the length of these muscles is described in Chapter 3.

Isometric muscle testing

Test trunk flexors, extensors, lateral flexors and rotators in resting position and, if indicated, in different parts of the physiological range. In addition the clinician observes the quality of the muscle contraction to hold this position (this can be done with the patient's eyes shut). The patient may, for example, be unable to prevent the joint from moving or may hold with excessive muscle activity; either of these circumstances would suggest a neuromuscular dysfunction.

Neurological tests

Neurological examination includes neurological integrity testing, neurodynamic tests and some other nerve tests.

Integrity of the nervous system

As a general guide, a neurological examination is indicated if the patient has symptoms below the level of the buttock crease.

Dermatomes/peripheral nerves. Light touch and pain sensation of the lower limb are tested using cotton wool and pinprick respectively, as described in Chapter 3. Knowledge of the cutaneous distribution of nerve roots (dermatomes) and peripheral nerves enables the clinician to distinguish the sensory loss due to a root lesion from that due to a peripheral nerve lesion. The cutaneous nerve distribution and dermatome areas are shown in Figure 3.21.

Myotomes/peripheral nerves. The following myotomes are tested (Fig. 3.27):

- L2: hip flexion
- L3: knee extension
- L4: foot dorsiflexion and inversion
- L5: extension of the big toe
- S1: eversion foot, contract buttock, knee flexion
- S2: knee flexion, toe standing
- S3–S4: muscles of pelvic floor, bladder and genital function.

A working knowledge of the muscular distribution of nerve roots (myotomes) and peripheral nerves enables the clinician to distinguish the motor loss due to a root lesion from that due to a peripheral nerve lesion. The peripheral nerve distributions are shown in Figure 3.25.

Reflex testing. The following deep tendon reflexes are tested (see Fig. 3.28):

- L3/4: knee jerk
- S1: ankle jerk.

Neurodynamic tests

The following neurodynamic tests may be carried out in order to ascertain the degree to which neural tissue is responsible for the production of the patient's symptom(s):

- Passive neck flexion (PNF)
- Straight leg raise (SLR)
- Passive knee bend (PKB)
- Slump.

These tests are described in detail in Chapter 3.

Other nerve tests

Plantar response to test for an upper motor neurone lesion (Walton 1989). Pressure applied from the heel along the lateral border of the plantar aspect of the foot produces flexion of the toes in the normal. Extension of the big toe with downward fanning of the other toes occurs with an upper motor neurone lesion.

Stoop test for intermittent cauda equina compression. The patient is asked to walk briskly for approximately 50 m. The test will produce the patient's buttock and leg pain, and causes lower limb muscle weakness. The test is considered positive – indicating cauda equina compression – if these symptoms are then eased by lumbar spine flexion (Dyck 1979).

Miscellaneous tests

Vascular tests

If the circulation is suspected of being compromised, the pulses of the femoral, popliteal and dorsalis pedis arteries are palpated. The state of the vascular system can also be determined by the response of symptoms to dependency and elevation of the lower limbs.

Leg length

True leg length is measured from the anterior superior iliac spine (ASIS) to the medial or lateral malleolus. Apparent leg length is measured from the umbilicus to the medial or lateral malleolus. A difference in leg length of up to 1–1.3 cm is considered normal. If there is a leg length difference then test the length of individual bones, the tibia with knees bent and the femurs in standing. Ipsilateral posterior rotation of the ilium (on the sacrum) or contralateral anterior rotation of the ilium will result in a decrease in leg length (Magee 1997).

Supine to sit test

The affected leg appears longer in supine and shorter in long sitting. This implicates anterior innominate rotation on the affected side (Wadsworth 1988).

Respiratory tests

These tests are appropriate for patients whose spinal dysfunction is such that respiration is affected and may include conditions such as severe scoliosis and ankylosing spondylitis.

Auscultation and examination of the patient's sputum may be required, as well as measurement of the patient's exercise tolerance.

Vital capacity can be measured using a hand-held spirometer. Normal ranges are 2.5–6 L for men and 2–5 L for women (Johnson 1990).

Maximum inspiratory and expiratory pressures (P_{Imax}/MIP, P_{Emax}/MEP) reflect respiratory muscle strength and endurance. A maximum static inspiratory or expiratory effort can be measured by a hand-held mouth pressure monitor (Micromedical Ltd, Chatham, Kent). Normal values (Wilson et al 1984) are:

P_{Imax} – > 100 cmH$_2$O for males
    > 70 cmH$_2$O for females
P_{Emax} – > 140 cmH$_2$O for males
    > 90 cmH$_2$O for females.

Palpation

The clinician palpates the lumbar spine and any other relevant areas. It is useful to record palpation findings on a body chart (see Fig. 2.3) and/or palpation chart (see Fig. 3.38).

The clinician notes the following:

- The temperature of the area
- Localized increased skin moisture
- The presence of oedema or effusion
- Mobility and feel of superficial tissues, e.g. ganglions, nodules and the lymph nodes in the femoral triangle
- The presence or elicitation of any muscle spasm
- Tenderness of bone, trochanteric and psoas bursae (palpable if swollen), ligaments, muscle (Baer's point, for tenderness/spasm of iliacus, lies a third of the way down a line from the umbilicus to the anterior superior iliac spine), tendon, tendon sheath, trigger points (shown in Fig. 3.39) and nerve. Palpable nerves in the lower limb are as follows:

  - The sciatic nerve can be palpated two-thirds of the way along an imaginary line between the greater trochanter and the ischial tuberosity with the patient in prone
  - The common peroneal nerve can be palpated medial to the tendon of biceps femoris and also around the head of the fibula
  - The tibial nerve can be palpated centrally over the posterior knee crease medial to the popliteal artery; it can also be felt behind the medial malleolus, which is more noticeable with the foot in dorsiflexion and eversion
  - The superficial peroneal nerve can be palpated on the dorsum of the foot along an imaginary line over the fourth metatarsal; it is more noticeable with the foot in plantar flexion and inversion
  - The deep peroneal nerve can be palpated between the first and second metatarsals, lateral to the extensor hallucis tendon
  - The sural nerve can be palpated on the lateral aspect of the foot behind the lateral malleolus, lateral to the tendocalcaneus
- Increased or decreased prominence of bones
- Pain provoked or reduced on palpation. Widespread, superficial, non-anatomical tenderness suggests illness behaviour.

Passive accessory intervertebral movements (PAIVMs)

It is useful to use the palpation chart and movement diagrams (or joint pictures) to record findings. These are explained in detail in Chapter 3.

The clinician notes the:

- Quality of movement
- Range of movement
- Resistance through the range and at the end of the range of movement
- Behaviour of pain through the range
- Provocation of any muscle spasm.

Lumbar spine (L1–L5) (Fig. 11.6), sacral (Fig. 11.7), and coccygeal (Fig. 11.8) accessory movements are listed in Table 11.6. Following accessory movements to the lumbar region, the clinician reassesses all the physical asterisks (movements or tests that have been found to reproduce the patient's symptoms) in order to establish the effect

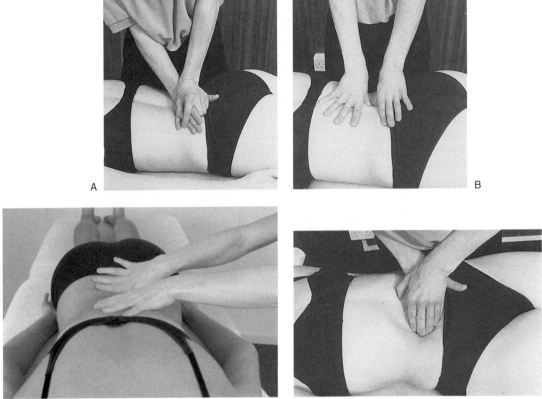

Figure 11.6 Lumbar spine accessory movements. **A** Central posteroanterior. The pisiform grip is used to apply a posteroanterior pressure on the spinous process. **B** Unilateral posteroanterior. Thumb pressure is applied to the transverse process. **C** Transverse. Thumb pressure is applied to the lateral aspect of the spinous process. **D** Unilateral anteroposterior. The fingers slowly apply pressure through the abdomen to the anterior aspect of the transverse process.

of the accessory movements on the patient's signs and symptoms. Accessory movements can then be tested for other regions suspected to be a source of, or contributing to, the patient's symptoms. Again, following accessory movements to any one region, the clinician reassesses all the asterisks. Regions likely to be examined are the sacroiliac, hip, knee, foot and ankle.

Sustained natural apophyseal glides (SNAGs)

The painful lumbar spine movements are examined in sitting and/or standing. Pressure to the spinous process or transverse process of the lumbar vertebrae is applied by the clinician as the patient moves slowly towards the pain. Figure 11.10 demonstrates a flexion SNAG on L3. The level chosen for treatment is the one that is pain-free. For further details on these techniques, see Chapter 3 and Mulligan (1999).

COMPLETION OF THE EXAMINATION

This completes the examination of the lumbar spine. The subjective and physical examinations produce a large amount of information, which needs to be recorded accurately and quickly. An outline examination chart may be useful for some clinicians and one is suggested in Figure 11.11. It is important, however, that the clinician does not

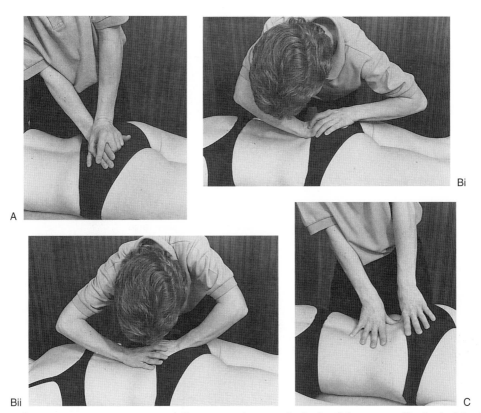

Figure 11.7   Sacrum accessory movements. **A** Posteroanterior over the body of the sacrum. The heel of the hand is used to apply the pressure. **B** (i) Sacral rock caudad. Pressure is applied to the base of the sacrum using the heel of the right hand in order to rotate the sacrum forwards in the sagittal plane, i.e. nutation. The left hand guides the movement. (ii) Sacral rock cephalad. Pressure is applied to the tip of the sacrum using the heel of the left hand in order to rotate the sacrum backwards in the sagittal plane, i.e. counternutation. The right hand guides the movement. **C** Posteroanterior pressure over the posterior superior iliac spine. Thumb or pisiform pressure can be used.

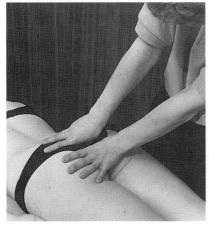

Figure 11.8   Posteroanterior pressure on the coccyx. Thumb pressure is used.

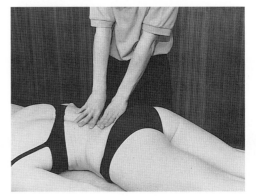

Figure 11.9   Palpation of the lumbar spine using a combined movement. A unilateral PA on the right of L3 is applied with the spine in left lateral flexion.

Table 11.6   Accessory movements, choice of application and reassessment of the patient's asterisks

Accessory movements	Choice of application	Identify any effect of accessory movements on patient's signs and symptoms

Lumbar spine (L1–L5) (Fig. 11.6)
↕   Central posteroanterior
⌐•˙⌐   Unilateral posteroanterior
⇄   Transverse
↑•˙↑   Unilateral anteroposterior
 	
Sacrum (Fig. 11.7)
↕   Posteroanterior pressure over base, body and apex
    Anterior gapping test (Fig. 12.7)
    Posterior gapping test (Fig. 12.8)
 	
Coccyx (Fig. 11.8)
↕   Posteroanterior
	Start position, e.g.
	– in flexion
	– in extension
	– in lateral flexion (Fig. 11.9)
	– in flexion and lateral flexion
	– in extension and lateral flexion
	Speed of force application
	Direction of the applied force
	Point of application of applied force
		Reassess all asterisks

?Sacroiliac joint	As above	Reassess all asterisks
?Hip	As above	Reassess all asterisks
?Knee	As above	Reassess all asterisks
?Foot and ankle	As above	Reassess all asterisks

examine in a rigid manner, simply following the suggested sequence outlined in the chart. Each patient presents differently and this needs to be

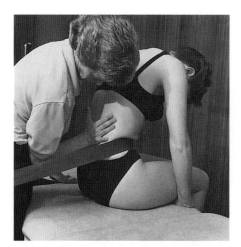

Figure 11.10   Flexion SNAG on L3. A seat belt around the patient's pelvis is used to stabilize the pelvis. The heel of the hand is then used to apply a posteroanterior pressure to L3 spinous process as the patient moves slowly into flexion.

reflected in the examination process. It is vital at this stage to highlight important findings from the examination with an asterisk (*). These findings must be reassessed at, and within, subsequent treatment sessions to evaluate the effects of treatment on the patient's condition.

The physical testing procedures which specifically indicate joint, nerve or muscle tissues, as a source of the patient's symptoms, are summarized in Table 3.10. The strongest evidence that a joint is the source of the patient's symptoms is that active and passive physiological movements, passive accessory movements and joint palpation all reproduce the patient's symptoms, and that following a treatment dose, reassessment identifies an improvement in the patient's signs and symptoms. Weaker evidence includes an alteration in range, resistance or quality of physiological and/or accessory movements and tenderness over the joint, with no alteration in signs and symptoms after treatment. One or more of these findings may indicate a dysfunction of a joint which may, or may not, be contributing to the patient's condition.

Body chart	Name
	Age
	Date
	24-hour behaviour
	Improving static worsening
	Special questions General health Weight loss RA Drugs Steroids Anticoagulants X-ray Cord symptoms Cauda equina symptoms VBI symptoms
Relationship of symptoms	
Aggravating factors and function	HPC
	PMH
Severe Irritable	
Easing factors	
	SH & FH (Patient's perspective, experience, expectations. Yellow, blue, black flags)

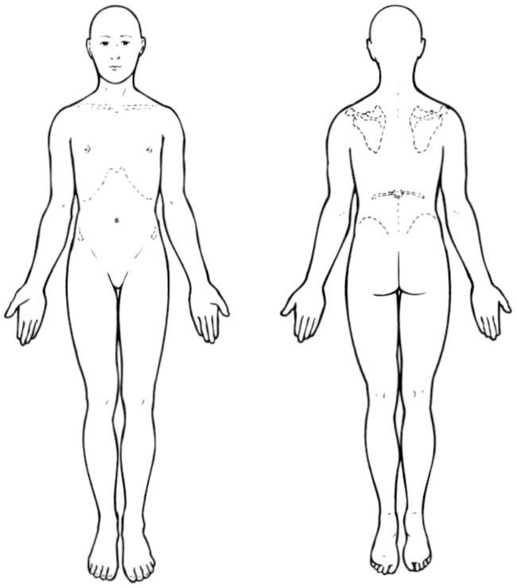

Figure 11.11   Lumbar spine examination chart.

Physical examination Observation	Isometric muscle testing
Joint integrity tests	Neurological integrity tests
Active and passive physiological movements of lumbar spine and other relevant regions	Neurodynamic tests
	Other nerve tests (stoop, plantar response)
	Miscellaneous tests (pulses, leg length, supine to sit, respiratory tests)
Muscle strength	Palpation
Muscle control	Accessory movements and reassessment of each relevant region
Muscle length	

Figure 11.11 *Continued*

The strongest evidence that a muscle is the source of a patient's symptoms is if active movements, an isometric contraction, passive lengthening and palpation of a muscle all reproduce the patient's symptoms, and that following a treatment dose, reassessment identifies an improvement in the patient's signs and symptoms. Further evidence of muscle dysfunction may be suggested by reduced strength or poor quality during the active physiological movement and the isometric contraction, reduced range, and/or increased/decreased resistance, during the passive lengthening of the muscle, and tenderness on palpation, with no alteration in signs and symptoms after treatment. One or more of these findings may indicate a dysfunction of a muscle which may or may not be contributing to the patient's condition.

The strongest evidence that a nerve is the source of the patient's symptoms is when active and/or passive physiological movements reproduce the patient's symptoms, which are then increased or decreased with an additional sensitizing movement, at a distance from the patient's symptoms. In addition, there is reproduction of the patient's symptoms on palpation of the nerve and neurodynamic testing, sufficient to be considered a treatment dose, results in an improvement in the above signs and symptoms. Further evidence of nerve dysfunction may be suggested by reduced range (compared to the asymptomatic side) and/or increased resistance to the various arm movements, and tenderness on nerve palpation.

On completion of the physical examination the clinician:

- Warns the patient of possible exacerbation up to 24–48 hours following the examination.
- Requests the patient to report details on the behaviour of the symptoms following examination at the next attendance.

- Explains the findings of the physical examination and how these findings relate to the subjective assessment. Any misconceptions patients may have regarding their illness or injury should be addressed.
- Evaluates the findings, formulates a clinical diagnosis and writes up a problem list. Clinicians may find the management planning forms shown in Figures 3.53 and 3.54 helpful in guiding them through what is often a complex clinical reasoning process.
- Determines the objectives of treatment.
- Devises an initial treatment plan.

In this way, the clinician will have developed the following hypotheses categories (adapted from Jones & Rivett 2004):

- Function: abilities and restrictions.
- Patients' perspectives on their experience.
- Source of symptoms. This includes the structure or tissue that is thought to be producing the patients' symptoms, the nature of the structure or tissues in relation to the healing process, and the pain mechanisms.
- Contributing factors to the development and maintenance of the problem. There may be environmental, psychosocial, behavioural, physical or heredity factors.
- Precautions/contraindications to treatment and management. This includes the severity and irritability of the patient's symptoms and the nature of the patient's condition.
- Management strategy and treatment plan.
- Prognosis – this can be affected by factors such as the stage and extent of the injury as well as the patient's expectation, personality and lifestyle.

References

Andersson G B J, Ortengren R, Nachemson A 1977 Intradiskal pressure, intra-abdominal pressure and myoelectric back muscle activity related to posture and loading. Clinical Orthopaedics and Related Research 129: 156–164

Clinical Standards Advisory Report 1994 Report of a CSAG committee on back pain. HMSO, London

Cole J H, Furness A L, Twomey L T 1988 Muscles in action, an approach to manual muscle testing. Churchill Livingstone, Edinburgh

Dyck P 1979 The stoop-test in lumbar entrapment radiculopathy. Spine 4(1): 89–92

Edwards B C 1994 Combined movements in the lumbar spine: their use in examination and treatment. In:

Boyling J D, Palastanga N (eds) Grieve's modern manual therapy, 2nd edn. Churchill Livingstone, Edinburgh, ch 54, p 745

Edwards B C 1999 Manual of combined movements: their use in the examination and treatment of mechanical vertebral column disorders, 2nd edn. Butterworth-Heinemann, Oxford

Grieve G P 1981 Common vertebral joint problems. Churchill Livingstone, Edinburgh

Grieve G P 1991 Mobilisation of the spine, 5th edn. Churchill Livingstone, Edinburgh

Grieve G P 1994 Counterfeit clinical presentations. Manipulative Physiotherapist 26: 17–19

Hides J A, Stokes M J, Saide M, Jull G A, Cooper D H 1994 Evidence of lumbar multifidus muscle wasting ipsilateral to symptoms in patients with acute/subacute low back pain. Spine 19(2): 165–172

Hislop H, Montgomery J 1995 Daniels and Worthingham's muscle testing, techniques of manual examination, 7th edn. W B Saunders, Philadelphia

Hodges P W, Richardson C A 1999 Altered trunk muscle recruitment in people with low back pain with upper limb movement at different speeds. Archives of Physical Medicine and Rehabilitation 80: 1005–1012

Janda V 1994 Muscles and motor control in cervicogenic disorders: assessment and management. In: Grant R (ed) Physical therapy of the cervical and thoracic spine, 2nd edn. Churchill Livingstone, Edinburgh, ch 10, p 195

Johnson N McL 1990 Respiratory medicine, 2nd edn. Blackwell Scientific Publications, Oxford, ch 3, p 37

Jones M A, Rivett D A 2004 Clinical reasoning for manual therapists. Butterworth-Heinemann, Edinburgh

Jull G A 1986 Examination of the lumbar spine. In: Grieve G P (ed) Modern manual therapy of the vertebral column. Churchill Livingstone, Edinburgh, ch 51, p 547

Jull G A, Janda V 1987 Muscles and motor control in low back pain: assessment and management. In: Twomey L T, Taylor J R (eds) Physical therapy of the low back. Churchill Livingstone, New York, ch 10, p 253

Kazarian L E 1975 Creep characteristics of the human spinal column. Orthopaedic Clinics of North America 6(1): 3–18

Kendall F P, McCreary E K, Provance P G 1993 Muscles testing and function, 4th edn. Williams & Wilkins, Baltimore, MD

Kendall N, Linton S, Main C 1997 Guide to assessing psychosocial yellow flags in acute low back pain: risk factors for long-term disability and work loss. Accident Rehabilitation & Compensation Insurance Corporation of New Zealand and the National Health Committee, Wellington, New Zealand, pp 1–22

Kirkaldy-Willis W H, Farfan H F 1982 Instability of the lumbar spine. Clinical Orthopaedics and Related Research 165: 110–123

McKenzie R A 1981 The lumbar spine mechanical diagnosis and therapy. Spinal Publications, New Zealand

Magee D J 1997 Orthopedic physical assessment, 3rd edn. W B Saunders, Philadelphia

Maitland G D, Hengeveld E, Banks K, English K 2001 Maitland's vertebral manipulation, 6th edn. Butterworth-Heinemann, Oxford

Mulligan B R 1995a Manual therapy 'NAGs', 'SNAGs', 'MWMs' etc., 4th edn. Plane View Services, New Zealand

Nachemson A 1992 Lumbar mechanics as revealed by lumbar intradiscal pressure measurements. In: Jayson M I V (ed) The lumbar spine and back pain, 4th edn. Churchill Livingstone, Edinburgh, ch 9, p 157

Pope M H, Hansson T H 1992 Vibration of the spine and low back pain. Clinical Orthopaedics and Related Research 279: 49–59

Richardson C, Hodges P W, Hides J 2004 Therapeutic exercise for lumbopelvic stabilization. A motor control approach for the treatment and prevention of low back pain, 2nd edn. Churchill Livingstone, Edinburgh

Sahrmann S A 2002 Diagnosis and treatment of movement impairment syndromes. Mosby, St Louis

Waddell G 2004 The back pain revolution, 2nd edn. Churchill Livingstone, Edinburgh

Wadsworth C T 1988 Manual examination and treatment of the spine and extremities. Williams & Wilkins, Baltimore, MD

Walton J H 1989 Essentials of neurology, 6th edn. Churchill Livingstone, Edinburgh

White A A, Panjabi M M 1990 Clinical biomechanics of the spine, 2nd edn. J B Lippincott, Philadelphia, PA

White S G, Sahrmann S A 1994 A movement system balance approach to musculoskeletal pain. In: Grant R (ed) Physical therapy of the cervical and thoracic spine, 2nd edn. Churchill Livingstone, Edinburgh, ch 16, p 339

Wilson S H, Cooke N T, Edwards R H T, Spiro S G 1984 Predicted normal values for maximal respiratory pressures in Caucasian adults and children. Thorax 39: 535–538

Chapter **12**

Examination of the pelvis

CHAPTER CONTENTS

POSSIBLE CAUSES OF PAIN AND/OR LIMITATION OF MOVEMENT

This region includes the sacroiliac joint, sacro-coccygeal joint and pubic symphysis with their surrounding soft tissues.

- Trauma and degeneration:
  - Fracture of the pelvis
  - Syndromes: arthrosis of the sacroiliac joint or pubic symphysis, osteitis condensans ilii, coccydynia, hypermobility, ilium on sacrum dysfunctions, sacrum on ilium dysfunctions
  - Ligamentous sprain
  - Muscular strain
- Inflammatory:
  - Ankylosing spondylitis
  - Rheumatoid arthritis
- Metabolic:
  - Osteoporosis
  - Paget's disease
- Infections
- Tumours, benign and malignant
- Piriformis syndrome
- Referral of symptoms from the lumbar spine
- Pregnancy is very often associated with low back pain – 88% of women studied by Bullock et al (1987) and 96% of those studied by Moore et al (1990).

The wealth of examination procedures documented for the sacroiliac joint and the frequency of isolated sacroiliac joint problems justify a chapter on the examination of the pelvis. The examination of the pelvic region is normally preceded by a detailed examination of the lumbar spine (see Ch. 11). Examination of the hip joint may also be required.

Further details of the questions asked during the subjective examination and the tests carried out in the physical examination can be found in Chapters 2 and 3 respectively.

The order of the subjective questioning and the physical tests described below can be altered as appropriate for the patient being examined.

SUBJECTIVE EXAMINATION

Body chart

The following information concerning the type and area of current symptoms can be recorded on a body chart (see Fig. 2.3).

Area of current symptoms

Be exact when mapping out the area of the symptoms. Pain localized over the sacral sulcus is indicative of sacroiliac joint dysfunction (Fortin et al 1994). Common areas of referral from the sacroiliac joint are to the groin, buttock, anterior and posterior thigh. Ascertain which is the worst symptom and record where the patient feels the symptoms are coming from. Pain is often unilateral with sacroiliac joint problems.

Areas relevant to the region being examined

All other relevant areas are checked for symptoms; it is important to ask about pain or even stiffness, as this may be relevant to the patient's main symptom. Mark unaffected areas with ticks (✓) on the body chart. Check for symptoms in the thoracic spine, lumbar spine, abdomen, groin and lower limbs.

Quality of pain

Establish the quality of the pain. Often the patient complains of a dull ache with sacroiliac joint problems.

Intensity of pain

The intensity of pain can be measured using, for example, a visual analogue scale (VAS) as shown in Figure 2.8. A pain diary may be useful for patients with chronic low back pain, to determine the pain patterns and triggering factors over a period of time.

Depth of pain

Establish the depth of the pain. Does the patient feel it is on the surface or deep inside?

Abnormal sensation

Check for any altered sensation over the lumbar spine and sacroiliac joint and any other relevant areas. Common abnormalities are paraesthesia and numbness.

Constant or intermittent symptoms

Ascertain the frequency of the symptoms, whether they are constant or intermittent. If symptoms are constant, check whether there is variation in the intensity of the symptoms, as constant unremitting pain may be indicative of neoplastic disease.

Relationship of symptoms

Determine the relationship between the symptomatic areas – do they come together or separately? For example, the patient could have buttock pain without back pain, or they may always be present together.

Behaviour of symptoms

Aggravating factors

For each symptomatic area, discover what movements and/or positions aggravate the patient's symptoms, i.e. what brings them on (or makes them worse), are they able to maintain this position or movement (severity), what happens to other symptom(s) when this symptom is produced (or is made worse), and how long does it take for symptoms to ease once the position or movement is stopped (irritability). These questions help to confirm the relationship of the symptoms one to another.

The clinician also asks the patient about theoretically known aggravating factors for structures that could be a source of the symptoms. Common aggravating factors for the sacroiliac joint are standing on one leg, turning over in bed, getting in or out of bed, sloppy standing with uneven weight distribution through the legs, habitual work stance, stepping up on the affected side and walking. Aggravating factors for other regions, which may need to be queried if they are suspected to be a source of the symptoms, are shown in Table 2.3.

The clinician ascertains how the symptoms affect function, such as: static and active postures, e.g. lying, sitting, standing, bending, standing on one leg, walking, walking on uneven ground and up and down stairs, running, washing, driving, lifting and digging, work, sport and social activities. Note details of training regimen for any sports activities. The clinician finds out if the patient is left- or right-handed as there may be increased stress on the dominant side.

Detailed information on each of the above activities is useful in order to help determine the structure(s) at fault and identify functional restrictions. This information can be used to determine the aims of treatment and any advice that may be required. The most notable functional restrictions are highlighted with asterisks (*), explored in the physical examination, and reassessed at subsequent treatment sessions to evaluate treatment intervention.

Easing factors

For each symptomatic area, the clinician asks what movements and/or positions ease the patient's symptoms, how long it takes to ease them and what happens to other symptoms when this symptom is relieved. These questions help to confirm the relationship between the symptoms.

The clinician asks the patient about theoretically known easing factors for structures that could be a source of the symptoms. For example, symptoms from the sacroiliac joint may be eased by lying supine, stooping forwards in standing and/or applying a wide belt around the pelvis. One study has found that a pelvic support gave some relief of pain in 83% of pregnant women

(Ostgaard et al 1994). The clinician can then analyse the position or movement that eases the symptoms to help determine the structure at fault.

Twenty-four-hour behaviour of symptoms

The clinician determines the 24-hour behaviour of symptoms by asking questions about night, morning and evening symptoms.

Night symptoms. The following questions may be asked:

- Do you have any difficulty getting to sleep?
- What position is most comfortable/uncomfortable?
- What is your normal sleeping position?
- What is your present sleeping position?
- Do your symptom(s) wake you at night? If so,
  - Which symptom(s)?
  - Is it because you moved?
  - How many times in the past week?
  - How many times in a night?
  - How long does it take to get back to sleep?
- How many and what type of pillows are used?
- Is the mattress firm or soft?
- Has the mattress been changed recently?

Morning and evening symptoms. The clinician determines the pattern of the symptoms first thing in the morning, through the day and at the end of the day. In ankylosing spondylitis, the cardinal and often earliest sign is erosion of the sacroiliac joints, which is often manifested by pain and stiffness around the sacroiliac joint and lumbar spine for the first few hours in the morning (Solomon et al 2001).

Stage of the condition

In order to determine the stage of the condition, the clinician asks whether the symptoms are getting better, getting worse or remaining unchanged.

Special questions

Special questions must always be asked, as they may identify certain precautions or contraindications to the physical examination and/or treatment (Table 2.4). As mentioned in Chapter 2, the clinician must differentiate between conditions that are suitable for conservative management and systemic, neoplastic and other non-neuromusculoskeletal conditions, which require referral to a medical practitioner. The reader is referred to Appendix 2.2 for details of various serious pathological processes that can mimic neuromusculoskeletal conditions (Grieve 1994).

The following information is routinely obtained from patients.

General health. Ascertain the general health of the patient – find out if the patient suffers from any malaise, fatigue, fever, nausea or vomiting, stress, anxiety or depression. In addition, ask, if necessary, whether the patient is pregnant. It is common for low back pain to be associated with pregnancy, although the underlying mechanism remains unclear. Recent research suggests that there may be a number of factors involved, including an increase in the load on the lumbar spine because of weight gain, hormonal changes causing hypermobility of the sacroiliac joint and pubic symphysis (Hagen 1974), and an increase in the abdominal sagittal diameter (Ostgaard et al 1993). Little evidence supports the hypothesis that the pain is related to alteration in posture (Bullock et al 1987, Ostgaard et al 1993).

Weight loss. Has the patient noticed any recent unexplained weight loss?

Rheumatoid arthritis. Has the patient (or a member of his/her family) been diagnosed as having rheumatoid arthritis?

Drug therapy. What drugs are being taken by the patient? Has the patient ever been prescribed long-term (6 months or more) medication/steroids? Has the patient been taking anticoagulants recently?

X-ray and medical imaging. Has the patient been X-rayed or had any other medical tests? Routine spinal X-rays are no longer considered necessary prior to conservative treatment as they only identify the normal age-related degenerative changes, which do not necessarily correlate with the patient's symptoms (Clinical Standards Advisory Report 1994). The medical tests may include blood tests, magnetic resonance imaging, myelography, discography or a bone scan.

Neurological symptoms. Has the patient experienced symptoms of spinal cord compression (i.e. compression of the spinal cord to L1 level), which are bilateral tingling in hands or feet and/or disturbance of gait?

Has the patient experienced symptoms of cauda equina compression (i.e. compression below L1), which are saddle anaesthesia/paraesthesia and bladder or bowel sphincter disturbance (loss of control, retention, hesitancy, urgency or a sense of incomplete evacuation) (Grieve 1991)? These symptoms may be due to interference of S3 and S4 (Grieve 1981). Prompt surgical attention is required to prevent permanent sphincter paralysis.

History of the present condition (HPC)

For each symptomatic area, the clinician needs to know how long the symptom has been present, whether there was a sudden or slow onset and whether there was a known cause that provoked the onset of the symptom, such as a fall. If the onset was slow, the clinician finds out if there has been any change in the patient's lifestyle, e.g. a new job or hobby or a change in sporting activity. If the patient is pregnant, she may develop associated symptoms as early as week 18 (Bullock et al 1987). To confirm the relationship of symptoms, the clinician asks what happened to other symptoms when each symptom began.

Past medical history (PMH)

The following information is obtained from the patient and/or the medical notes:

- The details of any relevant medical history, such as pelvic inflammatory disease or fractures of the lower limbs.
- The history of any previous attacks: how many episodes, when were they, what was the cause, what was the duration of each episode and did the patient fully recover between episodes? If there have been no previous attacks, has the patient had any episodes of stiffness in the thoracic or lumbar spine or any other relevant

region? Check for a history of trauma or recurrent minor trauma.

- Ascertain the results of any past treatment for the same or similar problem. Past treatment records may be obtained for further information.

Social and family history (SH, FH)

Social and family history that is relevant to the onset and progression of the patient's condition is recorded. This includes the patient's perspectives, experience and expectations, their age, employment, home situation, and details of any leisure activities. Factors from this information may indicate direct and/or indirect mechanical influences on the sacroiliac joint. In order to treat the patient appropriately, it is important that it is managed within the context of the patient's social and work environment.

The clinician may ask the following types of questions to elucidate psychosocial factors:

- Have you had time off work in the past with your pain?
- What do you understand to be the cause of your pain?
- What are you expecting will help you?
- How is your employer/co-workers/family responding to your pain?
- What are you doing to cope with your pain?
- Do you think you will return to work? When?

While these questions are described in relation to psychosocial risk factors for poor outcomes for patients with low back pain (Waddell 2004), they may be relevant to other patients.

Plan of the physical examination

When all this information has been collected, the subjective examination is complete. It is useful at this stage to highlight with asterisks (*), for ease of reference, important findings and particularly one or more functional restrictions. These can then be re-examined at subsequent treatment sessions to evaluate treatment intervention.

In order to plan the physical examination, the following hypotheses need to be developed from the subjective examination:

- The regions and structures that need to be examined as a possible cause of the symptoms, e.g. sacroiliac joint, pubic symphysis, lumbar spine, thoracic spine, cervical spine, hip, knee, ankle and foot, muscles and nerves. Often it is not possible to examine fully at the first attendance and so examination of the structures must be prioritized over subsequent treatment sessions.
- Other factors that need to be examined, e.g. working and everyday postures, leg length, etc.
- In what way should the physical tests be carried out? Will it be easy or hard to reproduce each symptom? Will it be necessary to use combined movements, repetitive movements, etc. to reproduce the patient's symptoms? Are symptom(s) severe and/or irritable? If symptoms are severe, physical tests may be carried out to just before the onset of symptom production or just to the onset of symptom production; no overpressures will be carried out, as the patient would be unable to tolerate this. If symptoms are irritable, physical tests may be examined to just before symptom production or just to the onset of provocation with less physical tests being examined to allow for rest period between tests.
- Are there any precautions and/or contraindications to elements of the physical examination that need to be explored further, such as neurological involvement, recent fracture, trauma, steroid therapy or rheumatoid arthritis; there may also be certain contraindications to further examination and treatment, e.g. symptoms of spinal cord or cauda equina compression.

A physical planning sheet can be useful for clinicians to help guide them through the clinical reasoning process (Fig. 2.10 and Appendix 2.1).

PHYSICAL EXAMINATION

The information from the subjective examination helps the clinician to plan an appropriate physical examination. The severity, irritability and nature of the condition are the major factors that will influence the choice and priority of physical testing procedures. The first and over-arching question the clinician might ask is: 'is this patient's condition suitable for me to manage as a therapist?' For example, a patient presenting with cauda equina compression symptoms may only need neurological integrity testing, prior to an urgent medical referral. The nature of the patient's condition has had a major impact on the physical examination. The second question the clinician might ask is: 'does this patient have a neuromusculoskeletal dysfunction that I may be able to help?' To answer that, the clinician needs to carry out a full physical examination; however, this may not be possible if the symptoms are severe and/or irritable. If the patient's symptoms are severe and/or irritable, the clinician aims to explore movements as much as possible, within a symptom-free range. If the patient has constant and severe and/or irritable symptoms, then the clinician aims to find physical tests that ease the symptoms. If the patient's symptoms are non-severe and non-irritable, then the clinician aims to find physical tests that reproduce each of the patient's symptoms.

Each significant physical test that either provokes or eases the patient's symptoms is highlighted in the patient's notes by an asterisk (*) for easy reference. The highlighted tests are often referred to as 'asterisks' or 'markers'.

The order and detail of the physical tests described below need to be appropriate to the patient being examined; some tests will be irrelevant, some tests will be carried out briefly, while others will need to be fully investigated. It is important that readers understand that the techniques shown in this chapter are some of many; the choice depends mainly on the relative size of the clinician and patient, as well as the clinician's preference. For this reason, novice clinicians may initially want to copy what is shown, but then quickly adapt to what is best for them.

Observation

Informal observation

The clinician needs to observe the patient in dynamic and static situations; the quality of movement is noted, as are the postural characteristics and facial expression. Informal observation will have begun from the moment the clinician begins

the subjective examination and will continue to the end of the physical examination.

Formal observation

Observation of posture. The clinician examines the patient's spinal and lower limb posture in standing from anterior, lateral and posterior views. Specific observation of the pelvis involves noting its position in the sagittal, coronal and horizontal planes: in the sagittal plane, there may be excessive anterior or posterior pelvic tilt; in the coronal plane there may be a lateral pelvic tilt; and in the horizontal plane there may be rotation of the pelvis. These abnormalities will be identified by observing the relative position of the iliac crest, the anterior and posterior iliac spines (ASIS and PSIS), ischial tuberosity, skin creases (particularly the gluteal crease) and the position of the pelvis relative to the lumbar spine and lower limbs.

The left and right ASIS and PSIS are compared for symmetry. In addition, the level of the ASIS and PSIS on the same side are compared; if the patient has an anterior pelvic tilt the PSIS will be higher than the ASIS on both left and right sides; however, if the patient has an anterior rotation dysfunction of the ilium on the sacrum (innominate anteriorly rotated on one side) then the PSIS will be higher than the ASIS on the affected side only. If the iliac crest and ischial tuberosity are higher on one side this would indicate an upslip (see the end of this chapter for further details). The patient may stand with unequal weight through the legs because of a short leg or in order to obtain pain relief. The clinician passively corrects any asymmetry to determine its relevance to the patient's problem.

In supine the clinician palpates the left and right pubic tubercles and pubic rami for symmetry in the transverse and coronal planes. Superoinferior asymmetry of the pubic tubercles or anteroposterior asymmetry of the pubic rami may indicate a pubic symphysis dysfunction. In prone the clinician palpates the relative position of the sacral base and inferior lateral angle (ILA) of the sacrum (Fig. 12.1). Asymmetry may indicate sacroiliac joint dysfunction; examples include a deep sacral base and ILA on one side indicative of a sacral torsion. The prone extension test (see later

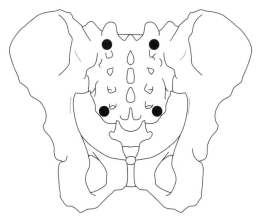

Figure 12.1 Palpation of sacral base and inferior lateral angle of the sacrum. (From Lee 1999, with permission.)

under passive physiological tests) is used to differentiate between an anterior or posterior sacral torsion; a deep sacral base and an inferior ILA on one side is indicative of a side bent sacrum.

Observation of muscle form. The clinician observes the muscle bulk and muscle tone of the patient, comparing left and right sides, and in particular notes the muscle bulk of gluteus maximus. It must be remembered that the level and frequency of physical activity, as well as the dominant side, may well produce differences in muscle bulk between sides.

Observation of soft tissues. The clinician observes the quality and colour of the patient's skin and any area of swelling or presence of scarring, and takes cues for further examination.

Observation of gait. The typical gait patterns that might be expected in patients with low back pain are the gluteus maximus gait, the Trendelenburg gait and the short leg gait (see Ch. 3 for further details).

Observation of the patient's attitudes and feelings. The age, gender and ethnicity of patients and their cultural, occupational and social backgrounds will all affect their attitudes and feelings towards themselves, their condition and the clinician. The clinician needs to be aware of and sensitive to these attitudes, and to empathize and communicate appropriately so as to develop a rapport with the patient and thereby enhance the patient's compliance with the treatment.

Active physiological movements

There are no active physiological movements at the sacroiliac joint. The movements of the sacroiliac joint are nutation (anterior rotation of the sacrum) and counternutation (posterior rotation of the sacrum), which occur during movement of the spine and hip joints. Sacroiliac joint movements are therefore tested using active physiological movements of the lumbar spine and hip joints, while the sacroiliac joint is palpated by the clinician; these are described under passive physiological movements.

Numerous differentiation tests (Maitland et al 2001) can be performed; the choice depends on the patient's signs and symptoms. For example, when the hip flexion/adduction test (see 'passive physiological movements' below for further details) reproduces the patient's groin pain, it may be necessary to differentiate between the sacroiliac joint and the hip joint as a source of the symptoms. The position of the sacroiliac joint is altered by placing a towel between the sacrum and the couch, and the test is then repeated. If the pain response is affected by this alteration, the sacroiliac joint is implicated as a source of the groin pain.

Other regions may need to be examined to determine their relevance to the patient's symptoms; they may be the source of the symptoms, or they may be contributing to the symptoms. The regions most likely are the thoracic spine, knee, ankle and foot. The joints within these regions can be tested fully (see relevant chapter) or partially with the use of joint clearing tests (Table 12.1).

Some functional ability has already been tested by the general observation of the patient during the subjective and physical examinations, e.g. the postures adopted during the subjective examination and the ease or difficulty of undressing prior to the examination. Any further functional testing can be carried out at this point in the examination and may include turning over in bed, sitting postures, sitting to standing, lifting, the bowling action for cricket, etc. Clues for appropriate tests can be obtained from the subjective examination findings, particularly aggravating factors.

Table 12.1   Joint clearing tests

Joint	Physiological movement	Accessory movement
Thoracic spine	Rotation and quadrants	All movements
Knee joint	All movements and squat	
Ankle joint	Plantarflexion/ dorsiflexion and inversion/eversion	
Patellofemoral joint		Medial/lateral glide and cephalad/ caudad glide

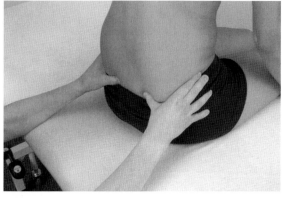

Figure 12.2   Sitting flexion test (Piedallu's test).

Passive physiological movements

The sitting flexion test, standing flexion test and standing hip flexion test are often referred to as kinetic tests.

Sitting flexion (Piedallu's test) (Fig. 12.2). In sitting, the patient flexes the trunk and the clinician palpates movement of the left and right posterior superior iliac spines. This tests the movement of the sacrum on the ilium. The left and right PSIS will normally move equally in a superior direction. If the PSIS rises more on one side during lumbar spine flexion, it is thought to indicate hypomobility of the sacroiliac joint on that side.

Standing flexion. In standing the patient flexes the trunk and the clinician palpates the movement of the left and right PSIS. This tests the movement of the ilium on the sacrum. The left and right PSIS will normally move equally in a superior direction. If the PSIS rises more on one side during lumbar spine flexion, it is thought to indicate hypomobility of the sacroiliac joint on that side.

Standing hip flexion (Gillet test). In standing, the patient flexes the hip and knee and the clinician palpates the inferior aspect of the PSIS and the sacrum (at the same horizontal level) on the same side as the movement – ipsilateral test (Fig. 12.3A). The test is repeated and compared to the opposite side. It tests the ability of the ilium to flex and posteriorly rotate, and the ability of the sacrum to rotate towards the side of movement (Lee 1999). If the PSIS does not move downwards and medially on the side of hip flexion, it may indicate hypomobility of the sacroiliac joint on that side. Abnormal findings may include hip hitching or movement of the PSIS in a superior direction.

For the contralateral test the patient flexes the hip and knee and the clinician palpates the inferior aspect of the PSIS and the sacrum (at the same horizontal level) on the opposite side as the movement; for example, the clinician palpates the left PSIS and sacrum while the patient flexes the right hip (Fig. 12.3B). The test is repeated and compared to the opposite side. It tests the ability of the sacrum to move on the ilium. Abnormal findings may be no movement or superior movement of the sacrum relative to the PSIS.

Prone trunk extension test (Greenman 1996). In prone the depth of the sacral base and inferior lateral angle of the sacrum are palpated and compared left to right sides. A sacral base and inferior lateral angle that are both deep on the same side may suggest a sacral torsion (see observation of posture). The prone extension test is used to differentiate between an anterior and posterior sacral torsion. The patient is asked to extend the lumbar spine while the clinician palpates the left and right sacral bases (Fig. 12.4). If the asymmetry increases on lumbar extension it

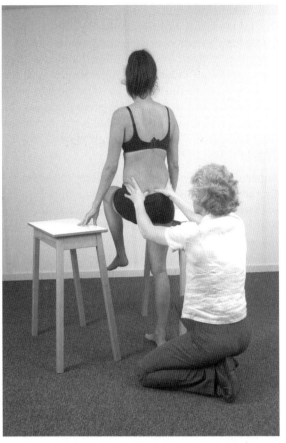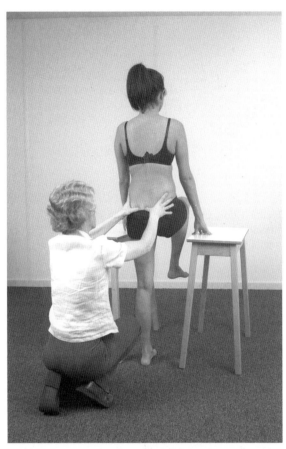

A   B

Figure 12.3   Standing hip flexion test.   **A** Ipsilateral.   **B** Contralateral.

may indicate a posterior sacral torsion; if the asymmetry reduces, this may indicate an anterior sacral torsion.

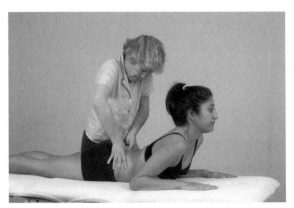

Figure 12.4   Prone extension test.

Anterior and posterior rotation (Lee 1999). With the patient in side lie, the clinician palpates the sacral sulcus just medial to the PSIS with the middle and ring fingers (to monitor movement between the innominate and sacrum) and palpates the lumbosacral junction with the index finger (Fig. 12.5). With the other hand the clinician anteriorly and posteriorly rotates the innominate on the sacrum. The clinician compares the movement and pain response on one side to the other. Normally the ilium would move first, followed by the lumbosacral junction. Typical abnormal findings on anterior/posterior rotation include no movement of the ilium; movement only occurring at the lumbosacral junction (hypomobility of the sacroiliac joint); and excessive movement of the ilium accompanied by little movement at the lumbosacral junction (hypermobility of the sacroiliac

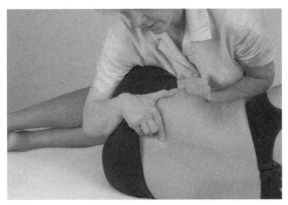

Figure 12.5 Clinician palpates the sacral sulcus and the lumbosacral junction while passively moving the innominate into anterior and posterior rotation.

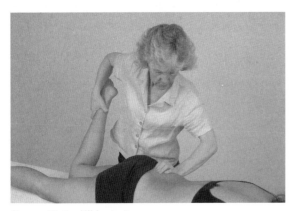

Figure 12.6 Hibbs test.

joint) – this is often accompanied with a lack of end-feel. This test thus compares the relative movement of the sacroiliac joint and the lumbosacral junction.

Hibbs test (Magee 1997). The patient lies prone with one knee in 90° of flexion. The clinician medially rotates the hip and palpates the sacroiliac joint via the posterior superior iliac spine (Fig. 12.6). The amount and quality of movement are compared on the left and right sides.

Anteroposterior translation: innominate/sacrum. With the patient in crook lying, the clinician palpates the sacral sulcus just medial to the PSIS with the middle and ring fingers (to monitor movement

between the innominate and sacrum) and palpates the lumbosacral junction with the index finger (same hand position as anterior/posterior rotation described above). With the other hand the clinician applies an anteroposterior force through the iliac crest, feels the range and the resistance to movement, and notes any reproduction of the patient's symptoms. End of range is reached when the pelvic girdle rotates as a unit beneath the L5 vertebra (Lee 1999).

Superoinferior/inferosuperior glide: innominate/sacrum. With the patient in side lie, the clinician palpates the sacral sulcus just medial to the PSIS with the middle and ring fingers (to monitor movement between the innominate and sacrum) and palpates the lumbosacral junction with the index finger (same hand position as above). With the other hand the clinician applies a superior or inferior pressure through the distal end of the femur, feels the range and the resistance to movement, and notes any reproduction of the patient's symptoms. A lack of translation of the innominate on the sacrum may indicate hypomobility of the sacroiliac joint.

Lumbar spine PPIVMs. It may be necessary to examine lumbar spine PPIVMs, particularly for the L5/S1 level. See Chapter 11 for further details.

It may be necessary to examine other regions to determine their relevance to the patient's symptoms; they may be the source of the symptoms, or they may be contributing to the symptoms. The regions most likely are the thoracic spine, knee, ankle and foot.

Muscle tests

Muscle control

The clinician may test the trunk muscles; readers are referred to Chapters 3 and 11 for further details.

Muscle length

The clinician tests the length of muscles, in particular those thought prone to shorten (Janda 1994, 2002, Sahrmann 2002). Description of muscle length tests is given in Chapter 3.

Neurological tests

The neurological tests are the same as those for the lumbar spine (see Ch. 11).

Miscellaneous tests

The vascular, leg length and respiratory tests are the same as those for the lumbar spine (see Ch. 11).

Palpation

The clinician palpates over the pelvis, including the sacrum, sacroiliac joints, pubic symphysis and any other relevant areas. It is useful to record palpation findings on a body chart (see Fig. 2.3) and/or palpation chart (Fig. 3.38).

The clinician notes the following:

- The temperature of the area
- Localized increased skin moisture
- The presence of oedema or effusion
- Mobility and feel of superficial tissues, e.g. ganglions, nodules and lymph nodes in the femoral triangle
- The presence or elicitation of any muscle spasm
- Tenderness of bone, trochanteric and psoas bursae (palpable if swollen), ligament, muscle (Baer's point, for tenderness/spasm of iliacus, lies a third of the way down a line from the umbilicus to the anterior superior iliac spine), tendon, tendon sheath, trigger points (shown in Fig. 3.39) and nerve. Palpable nerves in the lower limb are as follows:
  - The sciatic nerve can be palpated two-thirds of the way along an imaginary line between the greater trochanter and the ischial tuberosity with the patient in prone.
  - The common peroneal nerve can be palpated medial to the tendon of biceps femoris and also around the head of the fibula
  - The tibial nerve can be palpated centrally over the posterior knee crease medial to the popliteal artery; it can also be felt behind the medial malleolus, which is more noticeable with the foot in dorsiflexion and eversion
  - The superficial peroneal nerve can be palpated on the dorsum of the foot along an imaginary line over the fourth metatarsal; it

is more noticeable with the foot in plantar flexion and inversion
  - The deep peroneal nerve can be palpated between the first and second metatarsals, lateral to the extensor hallucis tendon
  - The sural nerve can be palpated on the lateral aspect of the foot behind the lateral malleolus, lateral to the tendocalcaneus
- Increased or decreased prominence of bones
- Pain provoked or reduced on palpation.

Accessory movements

It is useful to use the palpation chart and movement diagrams (or joint pictures) to record findings. These are explained in detail in Chapter 3. The following examination techniques will need to be adapted if the patient is pregnant and is unable to lie prone.

The clinician notes the:

- Quality of movement
- Range of movement
- Resistance through the range and at the end of the range of movement
- Behaviour of pain through the range
- Provocation of any muscle spasm.

Sacroiliac joint and coccygeal accessory movements are shown in Figures 12.7–12.11 and are listed in Table 12.2. Some of the accessory movements are described below.

Anterior gapping test (gapping test). In supine, the clinician applies a force that attempts to push the left and right ASIS apart (Fig. 12.7). Reproduction of the patient's symptom(s) indicates a sprain of the anterior sacroiliac joint or ligaments (Edwards 1999, Laslett & Williams 1994, Magee 1997, Maitland et al 2001).

Posterior gapping test (approximation test). In supine or side lying, the clinician applies a force that attempts to push the left and right ASIS towards each other (Fig. 12.8). Reproduction of the patient's symptom(s) indicates a sprain of the posterior sacroiliac joint or ligaments (Edwards 1999, Laslett & Williams 1994, Magee 1997, Maitland et al 2001).

Posterior shear test/femoral shear test (Porterfield & DeRosa 1998). In supine with the

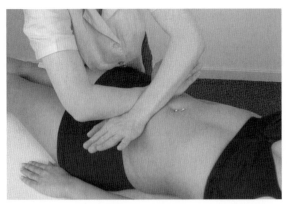

Figure 12.7 Anterior gapping test. The hands are crossed and the heels of the hands rest against the anteromedial aspect of the anterior superior iliac spines. The hands then apply a lateral force to the left and right ASIS.

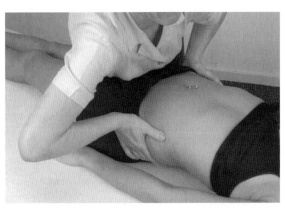

Figure 12.8 Posterior gapping test. The hands rest on the anterolateral aspect of the anterior superior iliac spines. The hands then apply a medial force to the left and right ASIS.

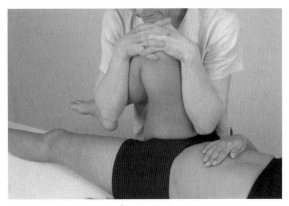

Figure 12.9 Posterior/femoral shear test. A longitudinal cephalad force is applied through the femur with the patient's hip flexed.

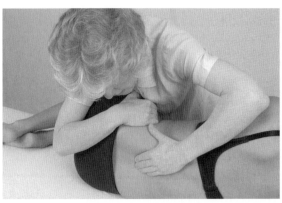

Figure 12.10 The clinician applies a longitudinal force to the innominate. The clinician may also feel the movement of the lumbar spine during this movement.

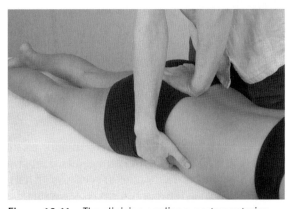

Figure 12.11 The clinician applies a posteroanterior pressure on the sacrum with the left hand and an anteroposterior pressure on the ASIS with the right hand.

hip slightly flexed, the clinician applies a longitudinal cephalad force through the femur to produce an anteroposterior shear at the sacroiliac joint (Fig. 12.9). Reproduction of the patient's symptom(s) may suggest a sacroiliac joint problem, although this test also stresses the hip joint.

Longitudinal caudad. With the patient in side lie and the knee slightly flexed, the clinician applies a longitudinal force to the ilium through the iliac crest (Fig. 12.10). Reproduction of pain or limited range of movement may suggest a sacroiliac joint problem.

Following accessory movements to the pelvis, the clinician reassesses all the physical asterisks (movements or tests that have been found to reproduce the patient's symptoms) in order to

Table 12.2   Accessory movements, choice of application and reassessment of the patient's asterisks

Accessory movements	Choice of application	Identify any effect of accessory movements on patient's signs and symptoms
Sacroiliac joint		
Anterior gapping test (gapping test)	Start position, e.g.	Reassess all asterisks
Posterior gapping test (approximation test)	– pelvis in anterior or posterior rotation	
Posterior shear test/femoral shear test	– hip in flexion	
↔ Caud longitudinal caudad	Speed of force application	
↕ PA pressure over base, body and apex (Maitland et al 2001)	Direction of the applied force	
	Point of application of applied force	
↕ PA pressure over the posterior superior iliac spine		
PA sacrum with AP to ASIS (Magee 1997) (Fig. 12.11).		
Coccyx (Fig. 11.8)		
↕ PA		
↔ Transverse		
↕ AP		
?Thoracic spine	As above	Reassess all asterisks
?Coccyx	As above	Reassess all asterisks
?Knee	As above	Reassess all asterisks
?Foot and ankle	As above	Reassess all asterisks

establish the effect of the accessory movements on the patient's signs and symptoms. Accessory movements can then be tested for other regions suspected to be a source of, or contributing to, the patient's symptoms. Again, following accessory movements to any one region, the clinician reassesses all the asterisks. Regions likely to be examined are the thoracic spine, coccyx, knee, foot and ankle (Table 12.2).

Sustained natural apophyseal glides (SNAGs)

Examination of the lumbar spine may involve the use of SNAGs, which are described in Chapter 11.

Dysfunctions of the sacroiliac joint (Fig. 12.12)

The reader may find it helpful to classify sacroiliac dysfunction using the following system.

Ilium on sacrum dysfunctions. Ilium on sacrum dysfunctions are categorized as an anterior rotation, posterior rotation, an upslip or a combination of a rotation (anterior or posterior) and an upslip.

Anterior rotation. The ilium is excessively anteriorly rotated relative to the sacrum; the ASIS is palpated inferior to the PSIS on the affected side. The standing flexion test and ipsilateral standing hip flexion tests are positive on examination. Anterior (and posterior) rotation dysfunctions are thought to be myofascial in origin and hence all accessory movement testing will be negative.

Posterior rotation. The ilium is excessively posteriorly rotated relative to the sacrum; the ASIS is palpated superior to the PSIS on the affected side. The standing flexion test and ipsilateral standing hip flexion tests are positive on examination.

Upslip. This is where the pelvis on one side has 'slipped upwards' relative to the sacrum. The iliac crest and ischial tuberosity are palpated superior to the corresponding bony prominences on the opposite side. The height of the ASIS may vary as upslip dysfunctions can occur in conjunction with anterior or posterior rotation dysfunctions. The standing flexion test and the ipsilateral standing hip flexion test are positive, as well as positive accessory joint findings.

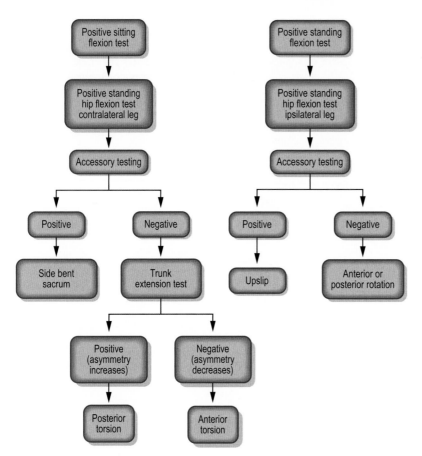

Figure 12.12 Developing a clinical diagnosis of sacroiliac joint dysfunction.

Sacrum on ilium dysfunctions. These are classified as anterior and posterior torsion and side-bent sacrum.

Torsion dysfunction. The depth of the sacral base and the inferior lateral angle on one side compared to the same prominences on the other side will be relatively superficial (posterior torsion) or relatively deep (anterior torsion). This is thought to be due to a rotation of the sacrum about an oblique axis (Greenman 1996). The prone extension test described earlier will differentiate between an anterior and posterior torsion.

Side-bent sacrum. The sacral base and inferior lateral angles are compared one side to another. A side-bent sacrum is where the sacral base is deep and the inferior lateral angle inferior on one side, so for a left side-bent sacrum the left sacral base would be deep and the left inferior lateral angle would be inferior, compared to the right sacral base, which would be superficial, and the right

inferior lateral angle, which would be superior; this is shown in Figure 12.1 (Greenman 1996). The sitting flexion test will be positive on the side of the dysfunction.

COMPLETION OF THE EXAMINATION

Having carried out the above tests, examination of the sacroiliac joint is now complete. The subjective and physical examinations produce a large amount of information, which needs to be recorded accurately and quickly. An outline examination chart may be useful for some clinicians and one is suggested in Figure 12.13. It is important, however, that the clinician does not examine in a rigid manner, simply following the suggested sequence outlined in the chart. Each patient presents differently and this needs to be reflected in the examination process. It is vital at this stage to highlight important findings from the

Body chart	Name
	Age
	Date
	24-hour behaviour
	Improving static worsening
	Special questions
	General health
	Weight loss
	RA
	Drugs
	Steroids
Relationship of symptoms	Anticoagulants
	X-ray
	Cord symptoms
	Cauda equina symptoms
	VBI symptoms
Aggravating factors and function	HPC
	PMH
Severe Irritable	
Easing factors	SH & FH
	(Patient's perspective, experience, expectations. Yellow, blue, black flags)

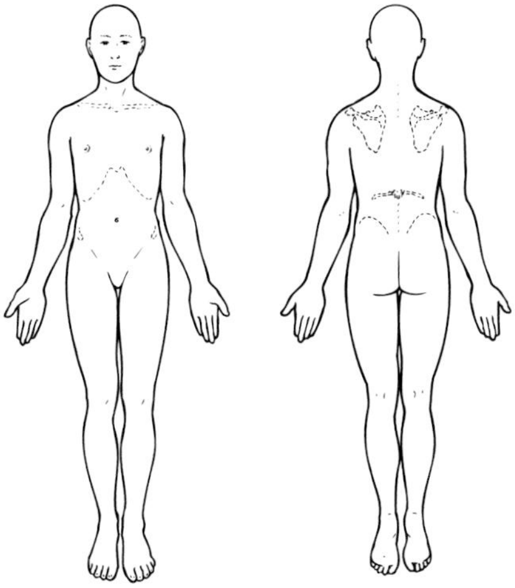

Figure 12.13   Pelvic examination chart.

Physical examination	Neurological integrity tests
Observation	
	Neurodynamic tests
Active and passive physiological movements of pelvis and other relevant regions	
	Other nerve tests (stoop, plantar response)
	Miscellaneous tests (pulses, leg length, respiratory tests)
	Palpation
	Accessory movements and reassessment of each relevant region
Muscle control	
Muscle length	

Figure 12.13 *Continued*

examination with an asterisk (*). These findings must be reassessed at, and within, subsequent treatment sessions to evaluate the effects of treatment on the patient's condition.

The physical testing procedures which specifically indicate joint, nerve or muscle tissues, as a source of the patient's symptoms, are summarized in Table 3.10. The strongest evidence that a joint is the source of the patient's symptoms is that active and passive physiological movements, passive accessory movements and joint palpation all reproduce the patient's symptoms, and that following a treatment dose, reassessment identifies an improvement in the patient's signs and symptoms. Weaker evidence includes an alteration in range, resistance or quality of physiological and/or accessory movements and tenderness over the joint, with no alteration in signs and symptoms after treatment. One or more of these findings may indicate a dysfunction of a joint which may or may not be contributing to the patient's condition.

The strongest evidence that a muscle is the source of a patient's symptoms is if active movements, an isometric contraction, passive lengthening and palpation of a muscle all reproduce the patient's symptoms, and that following a treatment dose, reassessment identifies an improvement in the patient's signs and symptoms. Further evidence of muscle dysfunction may be suggested by reduced strength or poor quality during the active physiological movement and the isometric contraction, reduced range, and/or increased/decreased resistance, during the passive lengthening of the muscle, and tenderness on palpation, with no alteration in signs and symptoms after treatment. One or more of these findings may indicate a dysfunction of a muscle which may or may not be contributing to the patient's condition.

The strongest evidence that a nerve is the source of the patient's symptoms is when active and/or passive physiological movements reproduce the patient's symptoms, which are then increased or decreased with an additional sensitizing movement, at a distance from the patient's symptoms. In addition, there is reproduction of the patient's symptoms on palpation of the nerve and neurodynamic testing, sufficient to be considered a treatment dose, results in an improvement in the above signs and symptoms. Further evidence of nerve dysfunction may be suggested by reduced range (compared to the asymptomatic side) and/or increased resistance to the various arm movements, and tenderness on nerve palpation.

On completion of the physical examination the clinician:

- Warns the patient of possible exacerbation up to 24–48 hours following the examination.
- Requests the patient to report details on the behaviour of the symptoms following examination at the next attendance.
- Explains the findings of the physical examination and how these findings relate to the subjective assessment. Any misconceptions patients may have regarding their illness or injury should be addressed.
- Evaluates the findings, formulates a clinical diagnosis and writes up a problem list. Clinicians may find the management planning forms shown in Figures 3.53 and 3.54 helpful in guiding them through what is often a complex clinical reasoning process.
- Determines the objectives of treatment.
- Devises an initial treatment plan.

In this way, the clinician will have developed the following hypotheses categories (adapted from Jones & Rivett 2004):

- Function: abilities and restrictions.
- Patients' perspectives on their experience.
- Source of symptoms. This includes the structure or tissue that is thought to be producing the patients' symptoms, the nature of the structure or tissues in relation to the healing process, and the pain mechanisms.
- Contributing factors to the development and maintenance of the problem. There may be environmental, psychosocial, behavioural, physical or heredity factors.
- Precautions/contraindications to treatment and management. This includes the severity and irritability of the patient's symptoms and the nature of the patient's condition.
- Management strategy and treatment plan.

- Prognosis – this can be affected by factors such as the stage and extent of the injury as well as the patient's expectation, personality and lifestyle.

References

Bullock J E, Jull G A, Bullock M I 1987 The relationship of low back pain to postural changes during pregnancy. Australian Journal of Physiotherapy 33(1): 10–17

Clinical Standards Advisory Report 1994 Report of a CSAG committee on back pain. HMSO, London

Edwards B C 1999 Manual of combined movements: their use in the examination and treatment of mechanical vertebral column disorders, 2nd edn. Butterworth-Heinemann, Oxford

Fortin J D, Aprill C N, Ponthieux B, Pier J 1994 Sacroiliac joint: pain referral maps upon applying a new injection technique. Part II: Clinical evaluation. Spine 19(13): 1483–1489

Greenman P E 1996 Principles of manual medicine, 2nd edn. Williams & Wilkins, Baltimore, MD

Grieve G P 1981 Common vertebral joint problems. Churchill Livingstone, Edinburgh

Grieve G P 1991 Mobilisation of the spine, 5th edn. Churchill Livingstone, Edinburgh

Grieve G P 1994 Counterfeit clinical presentations. Manipulative Physiotherapist 26: 17–19

Hagen R 1974 Pelvic girdle relaxation from an orthopaedic point of view. Acta Orthopaedica Scandinavica 45: 550–563

Janda V 1994 Muscles and motor control in cervicogenic disorders: assessment and management. In: Grant R (ed) Physical therapy of the cervical and thoracic spine, 2nd edn. Churchill Livingstone, New York, ch 10, p 195

Janda V 2002 Muscles and motor control in cervicogenic disorders. In: Grant R (ed) Physical therapy of the cervical and thoracic spine, 3rd edn. Churchill Livingstone, New York, ch 10, p 182

Jones M A, Rivett D A 2004 Clinical reasoning for manual therapists. Butterworth-Heinemann, Edinburgh

Laslett M, Williams M 1994 The reliability of selected pain provocation tests for sacroiliac joint pathology. Spine 19(11): 1243–1249

Lee D 1999 The pelvic girdle. An approach to the examination and treatment of the lumbo-pelvic-hip region, 2nd edn. Churchill Livingstone, Edinburgh

Magee D J 1997 Orthopedic physical assessment, 3rd edn. W B Saunders, Philadelphia

Maitland G D, Hengeveld E, Banks K, English K 2001 Maitland's vertebral manipulation, 6th edn. Butterworth-Heinemann, Oxford

Moore K, Dumas G A, Reid J G 1990 Postural changes associated with pregnancy and their relationship with low-back pain. Clinical Biomechanics 5(3): 169–174

Ostgaard H C, Andersson G B J, Schultz A B, Miller J A A 1993 Influence of some biomechanical factors in low-back pain in pregnancy. Spine 18(1): 61–65

Ostgaard H C, Zetherstrom G, Roos-Hansson E, Svanberg B 1994 Reduction of back and posterior pelvic pain in pregnancy. Spine 19(8): 894–900

Porterfield J A, DeRosa C 1998 Mechanical low back pain, perspectives in functional anatomy, 2nd edn. W B Saunders, Philadelphia

Sahrmann S A 2002 Diagnosis and treatment of movement impairment syndromes. Mosby, St Louis

Solomon L, Warwick D, Nayagam S 2001 Apley's system of orthopaedics and fractures, 8th edn. Arnold, London

Waddell G 2004 The back pain revolution, 2nd edn. Churchill Livingstone, Edinburgh

Chapter **13**

Examination of the hip region

POSSIBLE CAUSES OF PAIN AND/OR LIMITATION OF MOVEMENT

- Trauma:
    - Fracture of the neck or shaft of the femur
    - Dislocation
    - Contusion
    - Ligamentous sprain
    - Muscular strain
- Degenerative conditions: osteoarthrosis
- Inflammatory disorders: rheumatoid arthritis, acute pyogenic arthritis
- Childhood disorders:
    - Congenital dislocation of the hips (CDH)
    - Perthes' disease
    - Tuberculosis
- Adolescent disorders: slipped femoral epiphysis
- Ankylosing spondylitis
- Neoplasm: primary or secondary bone tumour
- Bursitis: subtrochanteric, ischiogluteal and iliopsoas
- Hypermobility
- Referral of symptoms from the lumbar spine, sacroiliac joint or pelvic organs.

Further details of the questions asked during the subjective examination and the tests carried out in the physical examination can be found in Chapters 2 and 3 respectively.

The order of the subjective questioning and the physical tests described below can be altered as appropriate for the patient being examined.

SUBJECTIVE EXAMINATION

Body chart

The following information concerning the type and area of current symptoms can be recorded on a body chart (see Fig. 2.3).

Area of current symptoms

Be exact when mapping out the area of the symptoms. Lesions of the hip joint commonly refer symptoms into the groin, anterior thigh and knee areas. Ascertain which is the worst symptom and record where the patient feels the symptoms are coming from.

Areas relevant to the region being examined

All other relevant areas are checked for symptoms; it is important to ask about pain or even stiffness, as this may be relevant to the patient's main symptom. Mark unaffected areas with ticks (✓) on the body chart. Check for symptoms in the lumbar spine, sacroiliac joint, knee joint and ankle joint.

Quality of pain

Establish the quality of the pain.

Intensity of pain

The intensity of pain can be measured using, for example, a visual analogue scale (VAS) as shown in Figure 2.8.

Depth of pain

Establish the depth of the pain. Does the patient feel it is on the surface or deep inside?

Abnormal sensation

Check for any altered sensation, such as paraesthesia or numbness, over the hip and other relevant areas.

Constant or intermittent symptoms

Ascertain the frequency of the symptoms, whether they are constant or intermittent. If symptoms are constant, check whether there is variation in the intensity of the symptoms, as constant unremitting pain may be indicative of neoplastic disease.

Relationship of symptoms

Determine the relationship between the symptomatic areas – do they come together or separately? For example, the patient could have thigh pain without back pain, or they may always be present together.

Behaviour of symptoms

Aggravating factors

For each symptomatic area, discover what movements and/or positions aggravate the patient's symptoms, i.e. what brings them on (or makes them worse), are they able to maintain this position or movement (severity), what happens to other symptom(s) when this symptom is produced (or is made worse), and how long does it take for symptoms to ease once the position or movement is stopped (irritability). These questions help to confirm the relationship of the symptoms one to another.

The clinician also asks the patient about theoretically known aggravating factors for structures that could be a source of the symptoms. Common aggravating factors for the hip are squatting, walking, stairs and side lying with the symptomatic side uppermost, which causes the hip to fall into adduction. Aggravating factors for other regions, which may need to be queried if they are suspected to be a source of the symptoms, are shown in Table 2.3.

The clinician ascertains how the symptoms affect function, such as: static and active postures, e.g. sitting, standing, lying, bending, walking, running, walking on uneven ground and up and down stairs, driving, work, sport and social activities. Note details of training regimen for any sports activities. The clinician finds out if the patient is left- or right-handed as there may be increased stress on the dominant side.

Detailed information on each of the above activities is useful in order to help determine the structure(s) at fault and identify functional restrictions. This information can be used to determine the aims of treatment and any advice that may be required. The most notable functional restrictions are highlighted with asterisks (*), explored in the physical examination, and reassessed at subsequent treatment sessions to evaluate treatment intervention.

Easing factors

For each symptomatic area, the clinician asks what movements and/or positions ease the patient's symptom, how long it takes to ease them and what happens to other symptom(s) when this symptom is relieved. These questions help to confirm the relationship between the symptoms.

The clinician asks the patient about theoretically known easing factors for structures that could be a source of the symptoms. For example, symptoms from the hip joint may be relieved by non-weight-bearing positions, whereas symptoms from the sacroiliac joint may be relieved by applying a wide belt around the pelvis. The clinician can then analyse the position or movement that eases the symptoms to help determine the structure at fault.

Twenty-four-hour behaviour of symptoms

The clinician determines the 24-hour behaviour of symptoms by asking questions about night, morning and evening symptoms.

Night symptoms. The following questions may be asked:

- Do you have any difficulty getting to sleep?
- What position is most comfortable/uncomfortable?
- What is your normal sleeping position?
- What is your present sleeping position?
- Are you able to lie on either side?
- Do your symptom(s) wake you at night? If so,
  - Which symptom(s)?
  - How many times in the past week?
  - How many times in a night?
  - How long does it take to get back to sleep?

- Is the mattress firm or soft?
- Has the mattress been changed recently?

Morning and evening symptoms. The clinician determines the pattern of the symptoms first thing in the morning, through the day and at the end of the day. Stiffness in the morning for the first few minutes might suggest arthrosis; stiffness and pain for a few hours are suggestive of an inflammatory process such as rheumatoid arthritis or ankylosing spondylitis.

Stage of the condition

In order to determine the stage of the condition, the clinician asks whether the symptoms are getting better, getting worse or remaining unchanged.

Special questions

Special questions must always be asked, as they may identify certain precautions or contraindications to the physical examination and/or treatment (Table 2.4). As mentioned in Chapter 2, the clinician must differentiate between conditions that are suitable for conservative management and systemic, neoplastic and other non-neuromusculoskeletal conditions, which require referral to a medical practitioner.

The following information is routinely obtained from patients.

General health. The clinician ascertains the state of the patient's general health and finds out if the patient suffers from any malaise, fatigue, fever, nausea or vomiting, stress, anxiety or depression. Check specifically whether the patient has had pelvic, lower abdominal or back surgery, or urogenital problems. Find out if a female patient is pregnant and whether an intrauterine device has been fitted, which may contraindicate the use of certain treatment modalities.

Weight loss. Has the patient noticed any recent unexplained weight loss?

Rheumatoid arthritis. Has the patient (or a member of his/her family) been diagnosed as having rheumatoid arthritis?

Drug therapy. What drugs are being taken by the patient? Has the patient ever been prescribed long-term (6 months or more) medication/ steroids? Has the patient been taking anticoagulants recently?

X-ray and medical imaging. Has the patient been X-rayed or had any other medical tests? Routine spinal X-rays are no longer considered necessary prior to conservative treatment as they only identify the normal age-related degenerative changes, which do not necessarily correlate with the patient's symptoms (Clinical Standards Advisory Report 1994). The medical tests may include blood tests, magnetic resonance imaging, myelography, discography or a bone scan.

Neurological symptoms. Has the patient experienced symptoms of spinal cord compression (i.e. compression of the spinal cord to L1 level), which are bilateral tingling in hands or feet and/or disturbance of gait?

Has the patient experienced symptoms of cauda equina compression (i.e. compression below L1), which are saddle anaesthesia/paraesthesia and bladder and/or bowel sphincter disturbance (loss of control, retention, hesitancy, urgency or a sense of incomplete evacuation) (Grieve 1991)? These symptoms may be due to interference of S3 and S4 (Grieve 1981). Prompt surgical attention is required to prevent permanent sphincter paralysis.

History of the present condition (HPC)

For each symptomatic area, the clinician needs to know how long the symptom has been present, whether there was a sudden or slow onset and whether there was a known cause that provoked the onset of the symptom. If the onset was slow, the clinician finds out if there has been any change in the patient's lifestyle, e.g. a new job or hobby or a change in sporting activity. To confirm the relationship between the symptoms, the clinician asks what happened to other symptoms when each symptom began.

Past medical history (PMH)

The following information is obtained from the patient and/or the medical notes:

- The details of any relevant medical history.
- The history of any previous attacks: how many episodes, when were they, what was the cause, what was the duration of each episode and did the patient fully recover between episodes? If there have been no previous attacks, has the patient had any episodes of stiffness in the lumbar spine, hip, knee, ankle, foot or any other relevant region? Check for a history of trauma or recurrent minor trauma.
- Ascertain the results of any past treatment for the same or similar problem. Past treatment records may be obtained for further information.

Social and family history (SH, FH)

Social and family history that is relevant to the onset and progression of the patient's problem is recorded. This includes the patient's perspectives, experience and expectations, their age, employment, home situation, and details of any leisure activities. Factors from this information may indicate direct and/or indirect mechanical influences on the hip. In order to treat the patient appropriately, it is important it is managed within the context of the patient's social and work environment.

The clinician may ask the following types of questions to elucidate psychosocial factors:

- Have you had time off work in the past with your pain?
- What do you understand to be the cause of your pain?
- What are you expecting will help you?
- How is your employer/co-workers/family responding to your pain?
- What are you doing to cope with your pain?
- Do you think you will return to work? When?

While these questions are described in relation to psychosocial risk factors for poor outcomes for patients with low back pain (Waddell 2004), they may be relevant to other patients.

Plan of the physical examination

When all this information has been collected, the subjective examination is complete. It is useful at this stage to highlight with asterisks (*), for ease of reference, important findings and particularly one or more functional restrictions. These can then be re-examined at subsequent treatment sessions to evaluate treatment intervention.

In order to plan the physical examination, the following hypotheses should be developed from the subjective examination:

- The regions and structures that need to be examined as a possible cause of the symptoms, e.g. lumbar spine, sacroiliac joint, pubic symphysis, hip, knee, muscles and nerves. Often it is not possible to examine fully at the first attendance and so examination of the structures must be prioritized over subsequent treatment sessions.
- Other factors that need to be examined, e.g. working and everyday postures, leg length, etc.
- In what way should the physical tests be carried out? Will it be easy or hard to reproduce each symptom? Will it be necessary to use combined movements, repetitive movements, etc. to reproduce the patient's symptoms? Are symptom(s) severe and/or irritable? If symptoms are severe, physical tests may be carried out to just before the onset of symptom production or just to the onset of symptom production; no overpressures will be carried out, as the patient would be unable to tolerate this. If symptoms are irritable, physical tests may be examined to just before symptom production or just to the onset of provocation with less physical tests being examined to allow for rest period between tests.
- Are there any precautions and/or contraindications to elements of the physical examination that need to be explored further, such neurological involvement, recent fracture, trauma, steroid therapy or rheumatoid arthritis; there may also be certain contraindications to further examination and treatment, e.g. symptoms of spinal cord or cauda equina compression.

A physical planning form can be useful for clinicians to help guide them through the clinical reasoning process (see Fig. 2.10 and Appendix 2.1).

PHYSICAL EXAMINATION

The information from the subjective examination helps the clinician to plan an appropriate physical examination. The severity, irritability and nature of

the condition are the major factors that will influence the choice and priority of physical testing procedures. The first and over-arching question the clinician might ask is: 'is this patient's condition suitable for me to manage as a therapist?' For example, a patient presenting with cauda equina compression symptoms may only need neurological integrity testing, prior to an urgent medical referral. The nature of the patient's condition has had a major impact on the physical examination. The second question the clinician might ask is: 'does this patient have a neuromusculoskeletal dysfunction that I may be able to help?' To answer that, the clinician needs to carry out a full physical examination; however, this may not be possible if the symptoms are severe and/or irritable. If the patient's symptoms are severe and/or irritable, the clinician aims to explore movements as much as possible, within a symptom-free range. If the patient has constant and severe and/or irritable symptoms, then the clinician aims to find physical tests that ease the symptoms. If the patient's symptoms are non-severe and non-irritable, then the clinician aims to find physical tests that reproduce each of the patient's symptoms.

Each significant physical test that either provokes or eases the patient's symptoms is highlighted in the patient's notes by an asterisk (*) for easy reference. The highlighted tests are often referred to as 'asterisks' or 'markers'.

The order and detail of the physical tests described below need to be appropriate to the patient being examined; some tests will be irrelevant, some tests will be carried out briefly, while it will be necessary to investigate others fully. It is important that readers understand that the techniques shown in this chapter are some of many; the choice depends mainly on the relative size of the clinician and patient, as well as the clinician's preference. For this reason, novice clinicians may initially want to copy what is shown, but then quickly adapt to what is best for them.

Observation

Informal observation

The clinician needs to observe the patient in dynamic and static situations; the quality of lower limb and general movement is noted, as are the postural characteristics and facial expression. Informal observation will have begun from the moment the clinician begins the subjective examination and will continue to the end of the physical examination.

Formal observation

Observation of posture. The clinician examines the patient's spinal and lower limb posture from anterior, lateral and posterior views in standing. Specific observation of the pelvis involves noting its position in the sagittal, coronal and horizontal planes: in the sagittal plane, there may be excessive anterior or posterior pelvic tilt; in the coronal plane there may be a lateral pelvic tilt; and in the horizontal plane there may be rotation of the pelvis. These abnormalities will be identified by observing the relative position of the iliac crest, the anterior and posterior iliac spines (ASIS and PSIS), skin creases (particularly the gluteal creases), and the position of the pelvis relative to the lumbar spine and lower limbs. In addition, the clinician notes whether there is even weight-bearing through the left and right leg. The clinician passively corrects any asymmetry to determine its relevance to the patient's problem.

Observation of muscle form. The clinician observes the muscle bulk and muscle tone of the patient, comparing left and right sides. It must be remembered that the level and frequency of physical activity as well as the dominant side may well produce differences in muscle bulk between sides. Some muscles are thought to shorten under stress, while other muscles weaken, producing muscle imbalance (see Table 3.2). Patterns of muscle imbalance are thought to produce the postures mentioned above.

Observation of soft tissues. The clinician observes the quality and colour of the patient's skin and any area of swelling or presence of scarring, and takes cues for further examination.

Observation of balance. Balance is provided by vestibular, visual and proprioceptive information. This rather crude and non-specific test is conducted by asking the patient to stand on one leg with the eyes open and then closed. If the patient's balance is as poor with the eyes open as with the eyes closed, this suggests a vestibular or proprioceptive dysfunction (rather than a visual dysfunction). The test is carried out on the affected and unaffected sides; if there is greater difficulty maintaining balance on the affected side, this may indicate some proprioceptive dysfunction.

Observation of gait. Analyse gait (including walking backwards) on even/uneven ground, slopes, stairs, running, etc. Note the stride length and weight-bearing ability. Inspect the feet, shoes and any walking aids. The typical gait patterns that might be expected in patients with hip pain are the gluteus maximus gait, the Trendelenburg gait and the short leg gait (see Ch. 3 for further details).

Observation of the patient's attitudes and feelings. The age, gender and ethnicity of patients and their cultural, occupational and social backgrounds will all affect their attitudes and feelings towards themselves, their condition and the clinician. The clinician needs to be aware of and sensitive to these attitudes, and to empathize and communicate appropriately so as to develop a rapport with the patient and thereby enhance the patient's compliance with the treatment.

Active physiological movements

For active physiological movements, the clinician notes the following:

- Quality of movement
- Range of movement
- Behaviour of pain through the range of movement
- Resistance through the range of movement and at the end of the range of movement
- Provocation of any muscle spasm.

A movement diagram can be used to depict this information. The active movements with overpressure listed below (Fig. 13.1) are tested with the patient lying supine. Movements are carried out on the left and right sides. The clinician establishes the patient's symptoms at rest, prior to each movement, and passively corrects any movement deviation to determine its relevance to the patient's symptoms.

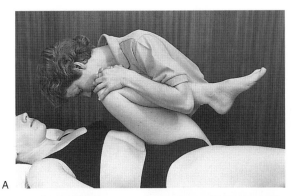

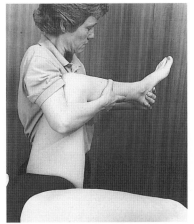

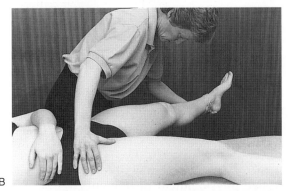

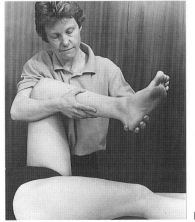

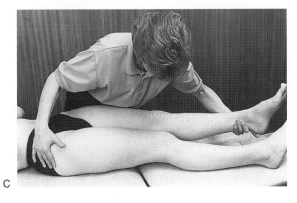

Figure 13.1   Overpressures to the hip joint. **A** Flexion. Both hands rest over the knee and apply overpressure to hip flexion. **B** Abduction. The right hand stabilizes the pelvis while the left hand takes the leg into abduction. **C** Adduction. The right hand stabilizes the pelvis while the left hand takes the leg into adduction. **D** Medial rotation. The clinician's trunk and right hand support the leg. The left hand and trunk then move to rotate the hip medially. **E** Lateral rotation. The clinician's trunk and right hand support the leg. The left hand and trunk then move to rotate the hip laterally. Alternatively, rotation can be examined in prone so that the hip is positioned in extension.

Active physiological movements of the hip with possible modifications are given in Table 13.1. Numerous differentiation tests (Maitland 1991) can be performed; the choice depends on the patient's signs and symptoms. For example, when trunk rotation with the patient standing on one leg (causing rotation in the lumbar spine and hip joint) reproduces the patient's buttock pain, differentiation between the lumbar spine and hip joint may be required. The clinician can increase and decrease the lumbar spine rotation and the pelvic rotation in turn, to find out what effect each movement has on the buttock pain. If the pain is coming from the hip then the lumbar spine

Table 13.1 Active physiological movements with possible modifications

Active physiological movements	Modifications
Hip movements	Repeated
Flexion	Speed altered
Extension	Combined, e.g.
Abduction	– flexion with rotation
Adduction	– rotation with flexion
Medial rotation	Compression or distraction, e.g.
Lateral rotation	– through greater tuberosity
?Lumbar spine	with flexion
?Sacroiliac joint	Sustained
?Knee	Injuring movement
?Ankle and foot	Differentiation tests
	Functional ability

Table 13.2 Joint clearing tests

Joint	Physiological movement	Accessory movement
Lumbar spine	Flexion and extension quadrants	All movements
Sacroiliac joint	Anterior and posterior gapping	
Knee joint	All movements and squat	
Patellofemoral joint	Medial/lateral glide and cephalad/caudad glide	
Ankle joint	Plantarflexion/ dorsiflexion and inversion/eversion	

movements will have no effect on the pain, but pelvic movements will alter the pain; conversely, if the pain is coming from the lumbar spine then lumbar spine movements will affect the pain but pelvic movement will have no effect.

It may be necessary to examine other regions to determine their relevance to the patient's symptoms; they may be the source of the symptoms, or they may be contributing to the symptoms. The regions most likely are the lumbar spine, sacroiliac joint, knee, ankle and foot. The joints within these regions can be tested fully (see relevant chapter) or partially with the use of clearing tests (Table 13.2).

Some functional ability has already been tested by the general observation of the patient during the subjective and physical examination, e.g. the postures adopted during the subjective examination and the ease or difficulty of undressing and changing position prior to the examination. Any further functional testing can be carried out at this point in the examination and may include lifting, sitting postures, dressing, etc. Clues for appropriate tests can be obtained from the subjective examination findings, particularly aggravating factors. There are a variety of functional scales that can be used for the hip; these are documented by Magee (1997).

Capsular pattern. The capsular pattern for the hip joint (Cyriax 1982) is gross limitation of

flexion, abduction and medial rotation, slight limitation of extension and no limitation of lateral rotation.

Passive physiological movements

All the active movements described above can be examined passively with the patient usually in supine, comparing left and right sides. Comparison of the response of symptoms to the active and passive movements can help to determine whether the structure at fault is non-contractile (articular) or contractile (extra-articular) (Cyriax 1982). If the lesion is non-contractile, such as ligament, then active and passive movements will be painful and/or restricted in the same direction. If the lesion is in a contractile tissue (i.e. muscle) then active and passive movements are painful and/or restricted in opposite directions.

In addition, the following tests can be carried out:

- Flexion/adduction (or quadrant) test (Maitland 1991)
- Faber's test.

Flexion/adduction (or quadrant) test (Maitland 1991)

The patient lies supine with one knee flexed. The clinician applies an adduction force to the hip and

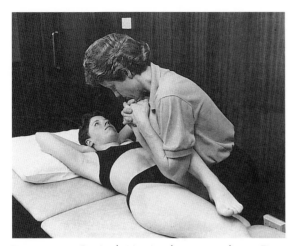

Figure 13.2 Flexion/adduction (or quadrant) test. The patient's thigh is fully supported by the clinician's arms and trunk. The clinician links the fingers of the hands over the top of the knee and rests the left forearm along the inner aspect of the patient's calf. This allows the clinician to add a longitudinal force and a medial rotation movement to the examination.

then moves the hip from just less than 90° flexion to full flexion (Fig. 13.2). The quality, range and pain behaviour of the movement are noted. Further information can be obtained by holding the hip in a position of hip flexion and adduction and adding medial rotation and/or a longitudinal cephalad.

Other regions may need to be examined to determine their relevance to the patient's symptoms; they may be the source of the symptoms, or they may be contributing to the symptoms. The regions most likely are the lumbar spine, sacroiliac joint, knee, ankle and foot. The joints within these regions can be tested fully (see relevant chapter) or partially with the use of clearing tests (Table 13.2).

Muscle tests

Muscle tests include those examining muscle strength, control and length and isometric muscle testing.

Muscle strength

The clinician tests the hip flexors, extensors, abductors, adductors, medial and lateral rotators and any other relevant muscle group. For details of these general tests readers are directed to Cole et al (1988), Hislop & Montgomery (1995) or Kendall et al (1993).

Greater detail may be required to test the strength of muscles, in particular those thought prone to become weak; that is, rectus abdominis, gluteus maximus, medius and minimus, vastus lateralis, medialis and intermedius, tibialis anterior and the peronei (Jull & Janda 1987, Sahrmann 2002). Testing the strength of these muscles is described in Chapter 3.

Muscle control

The relative strength of muscles is considered to be more important than the overall strength of a muscle group (Janda 1994, 2002, Sahrmann 2002, White & Sahrmann 1994). Relative strength is assessed indirectly by observing posture, as already mentioned, by the quality of active movement, noting any changes in muscle recruitment patterns, and by palpating muscle activity in various positions.

Muscle length

The clinician tests the length of muscles, in particular those thought prone to shorten (Janda 1994); that is: erector spinae, quadratus lumborum, piriformis, iliopsoas, rectus femoris, tensor fasciae latae, hamstrings, tibialis posterior, gastrocnemius and soleus (Jull & Janda 1987, Sahrmann 2002). Testing the length of these muscles is described in Chapter 3.

Isometric muscle testing

The clinician tests the hip joint flexors, extensors, abductors, adductors, medial and lateral rotators (and other relevant muscle groups) in resting position and, if indicated, in different parts of the physiological range. In addition the clinician observes the quality of the muscle contraction to hold this position (this can be done with the patient's eyes shut). The patient may, for example, be unable to prevent the joint from moving or may hold with excessive muscle activity; either of these circumstances would suggest a neuromuscular dysfunction.

Neurological tests

Neurological examination includes neurological integrity testing and neurodynamic tests.

Integrity of the nervous system

The integrity of the nervous system is tested if the clinician suspects that the symptoms are emanating from the spine or from a peripheral nerve.

Dermatomes/peripheral nerves. Light touch and pain sensation of the lower limb are tested using cotton wool and pinprick respectively, as described in Chapter 3. Knowledge of the cutaneous distribution of nerve roots (dermatomes) and peripheral nerves enables the clinician to distinguish the sensory loss due to a root lesion from that due to a peripheral nerve lesion. The cutaneous nerve distribution and dermatome areas are shown in Figure 3.21.

Myotomes/peripheral nerves. The following myotomes are tested (Fig. 3.27):

- L2: hip flexion
- L3: knee extension
- L4: foot dorsiflexion and inversion
- L5: extension of the big toe
- S1: eversion of the foot, contract buttock, knee flexion
- S2: knee flexion, toe standing
- S3–S4: muscles of pelvic floor, bladder and genital function.

A working knowledge of the muscular distribution of nerve roots (myotomes) and peripheral nerves enables the clinician to distinguish the motor loss due to a root lesion from that due to a peripheral nerve lesion. The peripheral nerve distributions are shown in Figure 3.25.

Reflex testing. The following deep tendon reflexes are tested (see Fig. 3.28):

- L3/4: knee jerk
- S1: ankle jerk.

Neurodynamic tests

The following neurodynamic tests may be carried out in order to ascertain the degree to which neural tissue is responsible for the production of the patient's symptom(s):

- Passive neck flexion (PNF)
- Straight leg raise (SLR)
- Passive knee bend (PKB)
- Slump.

These tests are described in detail in Chapter 3.

Miscellaneous tests

Vascular tests

If it is suspected that the circulation is compromised, the clinician palpates the pulses of the femoral, popliteal and dorsalis pedis arteries. The state of the vascular system can also be determined by the response of the symptoms to positions of dependency and elevation of the lower limbs.

Leg length

True leg length is measured from the ASIS to the medial or lateral malleolus. Apparent leg length is measured from the umbilicus to the medial or lateral malleolus. A difference in leg length of up to 1–1.3 cm is considered normal. If there is a leg length difference, test the length of individual bones; the tibia with knees bent and the femurs in standing. Ipsilateral posterior rotation of the ilium (on the sacrum) or contralateral anterior rotation of the ilium will result in a decrease in leg length (Magee 1997).

Supine to sit test

This is where one leg appears longer in supine and shorter in long sitting. This implicates anterior innominate rotation on the affected side (Wadsworth 1988).

Ortolani's sign tests

This tests for congenital dislocation of the hips in infants. The clinician applies pressure against the greater trochanter and moves the hip joints into abduction and lateral rotation while applying some gentle traction (Magee 1997). A hard clunk followed by an increased range of movement is a positive test indicating dislocating hips.

Palpation

The clinician palpates the hip region and any other relevant area. It is useful to record palpation findings on a body chart (see Fig. 2.3) and/or palpation chart (see Fig. 3.38).

The clinician notes the following:

- The temperature of the area.
- Localized increased skin moisture.
- The presence of oedema. This can be measured using a tape measure and comparing left and right sides.
- Mobility and feel of superficial tissues, e.g. ganglions, nodules, lymph nodes in the femoral triangle.
- The presence or elicitation of any muscle spasm.
- Tenderness of bone (the greater trochanter may be tender because of trochanteric bursitis and the ischial tuberosity because of ischiogluteal bursitis; inguinal area tenderness may be due to iliopsoas bursitis (Wadsworth 1988), ligaments, muscle (Baer's point, for tenderness/spasm of iliacus, lies a third of the way down a line from the umbilicus to the anterior superior iliac spine), tendon, tendon sheath, trigger points (shown in Fig. 3.39) and nerve. Palpable nerves in the lower limb are as follows:
  - The sciatic nerve can be palpated two-thirds of the way along an imaginary line between the greater trochanter and the ischial tuberosity with the patient in prone
  - The common peroneal nerve can be palpated medial to the tendon of biceps femoris and also around the head of the fibula
  - The tibial nerve can be palpated centrally over the posterior knee crease medial to the popliteal artery; it can also be felt behind the medial malleolus, which is more noticeable with the foot in dorsiflexion and eversion
  - The superficial peroneal nerve can be palpated on the dorsum of the foot along an imaginary line over the fourth metatarsal; it is more noticeable with the foot in plantar flexion and inversion
  - The deep peroneal nerve can be palpated between the first and second metatarsals, lateral to the extensor hallucis tendon
  - The sural nerve can be palpated on the lateral aspect of the foot behind the lateral malleolus, lateral to the tendocalcaneus.
- Increased or decreased prominence of bones.
- Pain provoked or reduced on palpation.

Accessory movements

It is useful to use the palpation chart and movement diagrams (or joint pictures) to record findings. These are explained in detail in Chapter 3.

The clinician notes the following:

- Quality of movement
- Range of movement
- Resistance through the range and at the end of the range of movement
- Behaviour of pain through the range
- Provocation of any muscle spasm.

Hip joint accessory movements (Fig. 13.3) are listed in Table 13.3. Following accessory movements to the hip region, the clinician reassesses all the physical asterisks (movements or tests that have been found to reproduce the patient's symptoms) in order to establish the effect of the accessory movements on the patient's signs and symptoms. Accessory movements can then be tested for other regions suspected to be a source of, or contributing to, the patient's symptoms. Again, following accessory movements to any one region, the clinician reassesses all the asterisks. Regions likely to be examined are the lumbar spine, sacroiliac joint, knee, foot and ankle (Table 13.3).

Mobilizations with movement (MWMs) (Mulligan 1999)

With the patient supine, the clinician stabilizes the pelvis and uses a seat belt to apply a lateral glide to the femur while the patient actively moves the

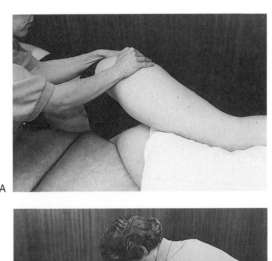

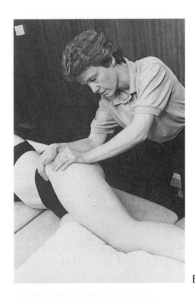

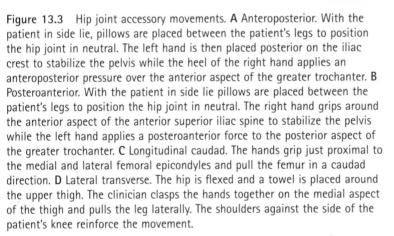

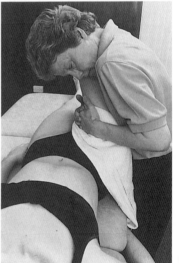

Figure 13.3 Hip joint accessory movements. **A** Anteroposterior. With the patient in side lie, pillows are placed between the patient's legs to position the hip joint in neutral. The left hand is then placed posterior on the iliac crest to stabilize the pelvis while the heel of the right hand applies an anteroposterior pressure over the anterior aspect of the greater trochanter. **B** Posteroanterior. With the patient in side lie pillows are placed between the patient's legs to position the hip joint in neutral. The right hand grips around the anterior aspect of the anterior superior iliac spine to stabilize the pelvis while the left hand applies a posteroanterior force to the posterior aspect of the greater trochanter. **C** Longitudinal caudad. The hands grip just proximal to the medial and lateral femoral epicondyles and pull the femur in a caudad direction. **D** Lateral transverse. The hip is flexed and a towel is placed around the upper thigh. The clinician clasps the hands together on the medial aspect of the thigh and pulls the leg laterally. The shoulders against the side of the patient's knee reinforce the movement.

hip into medial rotation or flexion (Fig. 13.4). An increase in the range of movement and no pain or reduced pain on active medial rotation or flexion of the hip joint in the lateral glide position are positive examination findings, indicating a mechanical joint problem.

COMPLETION OF THE EXAMINATION

Having carried out all of the above tests, the examination of the hip region is now complete. The subjective and physical examinations produce a large amount of information, which needs to be

Table 13.3   Accessory movements, choice of application and reassessment of the patient's asterisks

Accessory movements	Modifications	Identify any effect of accessory movements on patient's signs and symptoms
Hip joint (Fig. 13.3) ↕ anteroposterior ↕ posteroanterior ↔ Caud longitudinal caudad ⟶ Lat lateral transverse	Start position, e.g. – in flexion – in extension – in rotation (medial or lateral) – in flexion and internal rotation – in extension and lateral rotation Speed of force application Direction of the applied force Point of application of applied force	Reassess all asterisks
?Lumbar spine	As above	Reassess all asterisks
?Sacroiliac joint	As above	Reassess all asterisks
?Knee	As above	Reassess all asterisks
?Foot and ankle	As above	Reassess all asterisks

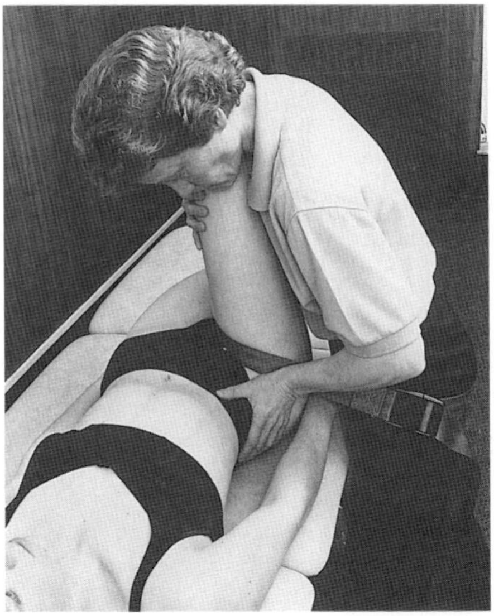

Figure 13.4 Mobilization with movement for hip flexion. The clinician stabilizes the pelvis with the left hand and uses a seat belt to apply a lateral glide to the femur while the patient actively flexes the hip.

recorded accurately and quickly. An outline examination chart may be useful for some clinicians and one is suggested in Figure 13.5. It is important, however, that the clinician does not examine in a rigid manner, simply following the suggested sequence outlined in the chart. Each patient pre-

sents differently and this needs to be reflected in the examination process. It is vital at this stage to highlight important findings from the examination with an asterisk (*). These findings must be reassessed at, and within, subsequent treatment sessions to evaluate the effects of treatment on the patient's condition.

The physical testing procedures which specifically indicate joint, nerve or muscle tissues, as a source of the patient's symptoms, are summarized in Table 3.10. The strongest evidence that a joint is the source of the patient's symptoms is that active and passive physiological movements, passive accessory movements and joint palpation all reproduce the patient's symptoms, and that following a treatment dose, reassessment identifies an improvement in the patient's signs and symptoms. Weaker evidence includes an alteration in range, resistance or quality of physiological and/or accessory movements and tenderness over the joint, with no alteration in signs and symptoms after treatment. One or more of these findings may indicate a dysfunction of a joint which may or may not be contributing to the patient's condition.

The strongest evidence that a muscle is the source of a patient's symptoms is if active movements, an isometric contraction, passive lengthening and palpation of a muscle all reproduce the patient's symptoms, and that following a treatment dose, reassessment identifies an

Body chart	Name
	Age
	Date
	24-hour behaviour
	Improving static worsening
	Special questions General health Weight loss RA Drugs Steroids Anticoagulants X-ray Cord symptoms Cauda equina symptoms VBI symptoms
Relationship of symptoms	
Aggravating factors and function	HPC
	PMH
Severe Irritable	
Easing factors	SH & FH (Patient's perspective, experience, expectations. Yellow, blue, black flags)

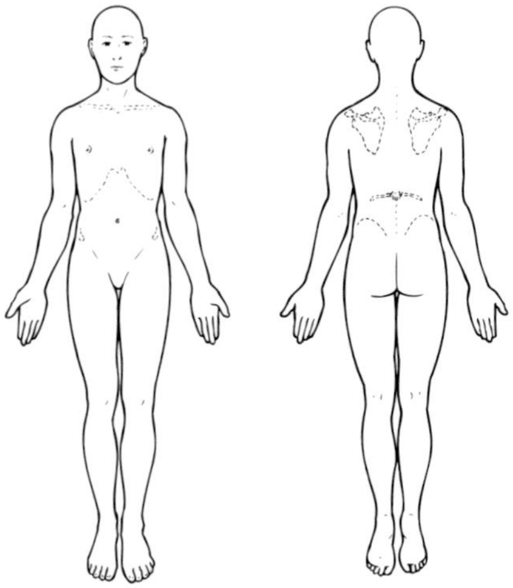

Figure 13.5   Hip examination chart.

Physical examination Observation	Isometric muscle testing
	Neurological integrity tests
Active and passive physiological movements of hip and other relevant regions	
	Neurodynamic tests
	Miscellaneous tests (pulses, leg length, supine to sit, Ortolani's, oedema)
Capsular pattern yes/no	Palpation
Muscle strength	
Muscle control	Accessory movements and reassessment of each relevant region
Muscle length	

Figure 13.5 *Continued*

improvement in the patient's signs and symptoms. Further evidence of muscle dysfunction may be suggested by reduced strength or poor quality during the active physiological movement and the isometric contraction, reduced range, and/or increased/decreased resistance, during the passive lengthening of the muscle, and tenderness on palpation, with no alteration in signs and symptoms after treatment. One or more of these findings may indicate a dysfunction of a muscle which may or may not be contributing to the patient's condition.

The strongest evidence that a nerve is the source of the patient's symptoms is when active and/or passive physiological movements reproduce the patient's symptoms, which are then increased or decreased with an additional sensitizing movement, at a distance from the patient's symptoms. In addition, there is reproduction of the patient's symptoms on palpation of the nerve and following neurodynamic testing, sufficient to be considered a treatment dose, results in an improvement in the above signs and symptoms. Further evidence of nerve dysfunction may be suggested by reduced range (compared to the asymptomatic side) and/or increased resistance to the various arm movements, and tenderness on nerve palpation.

On completion of the physical examination, the clinician:

- Warns the patient of possible exacerbation up to 24–48 hours following the examination.
- Requests the patient to report details on the behaviour of the symptoms following examination at the next attendance.
- Explains the findings of the physical examination and how these findings relate to the subjective assessment. Any misconceptions patients may have regarding their illness or injury need to be addressed.
- Evaluates the findings, formulates a clinical diagnosis and writes up a problem list. Clinicians may find the management planning forms shown in Figures 3.53 and 3.54 helpful in guiding them through what is often a complex clinical reasoning process.
- Determines the objectives of treatment.
- Devises an initial treatment plan.

In this way, the clinician will have developed the following hypothesis categories (adapted from Jones & Rivett 2004):

- Function: abilities and restrictions.
- Patients' perspectives on their experience.
- Source of symptoms. This includes the structure or tissue that is thought to be producing the patient's symptoms, the nature of the structure or tissues in relation to the healing process, and the pain mechanisms.
- Contributing factors to the development and maintenance of the problem. There may be environmental, psychosocial, behavioural, physical or heredity factors.
- Precautions/contraindications to treatment and management. This includes the severity and irritability of the patient's symptoms and the nature of the patient's condition.
- Management strategy and treatment plan.
- Prognosis – this can be affected by factors such as the stage and extent of the injury as well as the patient's expectation, personality and lifestyle.

References

Clinical Standards Advisory Report 1994 Report of a CSAG committee on back pain. HMSO, London

Cole J H, Furness A L, Twomey L T 1988 Muscles in action: an approach to manual muscle testing. Churchill Livingstone, Edinburgh

Cyriax J 1982 Textbook of orthopaedic medicine – diagnosis of soft tissue lesions, 8th edn. Baillière Tindall, London

Grieve G P 1981 Common vertebral joint problems. Churchill Livingstone, Edinburgh

Grieve G P 1991 Mobilisation of the spine, 5th edn. Churchill Livingstone, Edinburgh

Hislop H, Montgomery J 1995 Daniels and Worthingham's muscle testing, techniques of manual examination, 7th edn. W B Saunders, Philadelphia

Janda V 1994 Muscles and motor control in cervicogenic disorders: assessment and management. In: Grant R (ed) Physical therapy of the cervical and thoracic spine, 2nd edn. Churchill Livingstone, New York, ch 10, p 195

Janda V 2002 Muscles and motor control in cervicogenic disorders. In: Grant R (ed) Physical therapy of the cervical and thoracic spine, 3rd edn. Churchill Livingstone, New York, ch 10, p 182

Jones M A, Rivett D A 2004 Clinical reasoning for manual therapists. Butterworth-Heinemann, Edinburgh

Jull G A, Janda V 1987 Muscles and motor control in low back pain: assessment and management. In: Twomey L T, Taylor J R (eds) Physical therapy of the low back. Churchill Livingstone, New York, ch 10, p 253

Kendall F P, McCreary E K, Provance P G 1993 Muscles, testing and function, 4th edn. Williams & Wilkins, Baltimore, MD

Magee D J 1997 Orthopedic physical assessment, 3rd edn. W B Saunders, Philadelphia

Maitland G D 1991 Peripheral manipulation, 3rd edn. Butterworth-Heinemann, London

Mulligan B R 1999 Manual therapy 'NAGs', 'SNAGs', 'MWMs' etc., 4th edn. Plane View Services, New Zealand

Sahrmann S A 2002 Diagnosis and treatment of movement impairment syndromes. Mosby, St Louis

Waddell G 2004 The back pain revolution, 2nd edn. Churchill Livingstone, Edinburgh

Wadsworth C T 1988 Manual examination and treatment of the spine and extremities. Williams & Wilkins, Baltimore, MD

White S G, Sahrmann S A 1994 A movement system balance approach to musculoskeletal pain. In: Grant R (ed) Physical therapy of the cervical and thoracic spine, 2nd edn. Churchill Livingstone, Edinburgh, ch 16, p 339

Chapter 14

Examination of the knee region

CHAPTER CONTENTS

POSSIBLE CAUSES OF PAIN AND/OR LIMITATION OF MOVEMENT

This region includes the tibiofemoral, patello-femoral and superior tibiofibular joints with their surrounding soft tissues.

- Trauma:
  - Fracture of the lower end of the femur, upper end of the tibia or patella
  - Dislocation of the patella
  - Haemarthrosis
  - Traumatic synovitis
  - Ligamentous sprain
  - Muscular strain
  - Meniscal tear
  - Meniscal cyst
  - Damage to fat pads
  - Osgood–Schlatter disease
- Degenerative conditions:
  - Osteoarthrosis
  - Haemophilic arthritis
- Inflammatory conditions: rheumatoid arthritis
- Infection, e.g. acute septic arthritis (pyarthrosis), tuberculosis
- Chondromalacia patellae
- Osteochondritis desiccans
- Knee deformity: genu varum, genu valgum and genu recurvatum (hyperextension)
- Popliteal cyst
- Bursitis: semimembranosus, prepatellar and infrapatellar
- Loose bodies
- Plica syndrome
- Hypermobility

- Referral of symptoms from the lumbar spine, sacroiliac joint or hip joint.

Further details of the questions asked during the subjective examination and the tests carried out in the physical examination can be found in Chapters 2 and 3 respectively.

The order of the subjective questioning and the physical tests described below can be altered as appropriate for the patient being examined.

SUBJECTIVE EXAMINATION

Body chart

The following information concerning the type and area of the current symptoms can be recorded on a body chart (see Fig. 2.3).

Area of current symptoms

Be exact when mapping out the area of the symptoms. A lesion in the knee joint complex may refer symptoms proximally to the thigh or distally to the foot and ankle. Ascertain which is the worst symptom and record where the patient feels the symptoms are coming from.

Areas relevant to the region being examined

All other relevant areas are checked for symptoms; it is important to ask about pain or even stiffness, as this may be relevant to the patient's main symptom. Mark unaffected areas with ticks (✓) on the body chart. Check for symptoms in the lumbar spine, sacroiliac joint, hip, foot and ankle.

Quality of pain

Establish the quality of the pain. Symptoms may include swelling, weakness, crepitus, giving way, locking as well as pain.

Intensity of pain

The intensity of pain can be measured using, for example, a visual analogue scale (VAS) as shown in Figure 2.8.

Depth of pain

Establish the depth of the pain. Does the patient feel it is on the surface or deep inside? If appropriate, distinguish between pain felt underneath the patella and that felt in the tibiofemoral joint.

Abnormal sensation

Check for any altered sensation (such as paraesthesia or numbness) over the knee and other relevant areas.

Constant or intermittent symptoms

Ascertain the frequency of the symptoms, whether they are constant or intermittent. If symptoms are constant, check whether there is variation in the intensity of the symptoms, as constant unremitting pain may be indicative of neoplastic disease.

Relationship of symptoms

Determine the relationship between symptomatic areas – do they come together or separately? For example, the patient could have knee pain without back pain, or they may always be present together.

Behaviour of symptoms

Aggravating factors

For each symptomatic area, discover what movements and/or positions aggravate the patient's symptoms, i.e. what brings them on (or makes them worse), are they able to maintain this position or movement (severity), what happens to other symptom(s) when this symptom is produced (or is made worse), and how long does it take for symptoms to ease once the position or movement is stopped (irritability). These questions help to confirm the relationship between the symptoms.

The clinician also asks the patient about theoretically known aggravating factors for structures that could be a source of the symptoms. Common aggravating factors for the knee are walking, running, stairs, squatting and twisting on a flexed knee, sudden deceleration when running and various sporting activities. Patellofemoral pain is usually aggravated by stair climbing and prolonged sitting with the knee flexed, commonly referred to as the 'movie sign' (Jacobson & Flandry 1989). Aggravating factors for other regions, which may need to be queried if they are suspected to be a source of the symptoms, are shown in Table 2.3.

The clinician ascertains how the symptoms affect function, such as: static and active postures, e.g. sitting, standing, lying, bending, walking, running, walking on uneven ground and up and down stairs, driving, work, sport and social activities. Note details of training regimen for any sports activities. The clinician finds out if the patient is left- or right-handed as there may be increased stress on the dominant side.

Detailed information on each of the above activities is useful in order to help determine the structure(s) at fault and identify functional restrictions. This information can be used to determine the aims of treatment and any advice that may be required. The most notable functional restrictions are highlighted with asterisks (*), explored in the physical examination, and reassessed at subsequent treatment sessions to evaluate treatment intervention.

Easing factors

For each symptomatic area, the clinician asks what movements and/or positions ease the patient's symptoms, how long it takes to ease them and what happens to other symptoms when this symptom is relieved. These questions help to confirm the relationship between the symptoms.

The clinician asks the patient about theoretically known easing factors for structures that could be a source of the symptoms. For example, symptoms from the knee joint may be relieved by weight-relieving positions, whereas symptoms from the lumbar spine may be relieved by lying prone or in a crook lie. The clinician can then analyse the position or movement which eases the symptoms to help determine the structure at fault.

Twenty-four-hour behaviour of symptoms

The clinician determines the 24-hour behaviour of symptoms by asking questions about night,

morning and evening symptoms. It may give a clue as to the structure at fault; for example, patients with an injury to the medial meniscus often have trouble sleeping and lying with the symptomatic side uppermost as it compresses that side.

Night symptoms. The following questions may be asked:

- Do you have any difficulty getting to sleep?
- What position is most comfortable/uncomfortable?
- What is your normal sleeping position?
- What is your present sleeping position?
- Do your symptom(s) wake you at night? If so,
  - Which symptom(s)?
  - How many times in the past week?
  - How many times in a night?
  - How long does it take to get back to sleep?

Morning and evening symptoms. The clinician determines the pattern of the symptoms first thing in the morning, through the day and at the end of the day.

Stage of the condition

In order to determine the stage of the condition, the clinician asks whether the symptoms are getting better, getting worse or remaining unchanged.

Special questions

Special questions must always be asked, as they may identify certain precautions or contraindications to the physical examination and/or treatment (see Table 2.4). As mentioned in Chapter 2, the clinician must differentiate between conditions that are suitable for conservative treatment and systemic, neoplastic and other non-neuromusculoskeletal conditions, which require referral to a medical practitioner.

The following information is routinely obtained from patients.

General health. The clinician ascertains the state of the patient's general health and finds out if the patient suffers from any malaise, fatigue, fever, nausea or vomiting, stress, anxiety or depression.

Weight loss. Has the patient noticed any recent unexplained weight loss?

Rheumatoid arthritis. Has the patient (or a member of his/her family) been diagnosed as having rheumatoid arthritis?

Drug therapy. What drugs are being taken by the patient? Has the patient ever been prescribed long-term (6 months or more) medication/steroids? Has the patient been taking anticoagulants recently?

X-ray and medical imaging. Has the patient been X-rayed or had any other medical tests? The medical tests may include blood tests, arthroscopy, magnetic resonance imaging, myelography or a bone scan.

Neurological symptoms if a spinal lesion is suspected. Has the patient experienced symptoms of spinal cord compression (i.e. compression of the spinal cord to L1 level), which are bilateral tingling in hands or feet and/or disturbance of gait?

Has the patient experienced symptoms of cauda equina compression (i.e. compression below L1), which are saddle anaesthesia/paraesthesia and bladder and/or bowel sphincter disturbance (loss of control, retention, hesitancy, urgency or a sense of incomplete evacuation) (Grieve 1991)? These symptoms may be due to interference of S3 and S4 (Grieve 1981). Prompt surgical attention is required to prevent permanent sphincter paralysis.

History of the present condition (HPC)

For each symptomatic area the clinician needs to know how long the symptom has been present, whether there was a sudden or slow onset and whether there was a known cause that provoked the onset of the symptom. If the onset was slow, the clinician finds out if there has been any change in the patient's lifestyle, e.g. a new job or hobby or a change in sporting activity or training schedule. To confirm the relationship between the symptoms, the clinician asks what happened to other symptoms when each symptom began.

The mechanism of injury gives the clinician some important clues as to the injured structure in

Table 14.1 The possible diagnoses suspected from the mechanism of injury (McConnell, personal communication, 2000)

Mechanism of injury	Suspected diagnosis
Rotation of a fixed foot with a pop/crack with immediate swelling	Rupture of anterior cruciate ligament
Rotation of a fixed foot with a pop/crack with delayed swelling	Patellofemoral subluxation
Rapid knee extension and inferior patellar pain	Fat pad irritation
Eccentric loading of quadriceps and inferior patellar pain	Patellar tendinitis
Valgus stress	Medial collateral ligament sprain
Rotatory injury in younger patients with/without locking	Meniscal injury
Prolonged deep knee bend in older patients	Meniscal injury

the knee, particularly in the acute stage, when physical examination may be limited. An anterior cruciate ligament rupture may be suspected following an injury that involved rotation of the body on a fixed foot with a pop or crack sound, followed by immediate swelling of the knee (haemarthrosis); if the swelling appeared within the first 24 hours then acute patellofemoral subluxation (without osteochondral fracture) is the more likely diagnosis. The possible diagnoses suspected from the mechanism of injury are given in Table 14.1.

Past medical history (PMH)

The following information is obtained from the patient and/or the medical notes:

- The details of any relevant medical history.
- The history of any previous attacks: how many episodes, when were they, what was the cause, what was the duration of each episode and did the patient fully recover between episodes? If there have been no previous attacks, has the patient had any episodes of stiffness in the

lumbar spine, hip, knee, foot, ankle or any other relevant region? Check for a history of trauma or recurrent minor trauma.

- Ascertain the results of any past treatment for the same or similar problem. Past treatment records may be obtained for further information.

Social and family history (SH, FH)

Social and family history that is relevant to the onset and progression of the patient's problem is recorded. This includes the patient's perspectives, experience and expectations, their age, employment, home situation, and details of any leisure activities. Factors from this information may indicate direct and/or indirect mechanical influences on the knee. In order to treat the patient appropriately, it is important that the condition is managed within the context of the patient's social and work environment.

The clinician may ask the following types of questions to elucidate psychosocial factors:

- Have you had time off work in the past with your pain?
- What do you understand to be the cause of your pain?
- What are you expecting will help you?
- How is your employer/co-workers/family responding to your pain?
- What are you doing to cope with your pain?
- Do you think you will return to work? When?

While these questions are described in relation to psychosocial risk factors for poor outcomes for patients with low back pain (Waddell 2004), they may be relevant to other patients.

Plan of the physical examination

When all this information has been collected, the subjective examination is complete. It is useful at this stage to highlight with asterisks (*), for ease of reference, important findings and particularly one or more functional restrictions. These can then be re-examined at subsequent treatment sessions to evaluate treatment intervention.

In order to plan the physical examination, the following hypotheses should be developed from the subjective examination:

- The regions and structures that need to be examined as a possible cause of the symptoms, e.g. lumbar spine, sacroiliac joint, hip, knee, foot and ankle, muscles and nerves. Often it is not possible to examine fully at the first attendance and so examination of the structures must be prioritized over subsequent treatment sessions.
- Other factors that need to be examined, e.g. working and everyday postures, leg length.
- In what way should the physical tests be carried out? Will it be easy or hard to reproduce each symptom? Will it be necessary to use combined movements, repetitive movements, etc. to reproduce the patient's symptoms? Are symptom(s) severe and/or irritable? If symptoms are severe, physical tests may be carried out to just before the onset of symptom production or just to the onset of symptom production; no overpressures will be carried out, as the patient would be unable to tolerate this. If symptoms are irritable, physical tests may be examined to just before symptom production or just to the onset of provocation with less physical tests being examined to allow for rest period between tests.
- Are there any precautions and/or contraindications to elements of the physical examination that need to be explored further, such neurological involvement, recent fracture, trauma, steroid therapy or rheumatoid arthritis; there may also be certain contraindications to further examination and treatment, e.g. symptoms of spinal cord or cauda equina compression.

A physical planning form can be useful for clinicians to help guide them through the clinical reasoning process (see Fig. 2.10 and Appendix 2.1).

PHYSICAL EXAMINATION

The information from the subjective examination helps the clinician to plan an appropriate physical examination. The severity, irritability and nature of the condition are the major factors that will influence the choice and priority of physical testing procedures. The first and over-arching question the clinician might ask is: 'is this patient's condition suitable for me to manage as a therapist?' For example, a patient presenting with cauda equina compression symptoms may only need neurological integrity testing, prior to an urgent medical referral. The nature of the patient's condition has had a major impact on the physical examination. The second question the clinician might ask is: 'does this patient have a neuromusculoskeletal dysfunction that I may be able to help?' To answer that, the clinician needs to carry out a full physical examination; however, this may not be possible if the symptoms are severe and/or irritable. If the patient's symptoms are severe and/or irritable, the clinician aims to explore movements as much as possible, within a symptom-free range. If the patient has constant and severe and/or irritable symptoms, then the clinician aims to find physical tests that ease the symptoms. If the patient's symptoms are non-severe and non-irritable, then the clinician aims to find physical tests that reproduce each of the patient's symptoms.

Each significant physical test that either provokes or eases the patient's symptoms is highlighted in the patient's notes by an asterisk (*) for easy reference. The highlighted tests are often referred to as 'asterisks' or 'markers'.

The order and detail of the physical tests described below need to be appropriate to the patient being examined; some tests will be irrelevant, some tests will be carried out briefly, while it will be necessary to investigate others fully. It is important that readers understand that the techniques shown in this chapter are some of many; the choice depends mainly on the relative size of the clinician and patient, as well as the clinician's preference. For this reason, novice clinicians may initially want to copy what is shown, but then quickly adapt to what is best for them.

Observation

Informal observation

The clinician needs to observe the patient in dynamic and static situations; the quality of movement is noted, as are the postural characteristics and facial expression. Informal observation will have begun from the moment the clinician begins the subjective examination and will continue to the end of the physical examination.

Formal observation

This is particularly useful in helping to determine the presence of intrinsic predisposing factors.

Observation of posture. The clinician examines the patient's lower limb posture in standing and in sitting with the knee at 90°. Abnormalities include internal femoral rotation, enlarged tibial tubercle (seen in Osgood–Schlatter disease), genu varum/valgum/recurvatum, medial/lateral tibial torsion and excessive foot pronation. Genu valgum and genu varum are identified by measuring the distance between the ankles and the distance between the femoral medial epicondyles respectively. Normally, medial tibial torsion is associated with genu varum and lateral tibial torsion with genu valgum (Magee 1997).

Internal femoral rotation due to tight iliotibial band and poor functioning of the posterior gluteus medius muscle is a common finding with patients with patellofemoral pain and can cause squinting of the patella and an increased Q angle (see below). There may be abnormal positioning of the patella, such as a medial/lateral glide, a lateral tilt, an anteroposterior tilt, a medial/lateral rotation or any combination of these positions. An enlarged fat pad is usually associated with hyperextension of the knees and poor quadriceps control, particularly eccentric inner range (0–20° of flexion).

The clinician can palpate the talus medially and laterally; both aspects will normally be equally prominent in the mid position of the subtalar joint. If the medial aspect of the talus is more prominent this suggests that the subtalar joint is in pronation. The position of the calcaneus and talus can be examined: if the subtalar joint is pronated the calcaneus would be expected to be everted; if it is not, i.e. if it is straight or inverted, this would suggest a stiff subtalar joint. During gait the subtalar joint would pronate at mid-stance rather than at heel strike, as in the normal cycle.

Any abnormality will require further examination, as described in the section on palpation, below. In addition, the clinician notes whether there is even weight-bearing through the left and right legs. The clinician passively corrects any asymmetry to determine its relevance to the patient's problem.

It is worth remembering that pure postural dysfunction rarely influences one region of the body in isolation and it may be necessary to observe the patient more fully for a full postural examination.

The clinician examines dynamic postures such as gait, stair climbing, squatting, etc. Observation of gait may reveal, for example, excessive pelvic rotation (about a horizontal plane) associated with anterior pelvic tilt. This may be due to hyperextension of the knees and limited extension and external rotation of the hip.

Observation of muscle form. The clinician observes the muscle bulk and muscle tone of the patient, comparing left and right sides. It must be remembered that the level and frequency of physical activity as well as the dominant side may well produce differences in muscle bulk between sides. Some muscles are thought to shorten under stress, while other muscles weaken, producing muscle imbalance (see Table 3.2).

Observation of soft tissues. The clinician observes the quality and colour of the patient's skin, any area of swelling, joint effusion or presence of scarring, and takes cues for further examination.

Observation of balance. Balance is provided by vestibular, visual and proprioceptive information. This rather crude and non-specific test is conducted by asking the patient to stand on one leg with the eyes open and then closed. If the patient's balance is as poor with the eyes open as with the eyes closed, this suggests a vestibular or proprioceptive dysfunction (rather than a visual dysfunction). The test is carried out on the affected and unaffected side; if there is greater difficulty maintaining balance on the affected side, this may indicate some proprioceptive dysfunction.

Observation of gait. Analyse gait (including walking backwards) on even/uneven ground, slopes, stairs, running, etc. Note the stride length and weight-bearing ability. Inspect the feet, shoes and any walking aids.

Observation of the patient's attitudes and feelings. The age, gender and ethnicity of patients and their cultural, occupational and social backgrounds will all affect their attitudes and feelings towards themselves, their condition and the clinician. The clinician should be aware of and sensitive to these attitudes, and to empathize and communicate appropriately so as to develop a rapport with the patient and thereby enhance the patient's compliance with the treatment.

Joint integrity tests

For all of the tests below, a positive test is indicated by excessive movement relative to the unaffected side.

Abduction stress tests

With the patient supine, the clinician palpates the medial joint line of the knee and applies an abduction force to the lower leg. The clinician typically may examine this abduction movement with the knee in full extension and in 20–30° flexion (Fig 14.1); however, exploring this test with other angles of knee flexion, and with internal or external tibial rotation, may also be relevant and necessary for some patients. The clinician compares the left and right knee range of movement; excessive movement would be considered a positive test.

With the knee in full extension, the test is considered to stress the medial ligament, posterior oblique ligament, posteromedial capsule, anterior and posterior cruciate ligaments, medial quadriceps expansion and semimembranosus muscle; with knee flexion 20–30° the test is considered to stress the medial ligament, posterior oblique ligament and posterior cruciate ligament (Magee 1997).

Adduction stress tests

With the patient supine, the clinician palpates the lateral joint line and applies an adduction force to the lower leg (Fig. 14.2). The clinician may typically examine this adduction movement with the knee in full extension and in 20–30° flexion; however, exploring this test with other angles of

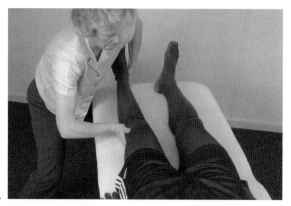
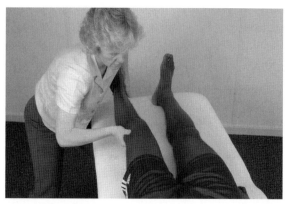

Figure 14.1 Abduction stress test with **A** the knee in extension and **B** in some flexion.

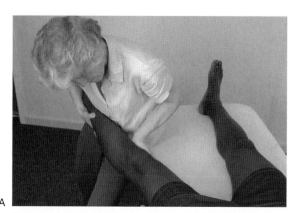
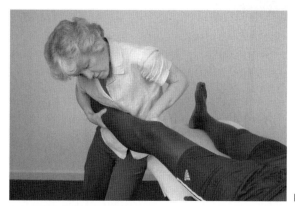

Figure 14.2 Adduction stress test with **A** the knee in extension and **B** in some flexion.

knee flexion, and with internal or external tibial rotation, may also be relevant and necessary for some patients. The clinician compares the left and right knee range of movement; excessive movement would be considered a positive test.

With the knee in extension, the test is considered to test the lateral ligament, posterolateral capsule, the arcuate–popliteus complex, anterior and posterior cruciate ligaments, and lateral gastrocnemius muscle; with the knee in 20–30° flexion, the test is considered to stress the lateral ligament, posterolateral capsule, arcuate–popliteus complex, iliotibial band and biceps femoris tendon (Magee 1997).

Anterior drawer tests

The anterior drawer test is typically carried out with the knee flexed at 0–30° (Lachman's test) and

at around 90°; however, exploring this test with other angles of knee flexion, and with internal or external tibial rotation, may be relevant and necessary for some patients. With the patient in supine and with the knee flexed (0–30°), the clinician stabilizes the femur and applies a posteroanterior force to the tibia (Fig. 14.3). With the knee flexed to 90°, the clinician applies a posteroanterior force to the tibia feeling the movement of the tibia anteriorly and any contraction of hamstring muscle group (Fig. 14.4). A positive test is indicated by a soft end-feel and excessive motion.

With the knee in 0–30°, the test is considered to stress the anterior cruciate ligament, posterior oblique ligament and the arcuate–popliteus complex; with the knee in 90° flexion, it is considered to stress the structures above, as well as the posteromedial and posterolateral joint capsules,

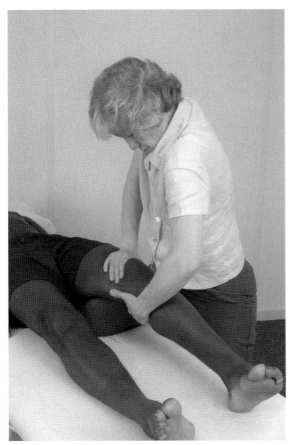

Figure 14.3   Lachman's test. The patient's knee rests over the clinican's thigh and is stabilized by the right hand. The left hand applies a posteroanterior force to the tibia.

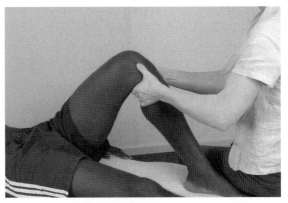

Figure 14.4   Anterior drawer test. With the knee around 90° flexion the clinician sits lightly on the patient's foot to stabilize the leg. The fingers grasp around the posterior aspect of the calf to apply the posteroanterior force, while the thumbs rest over the anterior joint line to feel the movement.

medial collateral ligament and the iliotibial band (Magee 1997).

Further variation of the anterior drawer test with the knee in 90° is with the addition of internal and external tibial rotation, known as the slocum test. With the addition of internal tibial rotation, excessive movement on the lateral aspect of the knee is thought to indicate anterolateral instability of the knee (Fig. 14.5), due to injury of one or more of the following structures: anterior cruciate ligament, posterolateral capsule, arcuate–popliteus complex, lateral ligament and iliotibial band (Magee 1997). With the addition of external tibial rotation, excessive movement on the medial aspect of the knee is thought to indicate anteromedial instability of the knee, due to injury of one or more of the following structures:

medial ligament, posterior oblique ligament, posteromedial capsule and anterior cruciate ligament (Magee 1997).

If anterolateral instability is suspected with the test above, this can be tested further, or alternatively tested by the lateral pivot shift test. The patient lies supine with the hip slightly flexed and medially rotated and with the knee flexed. In the first part of the test, the lower leg is medially rotated at the knee and the clinician moves the knee into extension while applying a posteroanterior force to the fibula. The tibia subluxes anteriorly when there is anterolateral instability. In the second part of the test, the clinician applies an abduction stress to the lower leg and passively moves the knee from extension to flexion while maintaining the medial rotation of the lower leg (Fig. 14.6). A positive test is indicated if at about 20–40° of knee flexion the tibia 'jogs' backward (reduction of the subluxation) and reproduces the patient's feeling of the knee 'giving way'. It is considered to test the anterior cruciate ligament, posterolateral capsule, arcuate–popliteus complex, lateral ligament and iliotibial band (Magee 1997).

Posterior drawer test

The posterior drawer test is typically carried out with the knee flexed to 90°; however, exploring

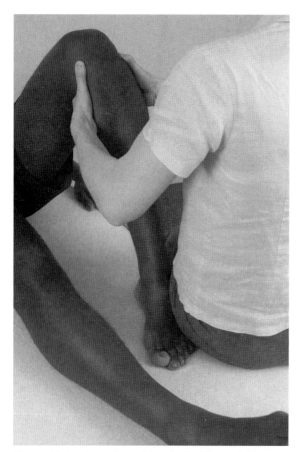

Figure 14.5 Anterolateral instability. The medially rotated lower leg is stabilized by the clinican sitting on the patient's foot. The hands grip around the posterior aspect of the tibia and the thumbs rest over the anterior joint space. A posteroanterior force is applied by both hands and the movement is palpated by the thumbs.

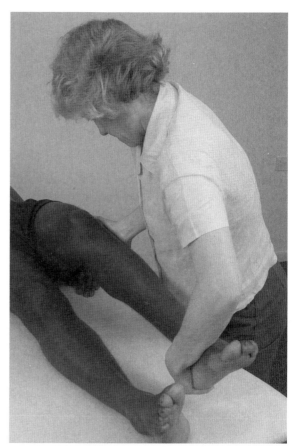

Figure 14.6 Lateral pivot shift. The clinician applies an abduction stress to the lower leg with the right hand and the left hand passively moves the knee from extension to flexion, while maintaining the medial rotation of the lower leg.

this test with other angles of knee flexion, and with internal or external tibial rotation, may be relevant and necessary for some patients. The clinician applies an anteroposterior force to the tibia (Fig. 14.7). A positive test is indicated by excessive motion due to injury of one or more of the following structures: posterior cruciate ligament, arcuate–popliteus complex, posterior oblique ligament and anterior cruciate ligament (Magee 1997).

Further variation of the posterior drawer test is with the addition of external tibial rotation (Hughston & Norwood 1980). Excessive movement on the lateral aspect of the tibia would indi-

cate posterolateral instability of the knee due to injury of one of more of the following structures: anterior and posterior cruciate ligaments, the arcuate–popliteus complex, the lateral ligament and the biceps femoris tendon, and posterolateral capsule.

Posterolateral instability of the knee can also be tested with the knee in extension, which may be more appropriate for some patients and may be named as the external rotational recurvatum test (Hughston & Norwood 1980). The patient lies supine and the clinician holds the heel and extends the knee from 30° flexion while palpating the posterolateral aspect of the knee (Fig. 14.8). Excessive hyperextension and external rotation of

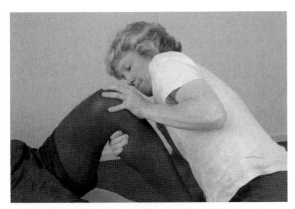

Figure 14.7   Posterior drawer test. The clinician sits lightly on the patient's foot to stabilize the leg. The right hand supports the calf posteriorly and the left hand applies an anteroposterior force to the tibia.

the tibia is considered to indicate posterolateral instability of the knee.

Meniscal tests

The medial meniscus is typically tested using a combination of knee flexion/extension with lateral rotation of the tibia. The clinician palpates the medial joint line and passively flexes and then laterally rotates the knee so that the posterior part of the medial meniscus is rotated with the tibia – a 'snap' of the joint may occur if the meniscus is torn. The knee is then moved from this fully flexed position to 90° flexion (to full extension for some patients), so the whole of the posterior part of the meniscus is tested (Fig. 14.9). A positive test occurs if the clinician feels a click, which may be heard, indicating a tear of the medial meniscus (McMurray 1942). Clinicians vary in performing this test; they may, for example, internally and externally rotate the tibia while moving the knee from full flexion to extension.

The lateral meniscus is typically tested using a combination of knee flexion/extension with medial rotation of the tibia. The clinician palpates the lateral joint line and passively flexes and then medially rotates the knee so that the posterior part of the lateral meniscus is rotated with the tibia – a 'snap' of the joint may occur if the meniscus is

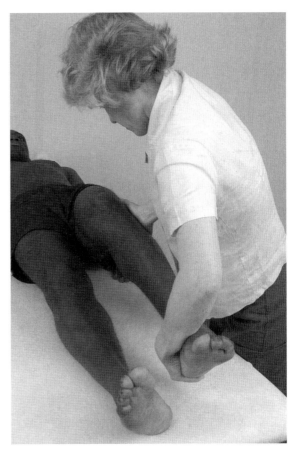

Figure 14.8   External rotational recurvatum test. The left hand holds the heel and extends the knee from 30° flexion while the right hand palpates the posterolateral aspect of the knee.

torn. The knee is then moved from this fully flexed position to 90° flexion (to full extension for some patients), so the whole of the posterior part of the meniscus is tested (Fig. 14.10). A positive test occurs if the clinician feels a click, which may be heard, indicating a tear of the lateral meniscus (McMurray 1942). Clinicians vary in performing this test; they may, for example, internally and externally rotate the tibia while moving the knee from full flexion to extension.

The menisci can also be tested with the patient in prone with the knee flexed to 90° (compression/ distraction test, Apley 1947). The clinician medially and laterally rotates the tibia with distraction

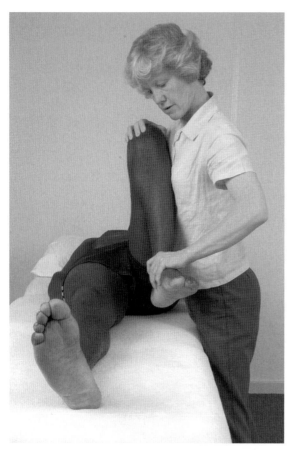

Figure 14.9 Medial meniscus. The right hand supports the knee and palpates the medial joint line. The left hand laterally rotates the lower leg and moves the knee from full flexion to extension.

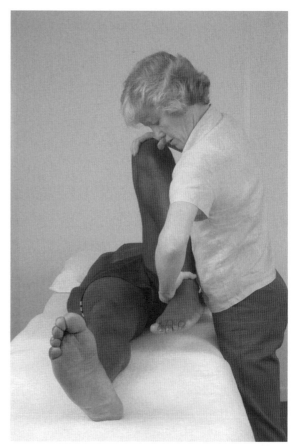

Figure 14.10 Lateral meniscus. The right hand supports the knee and palpates the lateral joint line. The left hand medially rotates the lower leg and moves the knee from full flexion to extension.

and then compression (Fig. 14.11). If symptoms are worse on compression, this suggests a meniscus injury; if symptoms are worse on distraction, this suggests a ligamentous injury (Apley 1947). Testing at other knee joint angles, apart from just at 90°, may be relevant and necessary for some patients.

Fairbank's apprehension test

This is considered to test for patellar subluxation or dislocation. It is typically carried out with the patient's knee in 30° of flexion; the clinician passively moves the patella laterally and a positive test is indicated by apprehension of the patient and/or excessive movement (Eifert-Mangine &

Bilbo 1995). It may be necessary and relevant for some patients to test the patella glide with the knee in other angles of knee flexion.

Active physiological movements

For active physiological movements, the clinician notes the following:

- Quality of movement
- Range of movement
- Behaviour of pain through the range of movement
- Resistance through the range of movement and at the end of the range of movement
- Provocation of any muscle spasm.

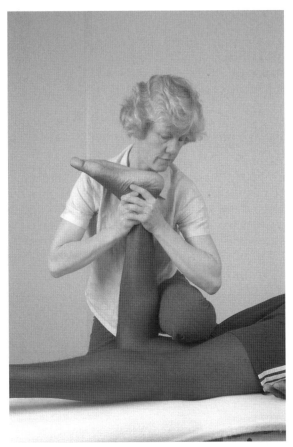

Figure 14.11 Apley compression/distraction test. The clinician gently rests his/her leg over the back of the patient's thigh to stabilize and then grasps around the lower calf to rotate and distract the knee. No stabilization is required for compression.

Table 14.2 Active physiological movements with possible modifications

Active physiological movements	Modifications
Knee flexion	Repeated
Knee extension	Speed altered
Medial rotation of the knee	Combined, e.g.
Lateral rotation of the knee	– Flexion with internal rotation
?Lumbar spine	Compression or distraction
?Sacroiliac joint	Sustained
?Hip	Injuring movement
?Foot and ankle	Differentiation tests
	Function

Table 14.3 Joint clearing tests

Joint	Physiological movement	Accessory movement
Lumbar spine	Flexion and extension quadrants	All movements
Sacroiliac joint	Anterior and posterior gapping	
Hip joint	Squat and hip quadrant	
Ankle joint	Plantarflexion/ dorsiflexion and inversion/eversion	

A movement diagram can be used to depict this information. The active movements with overpressure listed below (Fig. 14.12) are tested with the patient lying supine. Movements are carried out on the left and right sides. The clinician establishes the patient's symptoms at rest, prior to each movement, and passively corrects any movement deviation to determine its relevance to the patient's symptoms. Active physiological movements of the knee with possible modifications are shown in Table 14.2.

Numerous differentiation tests (Maitland 1991) can be performed; the choice depends on the patient's signs and symptoms. For example, when knee flexion in prone reproduces the patient's anterior knee pain, differentiation between knee joint, anterior thigh muscles and neural tissues may be required. Adding a compression force through the lower leg will stress the knee joint without particularly altering the muscle length or neural tissue. If symptoms are increased, this would suggest that the knee joint (patellofemoral or tibiofemoral joint) may be the source of the symptoms.

It may be necessary to examine other regions to determine their relevance to the patient's symptoms; they may be the source of the symptoms, or they may be contributing to the symptoms. The regions most likely are the lumbar spine, sacroiliac joint, hip, foot and ankle. The joints within these regions can be tested fully (see relevant chapter) or partially with the use of clearing tests (Table 14.3).

Some functional ability has already been tested by the general observation of the patient during the subjective and physical examination, e.g. the postures adopted during the subjective examination and the ease or difficulty of undressing and changing position prior to the examination. Any further functional testing can be carried out at this point in the examination and may include lifting, sitting postures, gait analysis, etc. Clues for appropriate tests can be obtained from the subjective examination findings, particularly aggravating factors. There are a variety of functional scales that can be used for the knee; these include the Cincinnati rating system for anterior cruciate ligament insufficiency (Noyes et al 1984) and the Knee Society rating scale (Insall et al 1989).

Capsular pattern

The capsular pattern for the knee joint (Cyriax 1982) is gross limitation of flexion with slight limitation of extension. Rotation is full and painless in the early stages.

Passive physiological movements

All of the active movements described above can be examined passively with the patient in supine, comparing left and right sides. Comparison of the response of symptoms to the active and passive movements can help to determine whether the structure at fault is non-contractile (articular) or contractile (extra-articular) (Cyriax 1982). If the

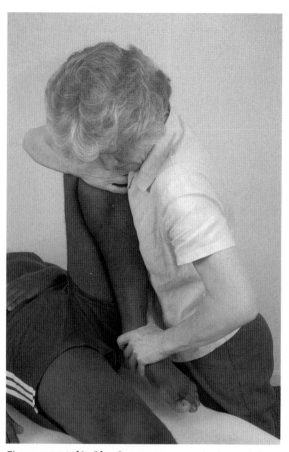
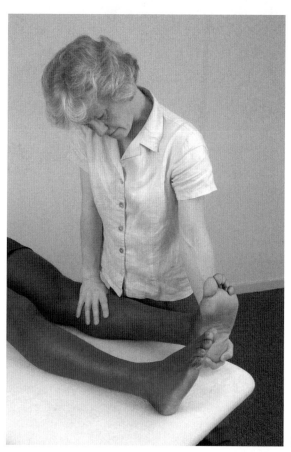

A   B

Figure 14.12 (A–D) Overpressures to the knee. **A** Flexion. One hand supports the knee while the other hand applies overpressure to flexion. **B** Extension. One hand stabilizes the tibia while the other hand lifts the lower leg into extension.

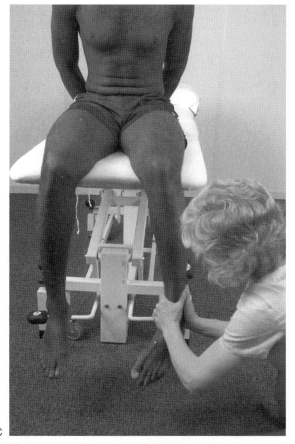
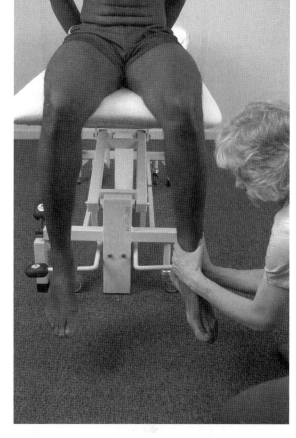

C

D

Figure 14.12 *Continued* **C** Medial rotation.

lesion is non-contractile, such as ligament, then active and passive movements will be painful and/or restricted in the same direction. If the lesion is in a contractile tissue (i.e. muscle) then active and passive movements are painful and/or restricted in opposite directions.

In addition, the following can be tested (Fig. 14.13) (Maitland 1991):

- Flexion/abduction
- Flexion/adduction
- Extension/abduction
- Extension/adduction.

It may be necessary to examine other regions to determine their relevance to the patient's symp-

toms; they may be the source of the symptoms, or they may be contributing to the symptoms. The regions most likely are the lumbar spine, sacro-iliac joint, hip, foot and ankle.

Muscle tests

Muscle tests include examining muscle strength, control, length and isometric muscle testing.

Muscle strength

The clinician tests the knee flexors/extensors and the ankle dorsiflexors/plantarflexors and any other relevant muscle groups. For details of these general tests, the reader is directed to Cole et al (1988), Hislop & Montgomery (1995) or Kendall et al (1993).

Greater detail may be required to test the strength of muscles, in particular those thought prone to become weak; that is: gluteus maximus, medius and minimus, vastus lateralis, medialis and intermedius, tibialis anterior and the peronei (Jull & Janda 1987, Sahrmann 2002). Testing the strength of these muscles is described in Chapter 3.

Muscle control

An imbalance of the vastus medialis oblique (VMO) and the vastus lateralis can occur in patients with patellofemoral pain (Mariani &

Caruso 1979, Voight & Wieder 1991). On quadriceps contraction, the patella may glide laterally as a result of weakness of VMO (McConnell 1996) and may contract after vastus lateralis (Voight & Wieder 1991). The timing of activation of VMO and vastus lateralis can be more objectively assessed using a dual-channel biofeedback machine. In addition, the inferior pole of the patella may be displaced posteriorly as the quadriceps contracts, which may result in fat pad irritation (McConnell 1996).

Muscle length

The clinician tests the length of muscles, in particular those thought prone to shorten (Janda 1994, 2002); that is: erector spinae, quadratus lumbo-

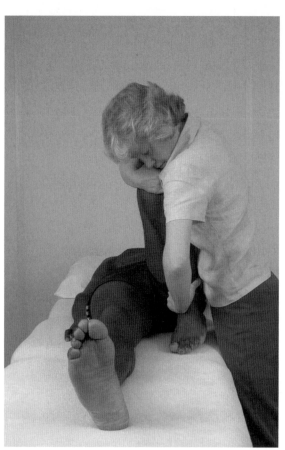
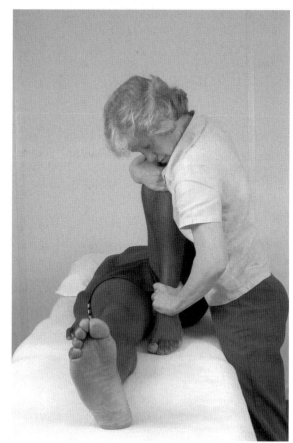

A   B

Figure 14.13 Passive physiological joint movements to the knee. **A** Flexion/abduction. The right hand supports the knee while the left hand moves the knee into flexion and abduction. **B** Flexion/adduction. The right hand supports the knee while the left hand moves the knee into flexion and adduction.

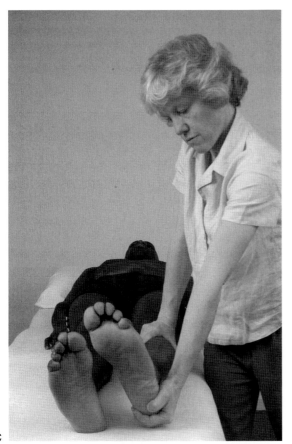
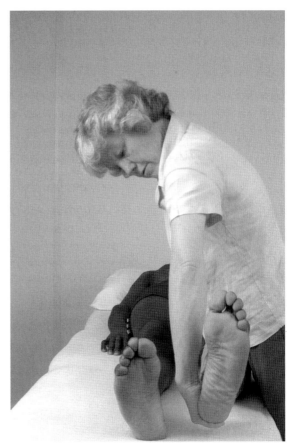

C   D

Figure 14.13 *Continued* **C** Extension/abduction. The right hand stabilizes the tibia while the left hand moves the knee into extension and abduction. **D** Extension/adduction. The right hand stabilizes the tibia while the left hand moves the knee into extension and adduction.

rum, piriformis, iliopsoas, rectus femoris, tensor fasciae latae, hamstrings, tibialis posterior, gastrocnemius and soleus (Jull & Janda 1987, Sahrmann 2002). Testing the length of these muscles is described in Chapter 3.

Isometric muscle testing

Test knee flexors (with tibia medially and laterally rotated to stress, in particular, the lateral and medial hamstrings, respectively), extensors and ankle dorsiflexors and plantarflexors in resting position and, if indicated, in different parts of the physiological range. In addition the clinician observes the quality of the muscle contraction to hold this position (this can be done with the patient's eyes shut). The patient may, for example,

be unable to prevent the joint from moving or may hold with excessive muscle activity; either of these circumstances would suggest a neuromuscular dysfunction.

The patient lies in high sitting with the femur laterally rotated. The patient isometrically contracts the quadriceps muscle for 10 seconds in various angles of knee flexion. If pain is produced, the test is repeated with the clinician holding a medial glide to the patella; if symptoms are eased this may indicate symptoms from the patellofemoral joint (McConnell 1986).

Neurological tests

Neurological examination includes neurological integrity testing and neurodynamic tests.

Integrity of the nervous system

The integrity of the nervous system is tested if the clinician suspects the symptoms are emanating from the spine or from a peripheral nerve.

Dermatomes/peripheral nerves. Light touch and pain sensation of the lower limb are tested using cotton wool and pinprick respectively, as described in Chapter 3. Knowledge of the cutaneous distribution of nerve roots (dermatomes) and peripheral nerves enables the clinician to distinguish the sensory loss due to a root lesion from that due to a peripheral nerve lesion. The cutaneous nerve distribution and dermatome areas are shown in Figure 3.21.

Myotomes/peripheral nerves. The following myotomes are tested and are shown in Figure 3.27:

- L2: hip flexion
- L3: knee extension
- L4: foot dorsiflexion and inversion
- L5: extension of the big toe
- S1: eversion of the foot, contract buttock, knee flexion
- S2: knee flexion, toe standing
- S3–S4: muscles of pelvic floor, bladder and genital function.

A working knowledge of the muscular distribution of nerve roots (myotomes) and peripheral nerves enables the clinician to distinguish the motor loss due to a root lesion from that due to a peripheral nerve lesion. The peripheral nerve distributions are shown in Figure 3.25.

Reflex testing. The following deep tendon reflexes are tested and are shown in Figure 3.28:

- L3/4: knee jerk
- S1: ankle jerk.

Neurodynamic tests

The following neurodynamic tests may be carried out in order to ascertain the degree to which neural tissue is responsible for the production of the patient's symptom(s):

- Passive neck flexion (PNF)
- Straight leg raise (SLR)
- Passive knee bend (PKB)
- Slump.

These tests are described in detail in Chapter 3.

Miscellaneous tests

Vascular tests

If the circulation is suspected of being compromised, the clinician palpates the pulses of the femoral, popliteal and dorsalis pedis arteries. The state of the vascular system can also be determined by the response of symptoms to positions of dependency and elevation of the lower limbs.

Leg length

True leg length is measured from the anterior superior iliac spine (ASIS) to the medial or lateral malleolus. Apparent leg length is measured from the umbilicus to the medial or lateral malleolus. A difference in leg length of up to 1–1.3 cm is considered normal. If there is a leg-length difference, test the length of individual bones, the tibia with knees bent and the femurs in standing. Ipsilateral posterior rotation of the ilium (on the sacrum) or contralateral anterior rotation of the ilium will result in a decrease in leg length (Magee 1997).

Supine to sit test

This is where one leg appears longer in supine and shorter in long sitting. This implicates anterior innominate rotation on the affected side (Wadsworth 1988).

Suprapatellar plica test (Hughston et al 1984)

Symptoms can arise from inflammation of the synovial fold around the supramedial pole of the patella, which is often caused by direct trauma to the knee. The patient lies supine and, with the knee flexed and medially rotated, the clinician applies a medial glide to the patella while palpating the medial femoral condyle (Fig. 14.14). The knee is flexed and extended; a 'popping' felt over the femoral condyle and tenderness are positive findings, indicating an inflamed suprapatellar plica.

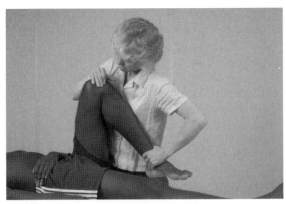

Figure 14.14   Test for suprapatellar plica. The left hand maintains medial rotation at the knee and moves the knee into flexion and extension, while the right hand applies a medial glide to the patella and palpates the medial femoral condyle.

Infrapatellar fat pad test (Wilson, personal communication, 1996)

With the patient's hip and knee flexed to 90° the clinician applies slight pressure to the fat pad (either side of the patellar tendon) and passively extends the knee (not hyperextension). A positive test, indicating fat pad irritation, is indicated when the patient's pain is reproduced towards the end of knee extension range of movement.

Palpation

The clinician palpates the knee region and any other relevant areas. It is useful to record palpation findings on a body chart (see Fig. 2.4) and/or palpation chart (see Fig. 3.37).

The clinician notes the following:

- The temperature of the area.
- Localized increased skin moisture.
- The presence of oedema or effusion – the clinician examines with the patella tap and fluid displacement test to assess if joint effusion is present. The circumference of the limb or joint can be measured with a tape measure and left and right sides compared.
- Mobility and feel of superficial tissues, e.g. ganglions, nodules, scar tissue.
- The presence or elicitation of any muscle spasm.

- Tenderness of bone (the upper pole of the patella and the femoral condyle may be tender in plica syndrome, while the undersurface of the patella may be tender with patellofemoral joint problems), bursae (prepatellar, infrapatellar), ligaments, muscle, tendon, tendon sheath, trigger points (shown in Fig. 3.38) and nerve. Palpable nerves in the lower limb are as follows:
    - The sciatic nerve can be palpated two-thirds of the way along an imaginary line between the greater trochanter and the ischial tuberosity with the patient in prone
    - The common peroneal nerve can be palpated medial to the tendon of biceps femoris and also around the head of the fibula
    - The tibial nerve can be palpated centrally over the posterior knee crease medial to the popliteal artery; it can also be felt behind the medial malleolus, which is more noticeable with the foot in dorsiflexion and eversion
    - The superficial peroneal nerve can be palpated on the dorsum of the foot along an imaginary line over the fourth metatarsal; it is more noticeable with the foot in plantar flexion and inversion
    - The deep peroneal nerve can be palpated between the first and second metatarsals, lateral to the extensor hallucis tendon
    - The sural nerve can be palpated on the lateral aspect of the foot behind the lateral malleolus, lateral to the tendocalcaneus.
- Increased or decreased prominence of bones – observe the position of the patella in terms of glide, lateral tilt, anteroposterior tilt and rotation on the femoral condyles (see below) (McConnell 1996). The quadriceps (Q) angle can be measured. It is 'the angle formed by the intersection of the line of pull of the quadriceps muscle and the patellar tendon measured through the centre of the patella' (McConnell 1986). The normal outer value is considered to be in the region of 15°.
- Pain provoked or reduced on palpation.

Increased or decreased prominence of bones. The optimal position of the patella is one where the patella is parallel to the femur in the frontal and sagittal planes and the patella is midway between the two condyles of the femur when the knee is slightly flexed (Grelsamer & McConnell 1998). In terms of the position of the patella, the following may be noted:

- The *base of the patella* normally lies equidistant (± 5 mm) from the medial and lateral femoral epicondyles when the knee is flexed 20°. If the patella lies closer to the medial or lateral femoral epicondyle, it is considered to have a medial or lateral glide respectively. The clinician also needs to test for any lateral glide of the patella on quadriceps contraction. The clinician palpates the left and right base of the patella and the vastus medialis oblique and vastus lateralis with thumbs and fingers respectively while the patient is asked to extend the knee. In some cases the patella is felt to glide laterally, indicating a dynamic problem, and vastus medialis oblique may be felt to contract after vastus lateralis; VMO is normally thought to be activated simultaneously with, or slightly earlier than, vastus lateralis. Quite a large difference will be needed to enable the clinician to feel a difference in the timing of muscle contraction.
- The *lateral tilt* is calculated by measuring the distance of the medial and lateral borders of the patella from the femur. The patella is considered to have a lateral tilt, for example, when the distance is decreased on the lateral aspect and increased on the medial aspect such that the patella faces laterally. A lateral tilt is considered to be due to a tight lateral retinaculum (superficial and deep fibres) and iliotibial band. When a passive medial glide is first applied (see below), the patellar tilt may be accentuated, indicating a dynamic tilt problem implicating a tight lateral retinaculum (deep fibres).
- The *anteroposterior tilt* is calculated by measuring the distance from the inferior and superior poles of the patella to the femur. Posterior tilt of the patella occurs if the inferior pole lies more posteriorly than the superior pole and may lead to fat pad irritation and inferior patellar pain. Dynamic control of a posterior patellar tilt is tested by asking the patient to brace the knee back and observing the movement of the tibia. With a positive patellar tilt the foot moves away

from the couch and the proximal end of the tibia is seen to move posteriorly; this movement is thought to pull the inferior pole of the patella into the fat pad.
- *Rotation* is the relative position of the long axis of patella to the femur, and is normally parallel. The patella is considered to be laterally rotated if the inferior pole of the patella is placed laterally to the long axis of the femur. A lateral or medial rotation of the patella is considered to be due to tightness of part of the retinaculum. The most common abnormality seen in patellofemoral pain is both a lateral tilt and a lateral rotation of the patella, which is thought to be due to an imbalance of the medial (weakness of vastus medialis oblique) and lateral structures (tightness of the lateral retinaculum and/or weakness of vastus lateralis) of the patella (McConnell 1996).
- *Testing the length of the lateral retinaculum.* With the patient in side lie and the knee flexed approximately 20°, the clinician passively glides the patella in a medial direction. The patella will normally move sufficient to expose the lateral femoral condyle; if this is not possible then tightness of the superficial retinaculum is suspected. The deep retinaculum is tested as above, but with the addition of an anteroposterior force to the medial border of the patella. The lateral border of the patella is normally able to move anteriorly away from the femur; inability may suggest tightness of the deep retinaculum.

Accessory movements

It is useful to use the palpation chart and movement diagrams (or joint pictures) to record findings. These are explained in detail in Chapter 3.

The clinician notes the following:

- Quality of movement
- Range of movement
- Resistance through the range and at the end of the range of movement
- Behaviour of pain through the range
- Provocation of any muscle spasm.

Patellofemoral joint (Figs 14.15 & 14.16), tibiofemoral joint (Fig. 14.17), superior tibiofibular

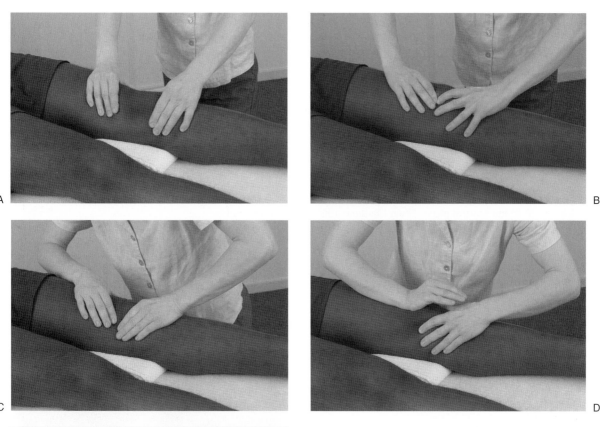

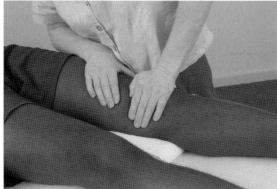

Figure 14.15 Patellofemoral joint accessory movements. **A** Medial transverse. The thumbs move the patella medially. **B** Lateral transverse. The fingers move the patella laterally. **C** Longitudinal cephalad. The right hand pushes the patella in a cephalad direction while the left hand helps to guide the movement. **D** Longitudinal caudad. The left hand pushes the patella in a caudad direction while the right hand helps to guide the movement. **E** Compression. The hands rest over the anterior aspect of the patella and push the patella towards the femur.

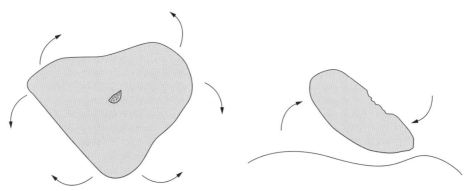

Figure 14.16 Rotation movements at the patellofemoral joint. **A** Medial and lateral rotation in the coronal plane. **B** Medial tilt in the sagittal plane. (From Maitland 1991, with permission.)

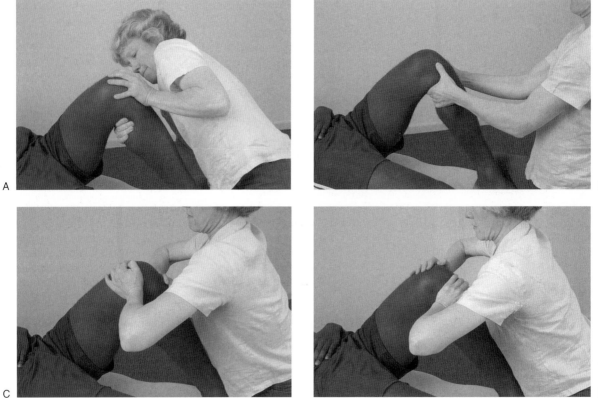

Figure 14.17 Tibiofemoral joint accessory movements. **A** Anteroposterior. The knee is placed in flexion and the clinician lightly sits on the patient's foot to stabilize this position. Both thumbs are then placed around the anterior aspect of the tibia to apply an anteroposterior force to the knee. **B** Posteroanterior. The knee is placed in flexion and the clinician lightly sits on the patient's foot to stabilize this position. The fingers grasp around the posterior aspect of the calf to apply the force, while the thumbs rest over the anterior joint line to feel the movement. **C** Medial transverse. The left hand stabilizes the medial aspect of the thigh while the right hand applies a medial force to the tibia. **D** Lateral transverse. The right hand stabilizes the lateral aspect to the thigh while the left hand applies a lateral force to the tibia.

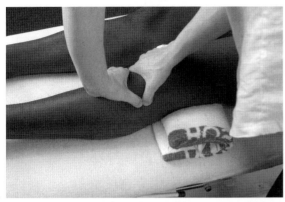
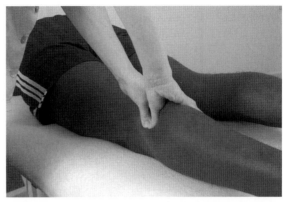

A   B

Figure 14.18   Superior tibiofibular joint accessory movements. **A** Anteroposterior. Thumb pressures are used to apply an anteroposterior force to the anterior aspect of the head of the fibula. **B** Posteroanterior. Thumb pressures are used to apply a posteroanterior force to the posterior aspect of the head of the fibula.

joint (Fig. 14.18) accessory movements are listed in Table 14.4. The clinician reassesses all the physical asterisks (movements or tests that have been found to reproduce the patient's symptoms) following accessory movements, in order to establish the effect of the accessory movements on the patient's signs and symptoms. Accessory movements can then be tested for other regions suspected to be a source of, or contributing to, the patient's symptoms. Again, following accessory movements, the clinician reassesses all the asterisks. Regions likely to be examined are the lumbar spine, sacroiliac joint, hip, foot and ankle (Table 14.4).

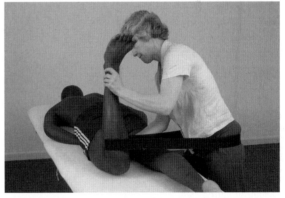

Figure 14.19   Mobilization with movement for knee flexion. The right hand stabilizes the thigh and the seat belt is used to apply a medial glide to the tibia, while the patient actively flexes the knee.

Mobilizations with movement (MWMs) (Mulligan 1999)

Tibiofemoral joint.   A medial glide is applied with medial joint pain and a lateral glide with lateral joint pain. The patient lies prone and the clinician stabilizes the thigh and applies a glide to the tibia using a seat belt around the tibia (Fig. 14.19). The glide is then maintained while the patient actively flexes or extends the knee. An increased range of movement which is pain-free would indicate a mechanical joint problem.

Another MWM can be used for patients who have at least 80° knee flexion. In supine, a posterior glide of the tibia is applied by the clinician

while the patient flexes the knee (Fig. 14.20). Increased range of movement which is pain-free would indicate a mechanical joint problem.

Superior tibiofibular joint.   This test is carried out if the patient has posterolateral knee pain. The patient in lying or standing actively flexes or extends the knee while the clinician applies an anteroposterior or posteroanterior glide to the fibula head (Fig. 14.21). Once again, increased range of movement that is pain-free would indicate a mechanical joint problem.

Table 14.4   Accessory movements, choice of application and reassessment of the patient's asterisks

Accessory movements	Choice of application	Identify any effect of accessory movements on patient's signs and symptoms
Patellofemoral joint (Fig. 14.15)	Start position, e.g.	Reassess all asterisks
→• Med medial transverse	– in flexion	
→• Lat lateral transverse	– in extension	
←•→ Ceph longitudinal cephalad	– in medial rotation	
←•→ Caud longitudinal caudad	– in lateral rotation	
⤸ medial rotation (Fig. 14.16)	– in flexion and lateral rotation	
medial tilt (Fig. 14.16)	– in extension and medial rotation	
⤿ lateral rotation	Speed of force application	
lateral tilt	Direction of the applied force	
Comp compression	Point of application of applied force	
Distr distraction		
Tibiofemoral joint (Fig. 14.17)		
↕ anteroposterior		
↕ posteroanterior		
→• Med medial transverse		
→• Lat lateral transverse		
Superior tibiofibular joint (Fig. 14.18)		
↕ anteroposterior		
↕ posteroanterior		
←•→ Ceph longitudinal cephalad by eversion of the foot		
←•→ Caud longitudinal caudad by inversion of the foot		
?Lumbar spine	As above	Reassess all asterisks
?Sacroiliac joint	As above	Reassess all asterisks
?Hip	As above	Reassess all asterisks
?Foot and ankle	As above	Reassess all asterisks

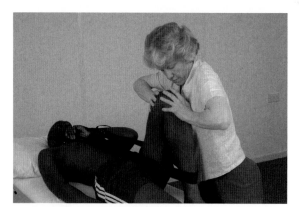

Figure 14.20 Mobilization with movement for knee flexion. The right hand supports the thigh and the left hand applies an anteroposterior glide to the tibia; the patient actively flexes the knee, which is reinforced by the seat belt.

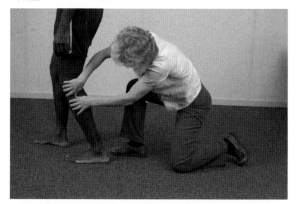

Figure 14.21 Mobilization with movement for the proximal tibiofibular joint. In standing the clinician applies a posteroanterior force to the fibula while the patient actively flexes the knee.

COMPLETION OF THE EXAMINATION

Having carried out all the above tests, the examination of the knee region is now complete. The subjective and physical examination produces a large amount of information, which needs to be recorded accurately and quickly. An outline examination chart may be useful for some clinicians and one is suggested in Figure 14.22. It is important, however, that the clinician does not examine in a rigid manner, simply following the suggested sequence outlined in the chart. Each patient presents differently and this needs to be reflected in the examination process. It is vital at this stage to highlight important findings from the examination with an asterisk (*). These findings must be reassessed at, and within, subsequent treatment sessions to evaluate the effects of treatment on the patient's condition.

The physical testing procedures which specifically indicate joint, nerve or muscle tissues, as a source of the patient's symptoms, are summarized in Table 3.10. The strongest evidence that a joint is the source of the patient's symptoms is that active and passive physiological movements, passive accessory movements and joint palpation all reproduce the patient's symptoms, and that following a treatment dose, reassessment identifies an improvement in the patient's signs and symptoms. Weaker evidence includes an alteration in range, resistance or quality of physiological and/or accessory movements and tenderness over the joint, with no alteration in signs and symptoms after treatment. One or more of these findings may indicate a dysfunction of a joint which may, or may not, be contributing to the patient's condition.

The strongest evidence that a muscle is the source of a patient's symptoms is if active movements, an isometric contraction, passive lengthening and palpation of a muscle all reproduce the patient's symptoms, and that following a treatment dose, reassessment identifies an improvement in the patient's signs and symptoms. Further evidence of muscle dysfunction may be suggested by reduced strength or poor quality during the active physiological movement and the isometric contraction, reduced range, and/or increased/decreased resistance, during the passive lengthen-

ing of the muscle, and tenderness on palpation, with no alteration in signs and symptoms after treatment. One or more of these findings may indicate a dysfunction of a muscle which may or may not be contributing to the patient's condition.

The strongest evidence that a nerve is the source of the patient's symptoms is when active and/or passive physiological movements reproduce the patient's symptoms, which are then increased or decreased with an additional sensitizing movement, at a distance from the patient's symptoms. In addition, there is reproduction of the patient's symptoms on palpation of the nerve and neurodynamic testing, sufficient to be considered a treatment dose, results in an improvement in the above signs and symptoms. Further evidence of nerve dysfunction may be suggested by reduced range (compared to the asymptomatic side) and/or increased resistance to the various arm movements, and tenderness on nerve palpation.

On completion of the physical examination the clinician:

- Warns the patient of possible exacerbation up to 24–48 hours following the examination.
- Requests the patient to report details on the behaviour of the symptoms following examination at the next attendance.
- Explains the findings of the physical examination and how these findings relate to the subjective assessment. Any misconceptions patients may have regarding their illness or injury should be addressed.
- Evaluates the findings, formulates a clinical diagnosis and writes up a problem list. Clinicians may find the management planning forms shown in Figures 3.53 and 3.54 helpful in guiding them through what is often a complex clinical reasoning process.
- Determines the objectives of treatment.
- Devises an initial treatment plan.

In this way, the clinician will have developed the following hypothesis categories (adapted from Jones & Rivett 2004):

- Function: abilities and restrictions.
- Patients' perspectives on their experience.
- Source of symptoms. This includes the structure or tissue that is thought to be producing the

Body chart	Name
	Age
	Date
	24-hour behaviour
	Improving static worsening
	Special questions
	General health
	Weight loss
	RA
	Drugs
	Steroids
Relationship of symptoms	Anticoagulants
	X-ray
	Cord symptoms
	Cauda equina symptoms
	VBI symptoms
Aggravating factors and function	HPC
	PMH
Severe Irritable	
Easing factors	SH & FH (Patient's perspective, experience, expectations. Yellow, blue, black flags)

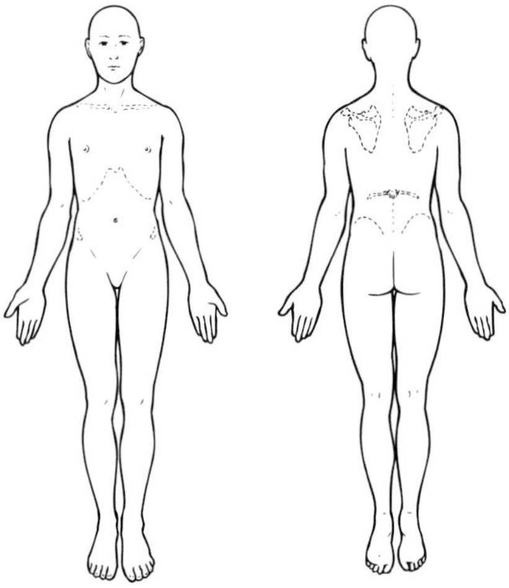

Figure 14.22   Knee examination chart.

Physical examination Observation	Isometric muscle testing
	Neurological integrity tests
Joint integrity tests (abduction/adduction, ant/post draw, meniscal tests, Fairbank's apprehension)	
	Neurodynamic tests
Active and passive physiological movements of knee and other relevant regions	
	Miscellaneous tests (pulses, leg length, supine to sit, plica, fat pad)
	Palpation
Capsular pattern yes/no	
Muscle strength	Accessory movements and reassessment of each relevant region
Muscle control	
Muscle length	

Figure 14.22 *Continued*

patients' symptoms, the nature of the structure or tissues in relation to the healing process, and the pain mechanisms.

- Contributing factors to the development and maintenance of the problem. There may be environmental, psychosocial, behavioural, physical or heredity factors.
- Precautions/contraindications to treatment and management. This includes the severity and

irritability of the patient's symptoms and the nature of the patient's condition.

- Management strategy and treatment plan.
- Prognosis – this can be affected by factors such as the stage and extent of the injury as well as the patient's expectation, personality and lifestyle.

References

Apley A G 1947 The diagnosis of meniscus injuries: some new clinical methods. Journal of Bone and Joint Surgery 29B: 78–84

Cole J H, Furness A L, Twomey L T 1988 Muscles in action, an approach to manual muscle testing. Churchill Livingstone, Edinburgh

Cyriax J 1982 Textbook of orthopaedic medicine – diagnosis of soft tissue lesions, 8th edn. Baillière Tindall, London

Eifert-Mangine M A, Bilbo J T 1995 Conservative management of patellofemoral chondrosis. In: Mangine R E (ed) Physical therapy of the knee, 2nd edn. Churchill Livingstone, New York, ch 5, p 113

Grelsamer R, McConnell J 1998 The patella in a team approach. Aspen, Gaithersburg, MD

Grieve G P 1981 Common vertebral joint problems. Churchill Livingstone, Edinburgh

Grieve G P 1991 Mobilisation of the spine, 5th edn. Churchill Livingstone, Edinburgh

Hislop H, Montgomery J 1995 Daniels and Worthingham's muscle testing, techniques of manual examination, 7th edn. W B Saunders, Philadelphia

Hughston J C, Norwood L A 1980 The posterolateral drawer test and external rotational recurvatum test for posterolateral rotary instability of the knee. Clinical Orthopaedics and Related Research 147: 82–87

Hughston J C, Walsh W M, Puddu G 1984 Patellar subluxation and dislocation. W B Saunders, Philadelphia, PA

Insall J N, Dorr L D, Scott R D, Scott W N 1989 Rationale of the Knee Society clinical rating system. Clinical Orthopaedics and Related Research 248: 13–14

Jacobson K E, Flandry F C 1989 Diagnosis of anterior knee pain. Clinics in Sports Medicine 8(2): 179–195

Janda V 1994 Muscles and motor control in cervicogenic disorders: assessment and management. In: Grant R (ed) Physical therapy of the cervical and thoracic spine, 2nd edn. Churchill Livingstone, New York, ch 10, p 195

Janda V 2002 Muscles and motor control in cervicogenic disorders. In: Grant R (ed) Physical therapy of the cervical and thoracic spine, 3rd edn. Churchill Livingstone, New York, ch 10, p 182

Jones M A, Rivett D A 2004 Clinical reasoning for manual therapists. Butterworth-Heinemann, Edinburgh

Jull G A, Janda V 1987 Muscles and motor control in low back pain: assessment and management. In: Twomey L T, Taylor J R (eds) Physical therapy of the low back. Churchill Livingstone, New York, ch 10, p 253

Kendall F P, McCreary E K, Provance P G 1993 Muscles testing and function, 4th edn. Williams & Wilkins, Baltimore, MD

McConnell J 1986 The management of chondromalacia patellae: a long term solution. Australian Journal of Physiotherapy 32(4): 215–223

McConnell J 1996 Management of patellofemoral problems. Manual Therapy 1(2): 60–66

McMurray T P 1942 The semilunar cartilages. British Journal of Surgery 29(116): 407–414

Magee D J 1997 Orthopedic physical assessment, 3rd edn. W B Saunders, Philadelphia

Maitland G D 1991 Peripheral manipulation, 3rd edn. Butterworth-Heinemann, London

Mariani P P, Caruso I 1979 An electromyographic investigation of subluxation of the patella. Journal of Bone and Joint Surgery 61B(2): 169–171

Mulligan B R 1999 Manual therapy 'NAGs', 'SNAGs', 'MWMs' etc., 4th edn. Plane View Services, New Zealand

Noyes F R, McGinniss G H, Mooar L A 1984 Functional disability in the anterior cruciate insufficient knee syndrome – review of knee rating systems and projected risk factors in determining treatment. Sports Medicine 1: 278–302

Sahrmann S A 2002 Diagnosis and treatment of movement impairment syndromes. Mosby, St Louis

Voight M L, Wieder D L 1991 Comparative reflex response times of vastus medialis obliquus and vastus lateralis in normal subjects and subjects with extensor mechanism dysfunction. American Journal of Sports Medicine 19(2): 131–137

Waddell G 2004 The back pain revolution, 2nd edn. Churchill Livingstone, Edinburgh

Wadsworth C T 1988 Manual examination and treatment of the spine and extremities. Williams & Wilkins, Baltimore, MD

Chapter **15**

Examination of the foot and ankle

POSSIBLE CAUSES OF PAIN AND/OR LIMITATION OF MOVEMENT

This region includes the inferior tibiofibular, talocrural, subtalar, midtarsal, tarsometatarsal, intermetatarsal, metatarsophalangeal, 1st and 5th rays and interphalangeal joints with their surrounding soft tissues. A ray is a functional unit formed by a metatarsal and its associated cuneiform; for the 4th and 5th rays it refers to the metatarsal alone (Norkin & Levangie 1992).

Ankle

- Trauma:
  - Fracture of the tibia, fibula, e.g. Pott's fracture
  - Ligamentous sprain, e.g. medial or lateral ligament of the ankle and inferior tibiofibular ligaments
  - Muscular strain, e.g. peritendinitis of tendocalcaneus and rupture of the tendocalcaneus
  - Tarsal tunnel syndrome
  - Tenosynovitis
- Osteochondritis dissecans of the talus
- Degenerative conditions: osteoarthrosis
- Inflammatory conditions: rheumatoid arthritis
- Infection, e.g. tuberculosis
- Endocrine diseases: diabetes.

Foot

Childhood foot

- Congenital talipes equinovarus (idiopathic club foot)

- Talipes calcaneovalgus
- In- and out-toeing (adducted and abducted stance respectively)
- Over-pronated foot
- Pes cavus and planus
- Köhler's disease (osteochondritis of the navicular)
- Freiberg's disease of lesser metatarsal heads (commonly second)
- Sever's disease causing a painful heel
- Retrocalcaneal bump (soft tissue or bony)
- Malignancy.

Adolescent foot

- Hallux valgus
- Exostoses
- Retrocalcaneal heel bumps (soft tissue or bony).

Adult foot

- Rheumatoid arthritis
- Gout
- Diabetic foot
- Paralysed foot, e.g. upper or lower motor neurone lesion, peripheral nerve injury
- Overuse syndrome and foot strain.

Hind foot

- Retrocalcaneal heel bumps (soft tissue or bony)
- Hindfoot varus and valgus
- Soft tissue conditions, e.g. bursitis, tendinitis, fat pad bruising.

Forefoot

- Brailsford's disease (osteochondritis of the navicular)
- Forefoot varus and valgus, forefoot adduction and abduction
- Over/excessive pronation
- Pes cavus and planus
- Plantar fasciitis and plantar calcaneal aesthesiopathy
- Anterior metatarsalgia
- March fracture
- Freiberg's disease (osteochondritis of second metatarsal head)

- Morton's metatarsalgia
- Verruca pedis
- Ligamentous strain/overuse injury.

Toes

- Hallux valgus
- Hallux rigidus
- Hallux flexus
- Ingrowing toenail
- Lesser toe deformity, e.g. hammer toe, mallet toe, claw toe
- Plantarflexion of big toe.

Other conditions

- Hypermobility
- Referral of symptoms from the lumbar spine, sacroiliac joint, hip or knee to the foot; or referral of foot structure and functional anomalies to more proximal structures in the locomotor system.

Further details of the questions asked during the subjective examination and the tests carried out in the physical examination can be found in Chapters 2 and 3 respectively.

The order of the subjective questioning and the physical tests described below can be altered as appropriate for the patient being examined.

SUBJECTIVE EXAMINATION

Body chart

The following information concerning the type and area of current symptoms can be recorded on a body chart (see Fig. 2.3).

Area of current symptoms

Be exact when mapping out the area of the symptoms. Lesions of the joints in this region usually produce localized symptoms over the affected joint. Ascertain which is the worst symptom and record where the patient feels the symptoms are coming from.

Areas relevant to the region being examined

All other relevant areas are checked for symptoms; it is important to ask about pain or even stiffness, as this may be relevant to the patient's main symptom. Mark unaffected areas with ticks (✓) on the body chart. Check for symptoms in the lumbar spine, hip joint and knee joint.

Quality of pain

Establish the quality of the pain.

Intensity of pain

The intensity of pain can be measured using, for example, a visual analogue scale (VAS) as shown in Figure 2.8.

Depth of pain

Establish the depth of the pain. Does the patient feel it is on the surface or deep inside?

Abnormal sensation

Check for any altered sensation (such as paraesthesia or numbness) over the ankle and foot and other relevant areas.

Constant or intermittent symptoms

Ascertain the frequency of the symptoms, whether they are constant or intermittent. If symptoms are constant, check whether there is variation in the intensity of the symptoms, as constant unremitting pain may be indicative of neoplastic disease.

Relationship of symptoms

Determine the relationship of the symptomatic areas to each other – do they come together or separately? For example, the patient could have ankle pain without back pain or they may always be present together.

Behaviour of symptoms

Aggravating factors

For each symptomatic area, discover what movements and/or positions aggravate the patient's symptoms, i.e. what brings them on (or makes them worse), are they able to maintain this position or movement (severity), what happens to other symptom(s) when this symptom is produced (or is made worse), and how long does it take for symptoms to ease once the position or movement is stopped (irritability). These questions help to confirm the relationship between the symptoms.

The clinician also asks the patient about theoretically known aggravating factors for structures that could be a source of the symptoms. Common aggravating factors for the foot and ankle are stair climbing, walking and running, especially on uneven ground. Aggravating factors for other regions, which may need to be queried if they are suspected to be a source of the symptoms, are shown in Table 2.3.

The clinician ascertains how the symptoms affect function, such as: static and active postures, e.g. standing, walking (even and uneven ground), running, going up and down stairs, work, sport and social activities. Note details of training regimen for any sports activities. The clinician finds out if the patient is left- or right-handed as there may be increased stress on the dominant side

Detailed information on each of the above activities is useful in order to help determine the structure(s) at fault and identify functional restrictions. This information can be used to determine the aims of treatment and any advice that may be required. The most notable functional restrictions are highlighted with asterisks (*), explored in the physical examination, and reassessed at subsequent treatment sessions to evaluate treatment intervention.

Easing factors

For each symptomatic area, the clinician asks what movements and/or positions ease the patient's symptoms, how long it takes to ease them and what happens to other symptoms when this symptom is relieved. These questions help to confirm the relationship of symptoms.

The clinician asks the patient about theoretically known easing factors for structures that could be a source of the symptoms. For example, symptoms from the foot and ankle may be relieved by weight-relieving positions, whereas symptoms from the lumbar spine may be relieved by lying prone or in a crook lie. The clinician can then analyse the position or movement that eases the symptoms to help determine the structure at fault.

Twenty-four-hour behaviour of symptoms

The clinician determines the 24-hour behaviour of symptoms by asking questions about night, morning and evening symptoms.

Night symptoms. The following questions may be asked:

- Do you have any difficulty getting to sleep?
- What position is most comfortable/uncomfortable?
- What is your normal sleeping position?
- What is your present sleeping position?
- Do your symptom(s) wake you at night? If so,
  – Which symptom(s)?
  – How many times in the past week?
  – How many times in a night?
  – How long does it take to get back to sleep?

Morning and evening symptoms. The clinician determines the pattern of the symptoms first thing in the morning, through the day and at the end of the day. Note whether the feet are painful on first getting out of bed, which suggests plantar fasciitis.

Stage of the condition

In order to determine the stage of the condition, the clinician asks whether the symptoms are getting better, getting worse or remaining unchanged.

Special questions

Special questions must always be asked, as they may identify certain precautions or contraindica-tions to the physical examination and/or treatment (see Table 2.4). As mentioned in Chapter 2, the clinician must differentiate between conditions that are suitable for manipulative therapy and systemic, neoplastic and other non-neuromusculoskeletal conditions, which are not suitable for such treatment and require referral to a medical practitioner.

The following information is routinely obtained from patients.

General health. The clinician ascertains the state of the patient's general health and finds out if the patient suffers from any malaise, fatigue, fever, nausea or vomiting, stress, anxiety or depression.

Weight loss. Has the patient noticed any recent unexplained weight loss?

Rheumatoid arthritis. Has the patient (or a member of his/her family) been diagnosed as having rheumatoid arthritis?

Drug therapy. What drugs are being taken by the patient? Has the patient been prescribed long-term (6 months or more) medication/steroids? Has the patient been taking anticoagulants recently?

X-rays and medical imaging. Has the patient been X-rayed or had any other medical tests? The medical tests may include blood tests, arthroscopy, magnetic resonance imaging, myelography or a bone scan.

Neuropathy secondary to the disorder. Has the patient any evidence of peripheral neuropathy – sensory, motor or autonomic – associated with a medical disorder such as diabetes (Armstrong 1999, McLeod-Roberts 1995)? Abnormality of skin and other structures will not necessarily be perceived or reported by the patient.

Neurological symptoms if a spinal lesion is suspected. Has the patient experienced symptoms of spinal cord compression (i.e. compression of the spinal cord to L1 level), which are bilateral tingling in hands or feet and/or disturbance of gait?

Has the patient experienced symptoms of cauda equina compression (i.e. compression below L1), which are saddle anaesthesia/paraesthesia and bladder and/or bowel sphincter disturbance (loss of control, retention, hesitancy, urgency or a sense of incomplete evacuation) (Grieve 1991)? These symptoms may be due to interference of S3 and S4 (Grieve 1981). Prompt surgical attention is required to prevent permanent sphincter paralysis.

History of the present condition (HPC)

For each symptomatic area the clinician needs to know how long the symptom has been present, whether there was a sudden or slow onset and whether there was a known cause that provoked the onset of the symptom. If the onset was slow, the clinician finds out if there has been any change in the patient's lifestyle, e.g. a new job or hobby or a change in sporting activity. To confirm the relationship between the symptoms, the clinician asks what happened to other symptoms when each symptom began.

Past medical history (PMH)

The following information is obtained from the patient and/or the medical notes:

- The details of any relevant medical history.
- The history of any previous attacks: how many episodes, when were they, what was the cause, what was the duration of each episode and did the patient fully recover between episodes? If there have been no previous attacks, has the patient had any episodes of stiffness in the lumbar spine, hip, knee, ankle, foot or any other relevant region? Check for a history of trauma or recurrent minor trauma.
- Ascertain the results of any past treatment for the same or similar problem. Past treatment records may be obtained for further information.

Social and family history (SH, FH)

Social and family history that is relevant to the onset and progression of the patient's problem is recorded. This includes the patient's perspectives, experience and expectations, their age, employment, home situation, and details of any leisure activities. Factors from this information may indicate direct and/or indirect mechanical influences on the foot and ankle. In order to treat the patient appropriately, it is important that the condition is managed within the context of the patient's social and work environment.

The clinician may ask the following types of questions to elucidate psychosocial factors:

- Have you had time off work in the past with your pain?
- What do you understand to be the cause of your pain?
- What are you expecting will help you?
- How is your employer/co-workers/family responding to your pain?
- What are you doing to cope with your pain?
- Do you think you will return to work? When?

While these questions are described in relation to psychosocial risk factors for poor outcomes for patients with low back pain (Waddell 2004), they may be relevant to other patients.

Plan of the physical examination

When all this information has been collected, the subjective examination is complete. It is useful at this stage to highlight with asterisks (*), for ease of reference, important findings and particularly one or more functional restrictions. These can then be re-examined at subsequent treatment sessions to evaluate treatment intervention.

In order to plan the physical examination, the following hypotheses need to be developed from the subjective examination:

- The regions and structures that need to be examined as a possible cause of the symptoms, e.g. lumbar spine, hip, knee, foot and ankle, muscles and nerves. Often it is not possible to examine fully at the first attendance and so examination of the structures must be prioritized over subsequent treatment sessions.
- Other factors that need to be examined, e.g. working and everyday postures, leg length.
- In what way should the physical tests be carried out? Will it be easy or hard to reproduce each symptom? Will it be necessary to use combined movements, repetitive movements, etc. to reproduce the patient's symptoms? Are

symptom(s) severe and/or irritable? If symptoms are severe, physical tests may be carried out to just before the onset of symptom production or just to the onset of symptom production; no overpressures will be carried out, as the patient would be unable to tolerate this. If symptoms are irritable, physical tests may be examined to just before symptom production or just to the onset of provocation with less physical tests being examined to allow for rest period between tests.

- Are there any precautions and/or contraindications to elements of the physical examination that need to be explored further, such neurological involvement, recent fracture, trauma, steroid therapy or rheumatoid arthritis; there may also be certain contraindications to further examination and treatment, e.g. symptoms of spinal cord or cauda equina compression.

A physical planning form can be useful for inexperienced clinicians to help guide them through the clinical reasoning process (Fig. 2.10 and Appendix 2.1).

PHYSICAL EXAMINATION

The information from the subjective examination helps the clinician to plan an appropriate physical examination. The severity, irritability and nature of the condition are the major factors that will influence the choice and priority of physical testing procedures. The first and over-arching question the clinician might ask is: 'is this patient's condition suitable for me to manage as a therapist?'. For example, a patient presenting with cauda equina compression symptoms may only need neurological integrity testing, prior to an urgent medical referral. The nature of the patient's condition has had a major impact on the physical examination. The second question the clinician might ask is: 'does this patient have a neuromusculoskeletal dysfunction that I may be able to help?'. To answer that, the clinician needs to carry out a full physical examination; however, this may not be possible if the symptoms are severe and/or irritable. If the patient's symptoms are severe and/or irritable, the clinician aims to explore movements as much as possible, within a symptom-free range. If the patient has constant and severe and/or irritable symptoms, then the clinician aims to find physical tests that ease the symptoms. If the patient's symptoms are non-severe and non-irritable, then the clinician aims to find physical tests that reproduce each of the patient's symptoms.

Each significant physical test that either provokes or eases the patient's symptoms is highlighted in the patient's notes by an asterisk (*) for easy reference. The highlighted tests are often referred to as 'asterisks' or 'markers'.

The order and detail of the physical tests described below need to be appropriate to the patient being examined; some tests will be irrelevant, some tests will be carried out briefly, while it will be necessary to investigate others fully. It is important that readers understand that the techniques shown in this chapter are some of many; the choice depends mainly on the relative size of the clinician and patient, as well as the clinician's preference. For this reason, novice clinicians may initially want to copy what is shown, but then quickly adapt to what is best for them.

Observation

Informal observation

The clinician needs to observe the patient in dynamic and static situations; the quality of movement is noted, as are the postural characteristics and facial expression. Informal observation will have begun from the moment the clinician begins the subjective examination and will continue to the end of the physical examination.

Formal observation

Observation of posture. The clinician examines the patient's posture in standing, noting the posture of the feet, lower limbs, pelvis and spine. Observation of the foot and ankle can also be carried out in a non-weight-bearing position. General lower limb abnormalities include uneven weight-bearing through the legs and feet, internal femoral rotation and genu varum/valgum or recurvatum (hyperextension). The foot may demonstrate a number of abnormalities, including forefoot varus/valgus and hindfoot varus/valgus. The toes may be deformed – claw toes, hallux rigidus, hammer toes, mallet toe, hallux valgus, Morton's foot, pes cavus or pes planus. Further details of these abnormalities can be found in a standard orthopaedic textbook. The clinician passively corrects any asymmetry to determine its relevance to the patient's problem.

It is worth remembering that pure postural dysfunction rarely influences one region of the body in isolation and it may be necessary to carry out a full postural examination.

Observation of alignment of foot and calf alignment

Leg–heel alignment. The patient lies prone with the foot over the end of the plinth and the clinician holds the foot with the subtalar joint in neutral. The clinician observes the position of the foot on the leg by using an imaginary line that bisects the calcaneus and the lower third of the leg (ignore the alignment of the tendocalcaneus). Normally, the calcaneus will be in slight varus (2–4°) (Roy & Irvin 1983). Excessive varus or presence of valgus alignment indicates hindfoot/rearfoot varus and valgus respectively; the latter is more likely to be observed following injury or disease process.

Forefoot–heel alignment. Test for forefoot varus and valgus with the patient in prone and the foot over the end of the plinth. The clinician holds the subtalar joint in neutral and the midtarsal joint in maximum eversion and observes the relationship between the vertical axis of the heel and the plane of the first to fifth metatarsal heads, which is normally perpendicular. The medial side of the foot will be raised if there is forefoot varus and the lateral side will be raised if there is forefoot valgus (Roy & Irvin 1983).

Tibial torsion. This test compares the alignment of the transverse axis of the knee with the ankle axis in the frontal plane. With the patient sitting, the clinician compares the ankle joint line (an imaginary line between the apex of the medial and lateral malleoli) and the knee joint line (Fig. 15.1) (Fromherz 1995). The tibia normally lies in 15–20° of lateral rotation (Wadsworth 1988).

Pes planus and over-pronation. Very high arched feet – pes cavus – may have a neurological

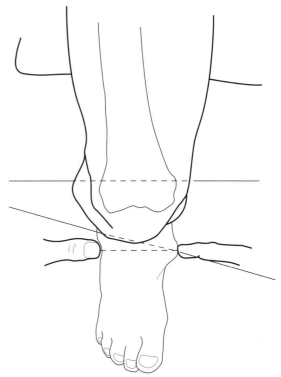

Figure 15.1 Tibial torsion. The line of the ankle joint is compared to a visual estimation of the knee joint axis. (From Fromherz 1995, with permission.)

or idiopathic aetiology and are invariably relatively rigid and cannot accommodate to uneven terrain, requiring other segments of the locomotor system to compensate. Feet that have an in-rolled appearance are termed over- or excessively pronated. On weight-bearing the vertical bisection of calcaneus is usually in a valgus alignment and medial bulging of the navicular is evident. Those feet that appear flattened with no longitudinal arch, but without inrolling, are called pes planus. This latter condition is not very common.

Observation of muscle form. The clinician observes the muscle bulk and muscle tone of the patient, comparing left and right sides. It must be remembered that the level and frequency of physical activity as well as the dominant side may well produce differences in muscle bulk between sides. Some muscles are thought to shorten under stress while other muscles weaken, producing muscle imbalance (see Table 3.2).

Observation of soft tissues. The clinician observes the quality and colour of the patient's skin, any area of swelling, exostosis, callosities, joint effusion or presence of scarring, and takes cues for further examination.

Observation of balance. Balance is provided by vestibular, visual and proprioceptive information. This rather crude and non-specific test is conducted by asking the patient to stand on one leg with the eyes open and then closed. If the patient's balance is as poor with the eyes open as with the eyes closed, this suggests a vestibular or proprioceptive dysfunction (rather than a visual dysfunction). The test is carried out on the affected and unaffected side; if there is greater difficulty maintaining balance on the affected side, this may indicate some proprioceptive dysfunction.

Observation of gait. Analyse gait (including walking backwards) on even/uneven ground and on toes, heels, and outer and inner borders of feet, as well as slopes, stairs and running, etc. Note the stride length and weight-bearing ability. Inspect the feet, shoes and any walking aids. The patient's gait is observed taking into account variations expected with age (Halliday et al 1998) and medical disorders or surgical interventions.

Working in a logical manner from head to toe, or vice versa, each body segment is observed. The clinician looks for asymmetry in each segment, e.g. arm swing, uneven stride length from left to right, as this may indicate tight musculature or structural anomaly, or even a habit such as carrying a bag on one shoulder. Leg alignment during the swing and stance phases of gait may provide useful indicators of the aetiology of problems; for example, a marked internal knee position increases the Q angle (Livingstone & Mandigo 1998) and thus the lateral pull of quadriceps. This could give rise to retropatellar pain as the patella is pulled laterally across the lateral femoral condyle. It is important to note the timing of the occurrence of the asymmetry as it may allow over-prolonged muscle contraction, for example, to be identified and related to the symptoms.

The angle of heel contact with the ground is usually slightly varus. Marked variations from this will cause abnormal foot function, with compensation attained either in the foot across the midtarsal joint and 1st and 5th rays or more proximally in the ankle, knee (less often hip) and sacroiliac joints. Early heel lift may indicate tight posterior leg muscles and causes a functional ankle equinus (Tollafield & Merriman 1995), a destructive functional condition of the lower limb.

Over-pronation or no pronation of the foot during midstance is observed and noted. Pronation is a normal part of gait that allows the foot to become a shock absorber and mobile adapter. At heel lift the foot changes to a more rigid lever for toe off. Limitation in range of motion of the metatarsophalangeal joints will affect gait also. Abnormality of function at any phase of gait may cause symptoms, varying from low-grade and cumulative to acute, in any structures of the locomotor system.

Summary of gait analysis:

- Observe alignment of head to toes during gait
- Look for asymmetry
- Look for abnormal alignment
- Look for timing of any malalignment during gait

Observation of the patient's attitudes and feelings. The age, gender and ethnicity of patients and their cultural, occupational and social backgrounds will all affect their attitudes and feelings towards themselves, their condition and the clinician. The clinician needs to be aware of and sensitive to these attitudes, and to empathize and communicate appropriately so as to develop a rapport with the patient and thereby enhance the patient's compliance with the treatment.

Joint integrity tests

Anterior drawer sign

This test is similar to the posteroanterior accessory movement to the ankle joint described below. The patient lies prone with the knee flexed (to relax gastrocnemius). The clinician applies a posteroanterior force to the talus with the ankle in dorsiflexion and then plantarflexion (Fig. 15.2), in order to test the integrity of the medial and lateral ligaments. Excessive anterior movement of the talus indicates insufficiency of the medial and lateral ligaments. If the movement only occurs on one

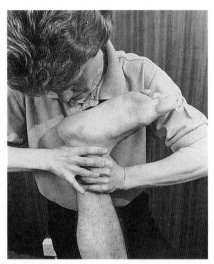

Figure 15.2 Anterior drawer sign. The left hand stabilizes the lower leg while the right hand applies a posteroanterior force to the talus.

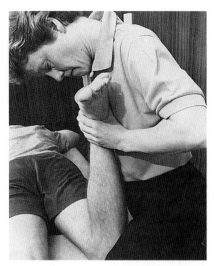

Figure 15.3 Talar tilt. The hands grip around the talus and move it into adduction.

side, this indicates insufficiency of the ligament on that side.

Talar tilt

The patient lies prone with the knee flexed (to relax gastrocnemius) and the ankle in neutral. The clinician moves the talus into abduction and then adduction (Fig. 15.3). Excessive adduction movement of the talus suggests that the calcaneofibular ligament is injured (Magee 1997).

Active physiological movements

For active physiological movements, the clinician notes the following:

- Quality of movement
- Range of movement
- Behaviour of pain through the range of movement
- Resistance through the range of movement and at the end of the range of movement
- Provocation of any muscle spasm.

A movement diagram can be used to depict this information. The active movements with overpressure listed below (Fig. 15.4) are tested with the patient lying prone. Movements are carried out on

Table 15.1 Active physiological movements and possible modifications

Active physiological movements	Modifications
Ankle dorsiflexion	Repeated
Ankle plantarflexion	Speed altered
Inversion	Combined, e.g.
Eversion	– inversion with plantarflexion
Metatarsophalangeal joints:	– metatarsophalangeal flexion and abduction
– Flexion	Compression or distraction
– Extension	Sustained
Interphalangeal joints:	Injuring movement
– Flexion	Differentiation tests
– Extension	Function
?Lumbar spine	
?Sacroiliac joint	
?Hip	
?Knee	

the left and right sides. The clinician establishes the patient's symptoms at rest, prior to each movement, and passively corrects any movement deviation to determine its relevance to the patient's symptoms. Active physiological movements of the foot and ankle and possible modifications are shown in Table 15.1.

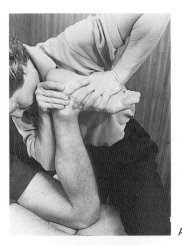

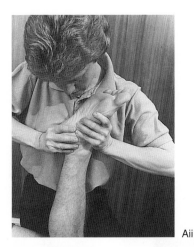

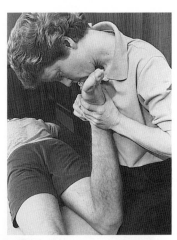

Ai

Aii

Aiii

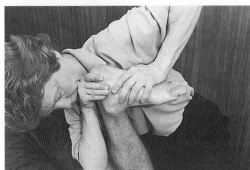

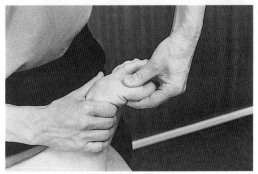

Aiv

B

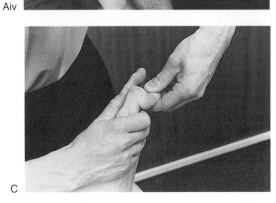

C

Figure 15.4 Overpressures to the foot and ankle.
A (i) Dorsiflexion. The right hand pulls the calcaneus upwards while the left hand applies overpressure to dorsiflexion. (ii) Plantarflexion. The left hand grips the forefoot and the right hand grips the calcaneus and both move the foot into plantarflexion. (iii) Inversion. The right hand adducts the calcaneus and reinforces the plantarflexion movement while the left hand plantarflexes the hindfoot and adducts, supinates and plantarflexes the forefoot. (iv) Eversion. The right hand abducts the calcaneus and reinforces the dorsiflexion while the left hand dorsiflexes the hindfoot and abducts, pronates and dorsiflexes the forefoot. **B** Metatarsophalangeal joint flexion and extension. The right hand stabilizes the metatarsal while the left hand flexes and extends the proximal phalanx. **C** Interphalangeal joint flexion and extension. The right hand stabilizes the proximal phalanx while the left hand flexes and extends the distal phalanx.

Numerous differentiation tests (Maitland 1991) can be performed; the choice depends on the patient's signs and symptoms. For example, when lateral ankle pain is reproduced on inversion, inversion consists of talocrural plantarflexion, subtalar adduction and transverse tarsal supination, and differentiation between these joints may therefore be required. The clinician takes the foot into inversion to reproduce the patient's pain and then systematically adds or releases talocrural plantarflexion, subtalar adduction and transverse tarsal supination and notes the effect this has on symptoms.

Other regions may need to be examined to determine their relevance to the patient's symptoms; they may be the source of the symptoms, or they may be contributing to the symptoms. The regions most likely are the lumbar spine, sacroiliac joint, hip and knee. The joints within these regions can be tested fully (see relevant chapter) or partially with the use of clearing tests (Table 15.1).

Some functional ability has already been tested by the general observation of the patient during the subjective and physical examination, e.g. the postures adopted during the subjective examination and the ease or difficulty of undressing and changing position prior to the examination. Any further functional testing can be carried out at this point in the examination and may involve further gait analysis over and above that carried out in the observation section earlier. Clues for appropriate tests can be obtained from the subjective examination findings, particularly aggravating factors.

Capsular pattern

Capsular patterns for these joints (Cyriax 1982) are as follows:

- Tibiofibular joints: pain when the joint is stressed
- Ankle joint: more limitation of plantarflexion than dorsiflexion
- Talocalcaneal joint: limitation of inversion
- Midtarsal joint: limitation of dorsiflexion, plantarflexion, adduction and medial rotation (abduction and lateral rotation are full range)
- Metatarsophalangeal joint of the big toe: more limitation of extension than flexion

- Metatarsophalangeal joint of the other four toes: variable, tend to fix in extension with interphalangeal joints flexed.

Passive physiological movements

All of the active movements described above can be examined passively with the patient in prone with the knee at 90° flexion, or supine with the knee flexed over a pillow, comparing left and right sides. Comparison of the response of symptoms to the active and passive movements can help to determine whether the structure at fault is non-contractile (articular) or contractile (extra-articular) (Cyriax 1982). If the lesion is non-contractile, such as ligament, then active and passive movements will be painful and/or restricted in the same direction. If the lesion is in a contractile tissue (i.e. muscle) then active and passive movements are painful and/or restricted in opposite directions.

Metatarsophalangeal abduction and adduction can be tested (Fig. 15.5).

It may be necessary to examine other regions to determine their relevance to the patient's symptoms; they may be the source of the symptoms, or they may be contributing to the symptoms. The

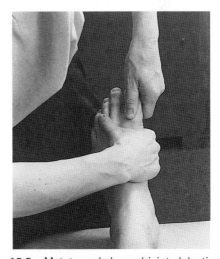

Figure 15.5 Metatarsophalangeal joint abduction and adduction. The right hand stabilizes the metatarsal while the left hand moves the proximal phalanx into abduction and adduction.

regions most likely are the lumbar spine, sacro-iliac joint, hip and knee.

Muscle tests

Muscle tests include examining muscle strength, length, isometric muscle testing and some other muscle tests.

Muscle strength

The clinician tests the ankle dorsiflexors, plantarflexors, foot inverters, everters and toe flexors, extensors, abductors and adductors and any other relevant muscle groups. For details of these general tests readers are directed to Cole et al (1988), Hislop & Montgomery (1995) or Kendall et al (1993).

Greater detail may be required to test the strength of muscles, in particular those thought prone to become weak; that is: gluteus maximus, medius and minimus, vastus lateralis, medialis and intermedius, tibialis anterior and the peronei (Jull & Janda 1987). Testing the strength of these muscles is described in Chapter 3.

Muscle length

The clinician tests the length of muscles, in particular those thought prone to shorten (Janda 1994, 2002); that is: erector spinae, quadratus lumborum, piriformis, iliopsoas, rectus femoris, tensor fasciae latae, hamstrings, tibialis posterior, gastrocnemius and soleus (Jull & Janda 1987). Testing the length of these muscles is described in Chapter 3.

Isometric muscle testing

The clinician tests the ankle dorsiflexors and plantarflexors and any other relevant muscle group in resting position and, if indicated, in different parts of the physiological range. In addition the clinician observes the quality of the muscle contraction to hold this position (this can be done with the patient's eyes shut). The patient may, for example, be unable to prevent the joint from moving or may hold with excessive muscle activity; either of these circumstances would suggest a neuromuscular dysfunction.

Table 15.2 Joint clearing tests

Joint	Physiological movement	Accessory movement
Lumbar spine	Flexion and extension quadrants	All movements
Sacroiliac joint	Anterior and posterior gapping	
Hip joint	Squat and hip quadrant	
Knee joint	All movements and squat	
Patellofemoral joint	Medial/lateral glide and cephalad/caudad glide	

Other muscle tests

Thompson's test for rupture of tendocalcaneus (Corrigan & Maitland 1994). With the patient prone and the feet over the end of the plinth or kneeling with the foot unsupported, the clinician squeezes the calf muscle; the absence of ankle plantarflexion indicates a positive test, suggesting rupture of tendocalcaneus.

Neurological tests

Neurological examination includes neurological integrity testing, neurodynamic tests and some other nerve tests.

Integrity of the nervous system

The integrity of the nervous system is tested if the clinician suspects that the symptoms are emanating from the spine or from a peripheral nerve.

Dermatomes/peripheral nerves. Light touch and pain sensation of the lower limb are tested using cotton wool and pinprick respectively, as described in Chapter 3. Knowledge of the cutaneous distribution of nerve roots (dermatomes) and peripheral nerves enables the clinician to distinguish the sensory loss due to a root lesion from that due to a peripheral nerve lesion. The cutaneous nerve distribution and dermatome areas are shown in Figure 3.21.

Myotomes/peripheral nerves. The following myotomes are tested and are shown in Figure 3.27:

- L2: hip flexion
- L3: knee extension
- L4: foot dorsiflexion and inversion
- L5: extension of the big toe
- S1: eversion of the foot, contract buttock, knee flexion
- S2: knee flexion, toe standing
- S3–S4: muscles of pelvic floor, bladder and genital function.

A working knowledge of the muscular distribution of nerve roots (myotomes) and peripheral nerves enables the clinician to distinguish the motor loss due to a root lesion from that due to a peripheral nerve lesion. The peripheral nerve distributions are shown in Figure 3.25.

Reflex testing. The following deep tendon reflexes are tested and are shown in Figure 3.28:

- L3/4: knee jerk
- S1: ankle jerk.

Neurodynamic tests

The following neurodynamic tests may be carried out in order to ascertain the degree to which neural tissue is responsible for the production of the patient's symptom(s):

- Passive neck flexion (PNF)
- Straight leg raise (SLR)
- Passive knee bend (PKB)
- Slump.

These tests are described in detail in Chapter 3.

Miscellaneous tests

Vascular tests

If it is suspected that the circulation is compromised, the clinician palpates the pulses of the dorsalis pedis artery. The state of the vascular system can also be determined by the response of symptoms to positions of dependency and elevation of the lower limbs.

Homans' sign for deep vein thrombosis. The clinician passively dorsiflexes the ankle joint. If the patient feels pain in the calf, this may indicate deep vein thrombosis.

Leg length

Leg length is measured if a difference in left and right sides is suspected (see Ch. 14 for details).

Palpation

The clinician palpates the foot and ankle and any other relevant areas. It is useful to record palpation findings on a body chart (see Fig. 2.3) and/or palpation chart (see Fig. 3.38).

The clinician notes the following:

- The temperature of the area
- Localized increased skin moisture
- The presence of oedema or effusion. A tape measure can be used around the circumference of the limb or joint and left side compared to right side
- Mobility and feel of superficial tissues, e.g. ganglions, nodules, scar tissue
- The presence or elicitation of any muscle spasm
- Tenderness of bone, ligament, muscle, tendon, tendon sheath, trigger points (shown in Fig. 3.39) or nerve. Palpable nerves in the lower limb are as follows:
  - The sciatic nerve can be palpated two-thirds of the way along an imaginary line between the greater trochanter and the ischial tuberosity with the patient in prone
  - The common peroneal nerve can be palpated medial to the tendon of biceps femoris and also around the head of the fibula
  - The tibial nerve can be palpated centrally over the posterior knee crease medial to the popliteal artery; it can also be felt behind the medial malleolus, which is more noticeable with the foot in dorsiflexion and eversion
  - The superficial peroneal nerve can be palpated on the dorsum of the foot along an imaginary line over the fourth metatarsal; it is more noticeable with the foot in plantar flexion and inversion
  - The deep peroneal nerve can be palpated between the first and second metatarsals, lateral to the extensor hallucis tendon

- – The sural nerve can be palpated on the lateral aspect of the foot behind the lateral malleolus, lateral to the tendocalcaneus
- Increased or decreased prominence of bones
- Pain provoked or reduced on palpation.

Accessory movements

It is useful to use the palpation chart and movement diagrams (or joint pictures) to record findings. These are explained in detail in Chapter 3.

The clinician notes the:

- Quality of movement
- Range of movement
- Resistance through the range and at the end of the range of movement
- Behaviour of pain through the range
- Provocation of any muscle spasm.

Accessory movements for the foot and ankle joints (Fig. 15.6) are listed in Table 15.3. Following accessory movements to the foot and ankle, the clinician reassesses all the physical asterisks (movements or tests that have been found to reproduce the patient's symptoms) in order to establish the effect of the accessory movements on the patient's signs and symptoms. Accessory movements can then be tested for other regions suspected to be a source of, or contributing to, the

patient's symptoms. Again, following accessory movements to any one region, the clinician reassesses all the asterisks. Regions likely to be examined are the lumbar spine, sacroiliac joint, hip and knee (Table 15.3).

Mobilizations with movement (MWMs) (Mulligan 1999)

Inferior tibiofibular joint. The patient lies supine and is asked to actively invert the foot while the clinician applies an anteroposterior glide to the fibula (Fig. 15.7). An increase in range and no pain or reduced pain are positive examination findings indicating a mechanical joint problem.

Plantarflexion of the ankle joint. The patient lies supine with the knee flexed and the foot over the end of the plinth. The clinician with one hand applies an anteroposterior glide to the lower end of the tibia and fibula and with the other hand rolls the talus anteriorly while the patient is asked to actively plantarflex the ankle (Fig. 15.8A). An increase in range and no pain or reduced pain are positive examination findings indicating a mechanical joint problem.

Dorsiflexion of the ankle joint. The patient lies supine with the foot over the end of the plinth. The clinician applies an anteroposterior glide to the

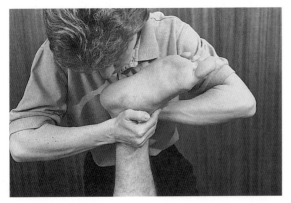

A (i) Anteroposterior. The heel of the right hand applies a posteroanterior force to the tibia while the left hand applies an anteroposterior force to the fibula.

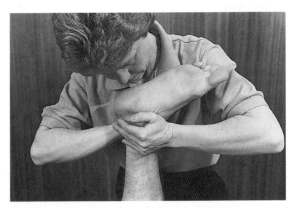

A (ii) Posteroanterior. The left hand applies an anteroposterior force to the tibia while the right hand applies a posteroanterior force to the fibula.

Figure 15.6 (A–G) Accessory movements for the foot and ankle joints. A Inferior tibiofibular joint.

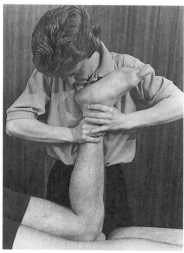

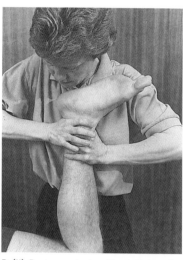

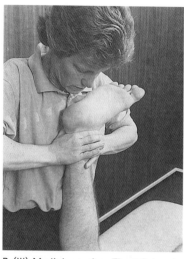

B (i) Anteroposterior. The right hand stabilizes the calf while the left hand applies an anteroposterior force to the anterior aspect of the talus.

B (ii) Posteroanterior. The left hand stabilizes the calf while the right hand applies a posteroanterior force to the posterior aspect of the talus.

B (iii) Medial rotation. The left hand grasps the malleoli anteriorly to stabilize the tibia while the right hand holds the talus posteriorly and rotates the talus medially.

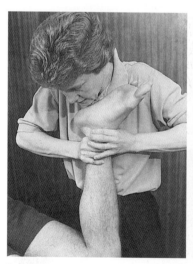

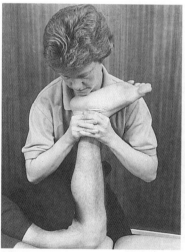

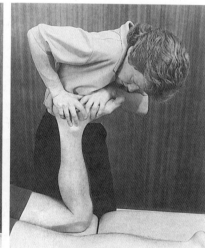

B (iv) Lateral rotation. The right hand grasps the malleoli posteriorly to stabilize the tibia while the left hand holds the talus anteriorly and rotates the talus laterally.

B (v) Longitudinal caudad. The clinican lightly rests the leg on the posterior aspect of the patient's thigh to stabilize and then grasps around the talus to pull upwards.

B (vi) Longitudinal cephalad. The left hand supports the foot in dorsiflexion while the right hand applies a longitudinal cephalad force through the calcaneus.

Figure 15.6 *Continued*   **B** Talocrural joint.

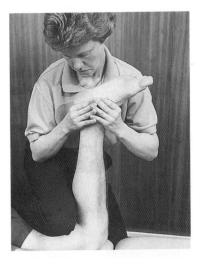

C Subtalar joint, longitudinal caudad. The clinician lightly rests his/her leg on the posterior aspect of the patient's thigh to stabilize it and then grasps around the calcaneus with the right hand and the forefoot with the left hand, and pulls the foot upwards.

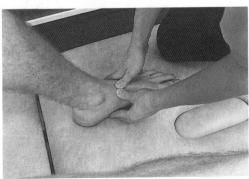

D (i) Anteroposterior to the navicular. Thumb pressure is applied to the anterior aspect of the navicular.

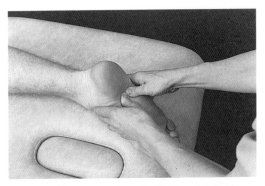

D (ii) Posteroanterior to the cuboid. Thumb pressure is applied to the posterior aspect of the cuboid.

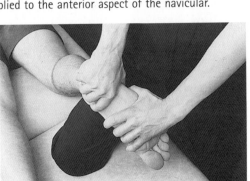

D (iii) Abduction. The calf is rested on the clinician's thigh. The right hand grasps the heel while the left hand grasps the forefoot. Both hands apply an abduction force to the foot.

Figure 15.6 *Continued* D Intertarsal joints.

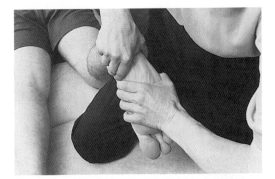

D (iv) Adduction. The calf is rested on the clinician's thigh. The right hand grasps the heel while the left hand grasps the forefoot. Both hands apply an adduction force to the foot.

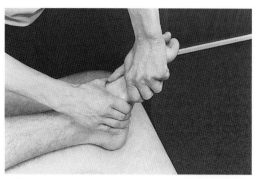

E (i) Anteroposterior and posteroanterior movement of the first tarsometatarsal joint. The right hand stabilizes the medial cuneiform while the left hand applies an anteroposterior and posteroanterior force to the base of the metatarsal.

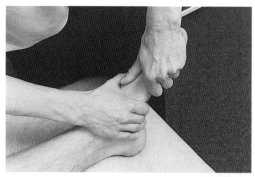

E (ii) Medial and lateral rotation of the second tarsometatarsal joint. The right hand stabilizes the intermediate cuneiform while the left hand rotates the second metatarsal medially and laterally.

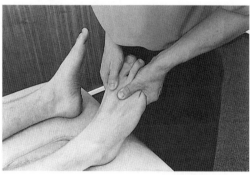

F (i) Anteroposterior and posteroanterior movement. The hands grasp adjacent metatarsal heads and apply a force in opposite directions to produce an anteroposterior and a posteroanterior movement at the distal intermetatarsal joint.

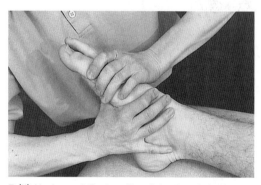

F (ii) Horizontal flexion. The right thumb is placed in the centre of the foot at the level of the metatarsal heads. The left hand grips around the dorsum of the metatarsal heads and curves them around the thumb to produce horizontal flexion.

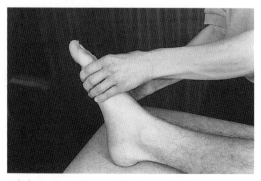

F (iii) Horizontal extension. Both thumbs are placed over the middle of the dorsum of the foot at the level of the metatarsal heads and the fingers grasp anteriorly around the foot. The fingers and thumbs then apply a force to produce horizontal extension.

Figure 15.6 *Continued* E Tarsometatarsal joints. F Proximal and distal intermetatarsal joints.

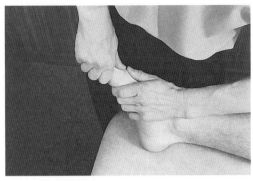

G (i) Anteroposterior and posteroanterior movement. The proximal phalanx is moved anteriorly and posteriorly.

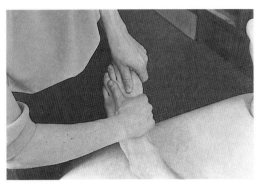

G (ii) Medial and lateral transverse movement. The proximal phalanx is moved medially and laterally.

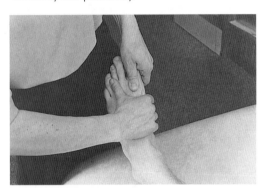

G (iii) Medial and lateral rotation. The proximal phalanx is moved into medial and lateral rotation.

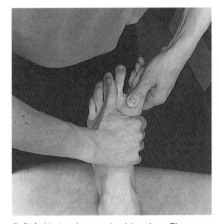

G (iv) Abduction and adduction. The proximal phalanx is moved into abduction and adduction.

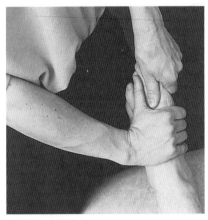

G (v) Longitudinal caudad and cephalad. The proximal phalanx is moved in a cephalad and caudad direction.

Figure 15.6 *Continued* **G** First metatarsophalangeal joint. For all these movements, one hand stabilizes the metatarsal head while the other hand moves the proximal phalanx.

Table 15.3   Accessory movements, choice of application and reassessment of the patient's asterisks

Accessory movements	Choice of application	Identify any effect of accessory movements on patient's signs and symptoms
Accessory movements for the foot and ankle joints (Fig. 15.6) **Inferior tibiofibular joint** ↕ AP ↕ PA ⇕ AP/PA glide	Start position, e.g. – in dorsiflexion – in plantarflexion – in inversion – in eversion Speed of force application Direction of applied force Point of application of applied force	Reassess all asterisks
Talocrural joint ↕ AP ↕ PA ↶ Med medial rotation ↷ Lat lateral rotation ↔ Caud longitudinal caudad ↔ Ceph longitudinal cephalad		
Subtalar joint ↔ Caud longitudinal caudad		

Intertarsal joints
↕   AP
↕   PA
⇕   AP/PA glide
    Abd   abduction
    Add adduction		

Tarsometatarsal joints ↕ AP ↕ PA ⇕ AP/PA glide ↶ Med medial rotation ↷ Lat lateral rotation		

Proximal and distal intermetatarsal joints
↕   AP
↕   PA
⇕   AP/PA glide
    HF   horizontal flexion
    HE horizontal extension		

MTP and IP joints ↕ AP ↕ PA ⇕ AP/PA glide → Med medial transverse → Lat lateral transverse		

Table 15.3 *Continued*

Accessory movements	Choice of application	Identify any effect of accessory movements on patient's signs and symptoms
MTP and IP joints *Continued*		
⌢ Med medial rotation		
⌢ Lat lateral rotation		
Abd abduction		
Add adduction		
←•→ Caud longitudinal caudad		
←•→ Ceph longitudinal cephalad		
Ten accessory movements of the tarsal bones (Kaltenborn 2002)		
Movements in the middle of the foot		
– Fix 2nd and 3rd cuneiform bones and mobilize 2nd metatarsal bone		
– Fix 2nd and 3rd cuneiform bones and mobilize 3rd metatarsal bone		
Movements on the medial side of the foot		
– Fix 1st cuneiform bone and mobilize 1st metatarsal bone		
– Fix the navicular bone and mobilize the 1st, 2nd and 3rd cuneiform bones		
– Fix the talus and mobilize the navicular bone		
Movements on the lateral side of the foot		
– Fix the cuboid bone and mobilize the 4th and 5th metatarsal bones		
– Fix the navicular and 3rd cuneiform bones and mobilize the cuboid bone		
– Fix the calcaneus and mobilize the cuboid bone		
Movement between talus and calcaneus		
– Fix the talus and mobilize the calcaneus		
Movements in the ankle joint		
– Fix the leg and move the talus or fix the talus and move the leg		
?Lumbar spine	As above	Reassess all asterisks
?Sacroiliac joint	As above	Reassess all asterisks
?Hip	As above	Reassess all asterisks
?Tibiofemoral joint	As above	Reassess all asterisks
?Patellofemoral joint	As above	Reassess all asterisks

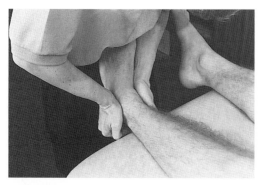

Figure 15.7   Mobilizations with movement for the inferior tibiofibular joint. The left hand supports the ankle while the heel of the right hand applies an anteroposterior glide to the fibula as the patient inverts the foot.

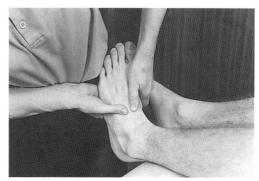

Figure 15.9   Mobilizations with movement for inversion of the foot and ankle. The left hand applies an anteroposterior glide to the base of the first metatarsal and the right hand applies a posteroanterior glide to the base of the second metatarsal while the patient actively inverts.

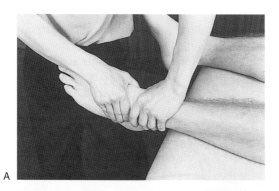

A

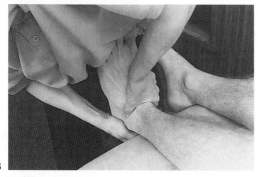

B

Figure 15.8   Mobilizations with movement for the ankle joint. **A** Plantarflexion. The left hand applies an anteroposterior glide to the tibia and fibula while the other hand rolls the talus anteriorly as the patient actively plantarflexes. **B** Dorsiflexion. The right hand holds the posterior aspect of the calcaneus and the left hand grips the anterior aspect of the talus. Both hands apply an anteroposterior glide as the patient actively dorsiflexes.

calcaneus and the talus while the patient is asked to actively dorsiflex the ankle (Fig. 15.8B). Since the extensor tendons lift the examiner's hand away from the talus, the patient is asked to contract repetitively and then relax. With relaxation, the clinician moves the ankle into the further range of dorsiflexion gained during the contraction.

Inversion of foot and ankle.   This test is carried out on patients with pain over the medial border of the foot on inversion due to a 'positional' fault of the first metatarsophalangeal joint. The patient actively inverts the foot while the clinician applies a sustained anteroposterior glide to the base of the first metatarsal and a posteroanterior glide on the base of the second metatarsal (Fig. 15.9). An increase in range and no pain or reduced pain are positive examination findings indicating a mechanical joint problem.

Metatarsophalangeal joints.   This test is carried out if the patient has pain under the transverse arch of the foot due to a positional fault of a metatarsal head. The patient actively flexes the toes while the clinician grasps the heads of adjacent metatarsals and applies a sustained posteroanterior glide to the head of the affected metatarsal (Fig 15.10). An increase in range and no pain or reduced pain are positive examination findings indicating a mechanical joint problem.

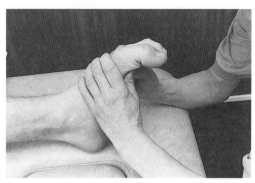

Figure 15.10 Metatarsophalangeal joints. The patient actively flexes the toes while the clinician uses thumb pressure to apply a posteroanterior glide to the head of a metatarsal.

COMPLETION OF THE EXAMINATION

Having carried out the above tests, the examination of the foot and ankle is complete. The subjective and physical examinations produce a large amount of information, which should be recorded accurately and quickly. An outline examination chart may be useful for some clinicians and one is suggested in Figure 15.11. It is important, however, that the clinician does not examine in a rigid manner, simply following the suggested sequence outlined in the chart. Each patient presents differently and this needs to be reflected in the examination process. It is vital at this stage to highlight important findings from the examination with an asterisk (*). These findings must be reassessed at, and within, subsequent treatment sessions to evaluate the effects of treatment on the patient's condition.

The physical testing procedures which specifically indicate joint, nerve or muscle tissues, as a source of the patient's symptoms, are summarized in Table 3.10. The strongest evidence that a joint is the source of the patient's symptoms is that active and passive physiological movements, passive accessory movements and joint palpation all reproduce the patient's symptoms, and that following a treatment dose, reassessment identifies an improvement in the patient's signs and symptoms. Weaker evidence includes an alteration in range, resistance or quality of physiological and/or accessory movements and tenderness over the joint, with no alteration in signs and symptoms after treatment. One or more of these findings may indicate a dysfunction of a joint which may or may not be contributing to the patient's condition.

The strongest evidence that a muscle is the source of a patient's symptoms is if active movements, an isometric contraction, passive lengthening and palpation of a muscle all reproduce the patient's symptoms, and that following a treatment dose, reassessment identifies an improvement in the patient's signs and symptoms. Further evidence of muscle dysfunction may be suggested by reduced strength or poor quality during the active physiological movement and the isometric contraction, reduced range, and/or increased/decreased resistance, during the passive lengthening of the muscle, and tenderness on palpation, with no alteration in signs and symptoms after treatment. One or more of these findings may indicate a dysfunction of a muscle which may or may not be contributing to the patient's condition.

The strongest evidence that a nerve is the source of the patient's symptoms is when active and/or passive physiological movements reproduce the patient's symptoms, which are then increased or decreased with an additional sensitizing movement, at a distance from the patient's symptoms. In addition, there is reproduction of the patient's symptoms on palpation of the nerve and following neurodynamic testing, sufficient to be considered a treatment dose, results in an improvement in the above signs and symptoms. Further evidence of nerve dysfunction may be suggested by reduced range (compared to the asymptomatic side) and/or increased resistance to the various arm movements, and tenderness on nerve palpation.

On completion of the physical examination the clinician:

- Warns the patient of possible exacerbation up to 24–48 hours following the examination.
- Requests the patient to report details on the behaviour of the symptoms following examination at the next attendance.
- Explains the findings of the physical examination and how these findings relate to the subjective assessment. Any misconceptions patients may have regarding their illness or injury should be addressed.

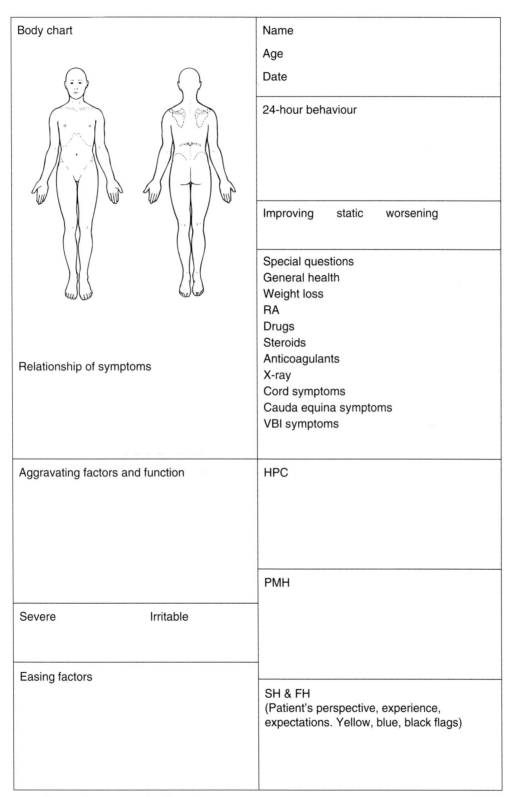

Body chart	Name
	Age
	Date
	24-hour behaviour
	Improving static worsening
	Special questions General health Weight loss RA Drugs Steroids Anticoagulants X-ray Cord symptoms Cauda equina symptoms VBI symptoms
Relationship of symptoms	
Aggravating factors and function	HPC
	PMH
Severe Irritable	
Easing factors	SH & FH (Patient's perspective, experience, expectations. Yellow, blue, black flags)

Figure 15.11   Foot and ankle examination chart.

Physical examination Observation	Isometric muscle testing
	Other muscle tests (Thompson's)
Joint integrity tests (anterior drawer, talar tilt)	
	Neurological integrity tests
Active and passive physiological movements of foot and ankle and other relevant regions	
	Neurodynamic tests
	Miscellaneous tests (pulses, Homan's sign, leg length)
Capsular pattern yes/no	Palpation
Muscle strength	
	Accessory movements and reassessment of each relevant region
Muscle length	

Figure 15.11 *Continued*

- Evaluates the findings, formulates a clinical diagnosis and writes up a problem list. Clinicians may find the management planning forms shown in Figures 3.53 and 3.54 helpful in guiding them through what is often a complex clinical reasoning process.
- Determines the objectives of treatment.
- Devises an initial treatment plan.

In this way, the clinician will have developed the following hypotheses categories (adapted from Jones & Rivett 2004):

- Function: abilities and restrictions.
- Patients' perspectives on their experience.
- Source of symptoms. This includes the structure or tissue that is thought to be producing the patients' symptoms, the nature of the structure or tissues in relation to the healing process, and the pain mechanisms.
- Contributing factors to the development and maintenance of the problem. There may be environmental, psychosocial, behavioural, physical or heredity factors.
- Precautions/contraindications to treatment and management. This includes the severity and irritability of the patient's symptoms and the nature of the patient's condition.
- Management strategy and treatment plan.
- Prognosis – this can be affected by factors such as the stage and extent of the injury as well as the patient's expectation, personality and lifestyle.

References

Armstrong D 1999 Loss of protective sensation: a practical evidence based definition. Journal of Foot and Ankle Surgery 38(10): 79–80

Cole J H, Furness A L, Twomey L T 1988 Muscles in action, an approach to manual muscle testing. Churchill Livingstone, Edinburgh

Corrigan B, Maitland G D 1994 Musculoskeletal and sports injuries. Butterworth-Heinemann, Oxford

Cyriax J 1982 Textbook of orthopaedic medicine – diagnosis of soft tissue lesions, 8th edn. Baillière Tindall, London

Fromherz W A 1995 Examination. In: Hunt G C, McPoil T G (eds) Physical therapy of the foot and ankle. Clinics in Physical Therapy, 2nd edn. Churchill Livingstone, New York, ch 4, p 81

Grieve G P 1981 Common vertebral joint problems. Churchill Livingstone, Edinburgh

Grieve G P 1991 Mobilisation of the spine, 5th edn. Churchill Livingstone, Edinburgh

Halliday S, Winter D, Frank J, Patla A, Prince P 1998 Initiation of gait in the young, elderly and in Parkinson's disease subjects. Gait and Posture 8(1): 8–14

Hislop H, Montgomery J 1995 Daniels and Worthingham's muscle testing, techniques of manual examination, 7th edn. W B Saunders, Philadelphia

Janda V 1994 Muscles and motor control in cervicogenic disorders: assessment and management. In: Grant R (ed) Physical therapy of the cervical and thoracic spine, 2nd edn. Churchill Livingstone, New York, ch 10, p 195

Janda V 2002 Muscles and motor control in cervicogenic disorders. In: Grant R (ed) Physical therapy of the cervical and thoracic spine, 3rd edn. Churchill Livingstone, New York, ch 10, p 182

Jones M A, Rivett D A 2004 Clinical reasoning for manual therapists. Butterworth-Heinemann, Edinburgh

Jull G A, Janda V 1987 Muscles and motor control in low back pain: assessment and management. In: Twomey L T, Taylor J R (eds) Physical therapy of the low back. Churchill Livingstone, New York, ch 10, p 253

Kaltenborn F M 2002 Manual mobilization of the joints, vol I. The extremities, 6th edn. Norli, Oslo

Kendall F P, McCreary E K, Provance P G 1993 Muscles testing and function, 4th edn. Williams & Wilkins, Baltimore, MD

Livingstone L, Mandigo J 1998 Bilateral Q angle asymmetry and anterior knee pain syndrome. Clinical Biomechanics 14(1): 7–13

McLeod-Roberts J 1995 Neurological assessment. In: Merriman L, Tollafield D (eds) Assessment of the lower limb. Churchill Livingstone, Edinburgh

Magee D J 1997 Orthopedic physical assessment, 3rd edn. W B Saunders, Philadelphia

Maitland G D 1991 Peripheral manipulation, 3rd edn. Butterworths, London

Mulligan B R 1999 Manual therapy 'NAGs', 'SNAGs', 'MWMs' etc., 4th edn. Plane View Services, New Zealand

Norkin C C, Levangie P K 1992 Joint structure and function, a comprehensive analysis, 2nd edn. F A Davis, Philadelphia, PA

Roy S, Irvin R 1983 Sports medicine: prevention, evaluation, management and rehabilitation. Prentice-Hall, Englewood Cliffs, NJ

Tollafield D, Merriman L 1995 Assessment of the locomotor system. In: Merriman L, Tollafield D (eds) Assessment of the lower limb. Churchill Livingstone, Edinburgh

Waddell G 2004 The back pain revolution, 2nd edn. Churchill Livingstone, Edinburgh

Wadsworth C T 1988 Manual examination and treatment of the spine and extremities. Williams & Wilkins, Baltimore, MD

Chapter 16

Epilogue

The aim of this text has been to make explicit the examination and assessment of patients with neuromusculoskeletal dysfunction; it has focused on the technical skills and clinical reasoning involved. It could be said that this text emphasizes a system of examination that focuses on the biological basis of symptoms, as opposed to the psychosocial factors. I have attempted to include the psychological and social aspects of the examination and assessment of patients; however, these aspects are not covered in detail and readers will need to draw on other literature to cover these gaps. In addition, readers are encouraged to further consider the diverse effects of pain on the neuromusculoskeletal system, and the mechanisms that underlie its clinical presentation.

The text has provided a step-by-step approach to the subjective and physical examination of the various regions in the body. The chapters have divided the body into regions: temporomandibular, upper cervical spine, cervicothoracic spine, thoracic spine, shoulder, elbow, wrist/hand, lumbar spine, pelvis, hip, knee and foot/ankle. Readers are reminded that functionally these are false divisions and a wider examination may be needed; for example, examination of the cervical–shoulder girdle–shoulder region or examination of the upper cervical spine–TMJ region may be needed.

I reiterate that the examination techniques shown in this text are carried out in a way that is possible for a small person! If you are larger than me, and you probably are, you may well want to adapt the techniques shown in this text. Another comment worth reiterating is that this text describes one way of doing a technique not the only way. For every technique shown here, there will be a number of other alternative ways in which it could be carried out. This text provides an example of how one clinician might perform a physical testing procedure; it is then left to readers to find alternative ways of carrying out the technique, making adaptations for themselves and for their patients. Clinicians can determine whether or not their adapted technique is effective and efficient by asking themselves whether it is easy and comfortable to perform, comfortable for the patient, and achieves what it intends to achieve.

It may be helpful here to summarize some of the main principles in clinical reasoning that are emphasized in this text, before the reader launches into the details of each chapter.

SUBJECTIVE EXAMINATION

- Understand the patient's perception of their problem.
- Obtain accurate unbiased subjective information.
- All structures under the symptoms and all structures/regions capable of referring to the area of symptoms are normally considered 'guilty until proven innocent'. In some cases, strong evidence of absence from the subjective examination may be all that is required to discount a structure/region as a source of the patient's symptoms. On other occasions it will

be necessary to obtain evidence of absence from both the subjective and physical examination.

- Find out the detailed information about the movements and postures that affect (aggravate and ease) each of the patient's symptoms. Ask about simple movements of all relevant regions, so that you can predict ahead, what and how movements need to be carried out for the patient in the physical examination.
- Predict the results of your physical tests by determining the severity and irritability of each symptom.
- Identify with asterisks (*) a wide range of subjective findings that will adequately summarize the subjective examination. These can then be used to judge the effectiveness of treatment and management strategies.

PHYSICAL EXAMINATION

- Underlying assumptions to physical testing:
  - When the patient's symptoms are reproduced during a physical test the structure at fault is somehow or other being affected. The word 'structure' is used in the widest sense of the word. The term 'somehow or other' aims to maintain a wide hypothesis as to the mechanism by which the patients' symptoms have been produced; this may be due to altered or abnormal neural activity as well as mechanical stress on structures.
  - It is worth remembering that the majority of the population will be asymmetrical and will display 'dysfunction'. The clinician needs to identify dysfunction that is relevant to their clinical presentation.
  - There is no pure joint, nerve or muscle test. A test that is called a 'muscle test', for example, might be said to bias muscle tissue, but will also affect a multitude of other tissues including joint and nerve. This is one reason why no one test determines the source of the patient's symptoms.
- Physical tests are carried out in as reliable a way as possible.
- Appropriate physical tests are carried out in an attempt to identify the source of the patient's symptoms.

- Detailed information is obtained about the behaviour of each symptom during every physical test. That is, where a symptom first comes on in range, what happens to that symptom as the movement continues, and what happens to that symptom on overpressure (if non-severe); this requires skilful communication with the patient. Imprecise information limits the ability to sensitively determine any change in that movement following treatment and therefore constrains clinical reasoning associated with treatment and management.
- There is accurate and comfortable handling.
- As a general guideline students are encouraged to examine neurological integrity when symptoms are below the acromion and below the buttock crease, and when spinal or neurological involvement is suspected.
- The patient is examined as fully as possible but without excessive symptom provocation.
- Identify with asterisks (*) a wide range of physical findings that will adequately summarize the physical examination. Along with the subjective asterisks, these can then be used to judge the effectiveness of treatment and management strategies.

At the end of the examination the clinician will develop the following hypotheses categories (adapted from Jones & Rivett 2004):

- Function: abilities and restrictions.
- Patients' perspectives on their experience.
- Source of symptoms. This includes the structure or tissue that is thought to be producing the patients' symptoms, the nature of the structure or tissues in relation to the healing process, and the pain mechanisms.
- Contributing factors to the development and maintenance of the problem. There may be environmental, psychosocial, behavioural, physical or heredity factors.
- Precautions/contraindications to treatment and management. This includes the severity and irritability of the patient's symptoms and the nature of the patient's condition.
- Management strategy and treatment plan.
- Prognosis – this can be affected by factors such as the stage and extent of the injury as well as the patient's expectation, personality and lifestyle.

It is perhaps worth mentioning at the outset that the clinician examining patients with neuromusculoskeletal dysfunction may not be able to identify a particular pathological process. In some patients it is possible, for example, for the clinician to suspect a meniscal tear or a medial collateral ligament tear of the knee, or a lateral ligament sprain of the ankle. However, in other patients, when one integrates current knowledge of pain mechanisms, and considers these effects on the presenting symptoms, the goal of identifying exact pathology is clouded. When the detailed analysis of movement dysfunction is considered in conjunction with the psychosocial factors highlighted previously, the clinician is then in a position to establish a reasoned treatment and management strategy. Readers are referred to the companion text for further information on the principles of treatment and management of patients with neuromusculoskeletal dysfunction (Petty 2004).

References

Jones M A, Rivett D A 2004 Clinical reasoning for manual therapists. Butterworth-Heinemann, Edinburgh

Petty N J 2004 Principles of neuromusculoskeletal treatment and management, a guide for therapists. Churchill Livingstone, Edinburgh

Index

Ankle dorsiflexion, 80, *378*, 382–9
Ankle inversion, 389
Ankle jerk, *80*
Ankle plantarflexion, 81, *378*, 382
Ankylosing spondylitis, 143, 165, 187, 283, 305, 323
Ankylosing vertebral hyperostosis, 283
Ankylosis, 125
Antalgic gait, 45
Anterior drawer test, 348–9, 376–7
Anterior gapping test, 315, *316*
Anterior iliac spine (ASIS), 310
Anterior interosseous syndrome, test for, 243
Anterior rotation
  ileum, 317
  sacrum, 313–14
Anterior sacral torsion, 312, 318
Anterior shoulder drawer test, 212, *213*
Anterior shoulder instability, 212, *213*
Anterior stability test, atlanto-occipital joint, 150
Anterior translation stress, atlas on the axis, 150
Anterolateral instability, knee, 349, *350*
Anteromedial instability, knee, 349
Anteroposterior glide
  acromioclavicular joint, *225*
  carpometacarpal joints, *273*
  costochondral joint, *201*
  glenohumeral joint, *224*
  hip joint, *334*
  inferior tibiofibular joint, *382*
  innominate/sacrum, 314
  intercarpal joints, *272*
  metatarsophalangeal joint, *386*
  navicular, *384*
  proximal and distal intermetacarpal joints, *274*
  proximal and distal intermetatarsal joints, *385*
  proximal phalanx, *274*
  radiocarpal joint, *271*
  sternoclavicular joint, *225*
  sternocostal joint, *201*
  superior radioulnar joint, *247*
  superior tibiofibular joint, *363*
  talocrural joint, *383*
  tarsometatarsal joints, *385*
  temporomandibular joint, *137*
  thoracic spine, *200*
  tibiofemoral joint, *362*
Anteroposterior tilt, patella, 360
Anticoagulants, 19

Apley compression/distraction test, 351–2, *353*
Approximation test, 315, *316*
Area of current symptoms, 7–10
  cervicothoracic spine, 166
  elbow region, 234
  foot and ankle, 370–1
  hip region, 324
  knee region, 342
  lumbar spine, 284
  pelvis region, 306
  shoulder region, 208
  temporomandibular region, 126
  thoracic spine, 188
  upper cervical spine, 144
  wrist and hand, 254
Areas relevant to the region being examined, 10
  cervicothoracic spine, 166
  elbow, 234
  foot and ankle, 371
  hip, 324
  knee, 342
  lumbar spine, 284
  pelvis, 306
  shoulder, 208
  temporomandibular joint, 126
  thoracic spine, 188
  upper cervical spine, 144
  wrist and hand, 254
Arm *see* upper limb
Arthrogenic gait, 45
Arthrosis, 143, 165, 187, 283, 305
Articular disc displacement, 125
Articular surfaces, physiological movements, *101*
Asymmetry, abnormal, 43
Atlanto-axial joint
  lateral stability test, 151
  PAIVMs, 157–9
  Sharp-Purser test, 150
Atlanto-occipital joint
  anterior stability test, 150
  PAIVMs, 157
  posterior stability test, 150
Auscultation, 198, 297
Axillary nerve, upper limb, *73*

B

Balance, observation
  foot and ankle examinations, 376
  hip examinations, 328
  knee examinations, 347
Barrel chest, 192
Behaviour of symptoms, 13–17
  see also specific regions
Biceps, rupture of long head of, 207

Biceps femoris, myofascial trigger point, *100*
Biceps jerk, *80*
Bicipital tendinitis, Speed's test, 220
Big toe, extension of, *78*
Bipupital line, checking, 130
Body charts, 7–13
  see also specific regions
Bouchard's nodes, 259
Boutonniere deformity, fingers or thumb, 258, *259*
Brachial plexus *see* upper limb
Bursitis, 207, 233, 323, 341

C

Calcification of tendons, 207, 233
Calf alignment, 375
Camptodactyly, 259
Capsular patterns, 53–4, 354
  cervicothoracic spine, 175
  elbow joint, 241–2
  foot and ankle, 379
  hip joint, 330
  lumbar spine, 294
  shoulder region, 217
  temporomandibular region, 133
  thoracic spine, 196
  wrist and hand, 267
Capsulitis, 125
Carpal tunnel syndrome, 253
Carpometacarpal joints
  accessory movements, *273*
  thumb, active physiological movements, *261, 265*
Cauda equina compression, 20, 211, 296, 308, 344
Central posteroanterior glide
  cervicothoracic spine, *179*
  lumbar spine, *298*
  thoracic spine, *199*
  upper cervical sine, *158*
Central sensitization, 10, *11*
Centralization of symptoms, 49–50
Cervical nerve roots, myotome testing, 76–7
Cervical rib, 165
Cervical rotation, SNAGS for, 160
Cervical spine
  common aggravating factors, *14*
  contralateral lateral flexion, 88, 90, 91, 93
  ipsilateral lateral flexion, 89, 91, 92, 94
  lateral flexion, 76
  pelvic tilt, 43
  temporomandibular symptoms, 133

Over-pronation, of foot, 375, 376
Overpressures, 47–9
    cervicothoracic spine, 171–3
    elbow complex, *240*
    foot and ankle, *378*
    hip joint, *329*
    knee region, *354*
    lumbar spine, *291, 292*
    shoulder girdle and glenohumeral
        joint, *214–15*
    temporomandibular region, 131,
        132, 136
    thoracic spine, *193–4*
    upper cervical spine, 152
    wrist and hand, *260–3*

P

Paget's disease, as cause of pain, 187,
    283, 305
Pain
    behaviour, 47
    dimensions of, 6
    distribution from visceral
        conditions, 33–4
    mechanisms, 10, *11*
    movement diagrams, 104
    possible causes *see specific regions*
    type, produced by various
        structures, *11*
    see also symptoms
Pain diaries, 126
Pain intensity scale, *12*
Palpation, 95–6
    chart, *95*
    hints on, *96*
    trigger points, 95–6, *97–100*
    see also specific regions
Paraesthesia, 12
Passive accessory intervertebral
        movements (PAIVMs), 42
    cervicothoracic spine, 175, 178–81
    lumbar spine, 294, 297–8
    thoracic spine, 196, 199
    upper cervical spine, 154, 157–60
Passive loading, temporomandibular
        joint, 136
Passive neck flexion (PNF), 75–80, *81*
Passive physiological intervertebral
        movements (PPIVMs), 42, 54–5
    cervicothoracic spine, 175
    lumbar spine, *294*
    recording, 55
    thoracic spine, 196
    upper cervical spine, 154
Passive physiological movements,
        54–5
    see also specific regions

Past medical history (PMH), 20
    see also specific regions
Patella
    dislocation as cause of pain, 341
    prominence of, 359–60
Patellofemoral joint, accessory
        movements, *361, 362*
Patellofemoral pain, 356
Patient's attitudes and feelings,
        observation, 4, 45
    cervicothoracic spine
        examinations, 171
    elbow examinations, 238
    foot and ankle examinations,
        376
    hip examinations, 328
    knee examinations, 347
    lumbar spine examinations, 290
    pelvis examinations, 311
    shoulder examinations, 212
    temporomandibular examinations,
        131
    thoracic spine examinations, 193
    upper cervical spine examinations,
        149
    wrist and hand examinations, 259
Pectoralis major
    myofascial trigger point, *99*
    testing, *61*
    tightness, *171*
Pectoralis minor
    myofascial trigger point, *99*
    testing, *62*
    tightness, *171*
Pelvic crossed syndrome, 39, *40*
Pelvic tilt, cervical spine posture, *43*
Pelvis, 305–22
    completion of the examination,
        318–22
    physical examination, 309–18
        accessory movements, 315–18
        active physiological
            movements, 311
        muscle tests, 314–15
        neurological tests, 315
        observation, 310–11
        palpation, 313, *314,* 315
        passive physiological
            movements, 312–14
    possible causes of pain/movement
        limitation, 305–6
    subjective examination, 306–9
        behaviour of symptoms, *14,*
            306–7
        body chart, 306
        history of the present condition,
            308
        past medical history, 308–9

plan of the physical
    examination, 309
social and family history, 309
special questions, 307–8
Peripheral nerve lesions, 45, 65, 253
Peripheral nerves
    brachial plexus, *66*
    cutaneous distribution, 65
    referred pain, 7, *8*
    tests
        cervicothoracic spine, 177
        elbow region, 243
        foot and ankle, 380, 381
        hip region, 332
        knee region, 358
        lumbar spine, 296
        shoulder region, 221
        temporomandibular region,
            134–5
        thoracic spine, 197–8
        upper cervical spine, 155–6
        wrist and hand, 269
Peripheral nervous system, effects of
        compression, 65–73
Peripheral neurogenic pain, 10, *11*
Peripheralization, of symptoms, 49–50
Permeable brick wall, 3–4
Peroneus longus and brevis
    myofascial trigger points, *100*
    testing, *59*
Perthes' disease, 323
Pes planus, 375
Phalen's wrist flexion test, 270
Phasic muscles, reaction to stress, 44
Physical examinations, 37–120
    accessory movements, 96–109
    active physiological movements,
        45–54
    aim, 37
    assumptions, 37–8
    clinical reasoning form, *114–19*
    joint integrity tests, 45
    management planning form, *113*
    muscle tests, 55–65
    neurological tests, 65–95
    observation, 38–45
    outline examination charts, *110*
    passive physiological movements,
        54–5
    plan, 21
    planning form, *23*
    summary, *38*
    see also specific regions
Physiological movement
    defined, 45
    see also active physiological
        movements; passive
        physiological movements